THE LITTLE Herb ENCYCLOPEDIA
Third Edition

By: Jack Ritchason, N.D.

Woodland Health Books
P.O. Box 160
Pleasant Grove, Utah 84062

© Copyright 1995 by Jack Ritchason

ISBN 0-913923-89-3
Woodland Health Books
P.O. Box 160
Pleasant Grove, Utah 84062

ACKNOWLEDGMENT

I would like to acknowledge the expert help and research, Linda Terrell has given in the completion of this project.

I would also like to thank my wife, Verlyn, for her help and support in working on this book.

Jack Ritchason

DEDICATION

This book is dedicated to my very dear and loving wife who has always inspired me to continue seeking knowledge in all fields, especially health. It is my hope that this book will become a guideline to my posterity and others in their search for a better and healthier life. I am thankful that I have an all-just and merciful Heavenly Father who has given us the answer already for our physical problems on this earth. We simply need to search for the knowledge that is already here, for without health, we have nothing.

"I have been given a gift of knowledge from my Heavenly Father and if I do not share this with my fellow man, the gift will be taken away from me."

THE PARABLE OF THE TEN TALENTS

"Again, it will be like a man going on a journey, who called his servants and entrusted his property to them. To one he gave five talents of money, to another two talents, and to another one talent, each according to his ability. Then he went on his journey. The man who had received the five talents went at once and put his money to work and gained five more. So also, the one with the two talents gained two more. But the man who had received the one talent went off, dug a hole in the ground and hid his master's money."

"After a long time the master of those servants returned and settled accounts with them. The man who had received the five talents brought the other five. "Master," he said, "you entrusted me with five talents. See, I have gained five more.""

"His master replied, "Well done, good and faithful servant! You have been faithful with a few things; I will put you in charge of many things. Come and share your master's happiness!"

"The man with the two talents also came. "Master," he said, "you entrusted me with two talents; see, I have gained two more."

"His master replied, "Well done, good and faithful servant! You have been faithful with a few things; I will put you in charge of many things. Come and share your master's happiness!"

"Then the man who had received the one talent came. "Master," he said, "I knew that you are a hard man, harvesting where you have not sown and gathering where you have not scattered seed. So I was afraid and went out and hid your talent in the ground. See, here is what belongs to you."

"His master replied, "You wicked, lazy servant! So you knew that I harvest where I have not sown and gather where I have not scattered seed? Well then, you should have put my money on deposit with the bankers, so that when I returned I would have received it back with interest.

"Take the talent from him and give it to the one who has the ten talents. For everyone who has will be given more, and he will have abundance. Whoever does not have, even what he has will be taken from him."

(NIV) Matthew 25:14-29.

"I have been given a gift of knowledge from my Heavenly Father and if I do not share this with my fellow man, the gift will be taken away from me."

It is my deepest desire to invest the Lord's gift.

Jack Ritchason, N.D., Ph.D., I.D.

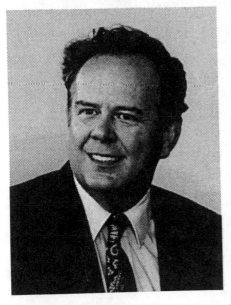

Dr. John (Jack) Ritchason has been in the health field since 1963 and has lectured nationally and internationally on herbs, vitamins, minerals, nutrition, and Iridology. He graduated in 1979, as a Naturopathic Doctor from the Arizona College of Naturopathic Medicine, a branch of the American University of Natural Therapeutics and Preventive Medicine.

He has his Ph.D. in Nutrition from Donsbach University and has done graduate work in Homeopathy in Missouri and also Florida Institute of Technology in Florida. Dr. Ritchason is a charter board member of Iridologists International. He is a member of the State Society of Homeopathic Physicians, is a Master Herbalist and (was the Dean of the Herbal Institute in Huntington Beach, California.)

Dr. Ritchason is a Life Member of the National Health Federation (NHF) and for a number of years held such positions as Vice President, Vice Chairman and Chairman.

Dr. Ritchason is a Registered Healthologist, Iridologist, Touch-for-Health Instructor and is certified in five different areas of Kinesiology. He has also completed his two year tutorial in Acupuncture. He is certified in both Colon Therapy and Reflexology. He has been involved as a teacher in all these sciences for 30 years. He is considered to be one of the top Iridologists and teachers of Iridology today. He is dedicated to the teaching of these principles. He has attempted to expand the knowledge to his fellow man to be able to help themselves and others. Since 1963, he has been sharing this knowledge with everyone who is willing to listen and the teaching aspect of it has been the most important part of his life.

CONTENTS

INDIVIDUAL HERBS

The recent emphasis on the use of herbs for health and well-being may seem to be new to you, but they are not. They are rather a renewal of the ancient medicinal methods of healing. We have all had experiences with herbs. As an example, everyone, has sneezed from a whiff of black pepper or cried while chopping an onion. In this book, spices (peppers), vegetables (onions) etc., will be referred to as herbs, because, we are dealing with their medicinal values.

You will note that we list an herb as a treatment for several ailments. That's the beauty of herbs. They are amazingly versatile. Our bodies are uniquely individual and what has achieved results for one, may not be successful for others.

There are many herbs that will work equally as well on one particular disease; some work better for one person than for another, thus many alternatives are given. This has been taken into account by Herbalists worldwide and especially by those cultures that have traditionally used herbs as a part of dealing with health problems.

It is not our intent, however, in this book to diagnose or prescribe. We offer only advice that has worked for others. An exciting new adventure in better health is about to unfold before you. You will find listed in this book, the most common herbs that have the potential to immeasurably improve the quality of your life when combined with proper diet, rest, exercise and a healthy mental, emotional, spiritual and physical approach to living. An important factor for health and well being, in addition to our general life style, is our attitude toward life. This can have a good or bad effect on our health and needs to be considered by each of us.

ABOUT GOLDEN SEAL

A women writes, my daughter cut her heel on a nail on our carpeted stair step. Infection soon set in with a red streak going up her leg. Golden Seal powder and distilled water were used in paste form on the cut, then wrapped with plastic and left on overnight. The next morning the infection area was back to the normal pink color, the red streak was gone and within two days a light scab had healed over the cut.

ABOUT COMFREY AND THE CALCIUM RICH
FORMULA AND POULTICE FORMULA

A father relates, "My son had a motorcycle wreck and broke his leg and arm and cut his forehead quite badly. After the casts were placed on his leg and arm. After he was taken home, we started giving him a pain formula, of about 4 capsules every 12 hours and within 2 to 3 hours the pain had subsided. Then I give him 9 capsules of Comfrey, 9 capsules of the calcium rich formula, and 9 capsules of the poultice formula every day. The doctors said it would take 12 weeks for the bone to heal and the casts to be taken off. With using the above, the casts were taken off in 5 weeks and he was playing football in 6 weeks. Hooray for herbs!"

ABOUT EYE-WASH FORMULA

The story is told by a young woman, "My mother was to have a cataract operation, but did not want to. We introduced her to the eye-wash formula and instructed her on how to use it. She used the eye-wash externally in her eyes two to three times a day. She took several capsules a day internally and within three weeks she could thread a needle. When she was later examined by her doctor, he told her she did not need an operation!"

ABOUT CAPSICUM AND GARLIC

From an acquaintance, I learned that, as he states, "I had very high blood pressure and had been doctoring for it for about 12 years to no avail. After using 6 capsules of Capsicum and Garlic a day for 2 weeks, my blood pressure was down to normal for the first time in 12 years. I also switched to the thyroid formula using about six a day instead of 4 grains of thyroid medicine a day and shortly thereafter, my thyroid problem was under control."

ABOUT BLACK COHOSH

A women friend relates, "I was having lumps reoccur in my breasts and after having surgery 3 previous times, I was fearful, and did not desire this again. I used 6 Black Cohosh a day for one month, then cut back to 2 to 3 capsules a day and within two months all the lumps disappeared and the accompanying dryness in the vaginal area was gone."

Many different herb remedies have been successfully used to cure health problems. The uses of herbs explained in this book are common often used herb applications, but they are not the only uses for these herbs. We believe that the descriptions, give an accurate account of the most accepted uses for each herb listed. We offer only advice that has worked for others. It is not our intent to diagnose or prescribe.

ACACIA (Acacia spp.,)
A.K.A.,: Gum Arabic.

BODILY INFLUENCE: Alterative, Anti-inflammatory, Anti-rheumatic, Anti-spasmodic, Astringent, Demulcent, Emollient, Febrifuge, Mucilant, Nutritive, Stimulant, Tonic.
PART USED: Gum, Flowers, Bark, Beans, Leaves.

Historically, Gum Arabic was harvested from the Acacia tree, native to the Middle East, by the Bedouin tribes. They used it as a food and also used it medicinally to soothe irritated areas of the digestive tract. Later, it is was found it could be used as a binder for pill and tablets. It also has been used in paints and as a compound for wax to improve polishing and to act as a glue for envelopes and postage stamps.

Used in ancient Egypt, the Gum Acacia was considered a prized herb.

Gum Arabic is very good for treating inflammation. It is effective as a demulcent, softening irritation of the stomach and throat. It is also effective to soften the harshness of pills when used as a coating over bitter or difficult to digest medicine. When used as a salve or in a poultice, it is beneficial in the treatment of burns, nodular leprosy and for women who are suffering from over-nursing and are experiencing painful nipples.

• The gum from the Acacia, also called "Gum Arabic," exudes resins naturally and by adding those resins to boiling water, it is transformed into a mucilage. It is edible and nutritive. As a mucilage, it acts as a demulcent, supplying a soothing protective coat on the respiratory, gastrointestinal and urinary linings. It acts also to soothe irritated mucous membranes, including the stomach, bowels, uterus and vaginal area. It is evident that Gum Arabic's main effect is to form a protective, soothing coating over inflammations.

• Gum Arabic proves relaxing, as it retains its warmth and moisture, when used in poultices or other external applications.

• Gum Arabic also soothes irritated mucous membranes for sore throats, coughs, catarrh, and diarrhea and as such, is one of the main ingredients in many products for these conditions. It has also been used in throat lozenges for the soothing of the throat.

Catarrh
Coughs
Diarrhea
INFLAMMATION
MUCOUS MEMBRANES
Nipples (sore)
Sore throat

AGRIMONY   (Agrimonia eupatoria)
A.K.A.,: Stickwort, Cocklebur.

BODILY INFLUENCE: Analgesic, Anti-inflammatory, Astringent, Cholagogue, Coagulant, Depurative, Diuretic, Emmenagogue, Hemostatic, Tonic, Vermifuge, Vulnerary.
PART USED: The whole plant.

Historically, Agrimony was known by the ancient Greeks who made use of it for ailments of the eye. In northern Europe, it was used by the Anglo-Saxons to treat wounds. Late in the sixteenth century, it was used to treat gout, fevers and rheumatism. It was referred to by the English poet Michael Dayton as an "all-heal" herb.

The plants' medicinal properties are due to the large amounts of tannin. Herbalists use the flowering stem tips to create an elixir as a diuretic and for digestive problems.

• Agrimony is high in the nutrients which are necessary for normal healthy functioning of the body especially of benefit to the colon, intestines, kidneys, liver and stomach.

• Agrimony functions as a tonic to treat general conditions, as it absorbs into the various systems of the body, working to tone the muscles.

• When applied as a diuretic, Agrimony is useful in the treatment of gravel or stones in the bladder or kidneys.

• Agrimony is also known for its throat soothing properties. Singers have used Agrimony as a gargle to help cut the mucus in their throats before singing.

• Agrimony has also been used in Homeopathic medicine such as in Bach Flower Remedies. (See "Vitamin and Health Encyclopedia", by Dr. Jack Ritchason, N.D.

Appendicitis
Bladder problems
Bleeding (general)
Cancer (stomach)
Colitis (mucus)
DIARRHEA (suppository)
Diarrhea, child (suppository)
Enuresis
Fevers
Gallbladder (chronic)
GASTRIC DISORDERS
Hematuria (blood in urine)
Hemorrhoids (suppository)
INCONTINENCE (URINATION)
INTESTINES

JAUNDICE
KIDNEY STONES
LIVER DISORDERS
Rheumatism
SKIN DISEASES
Sore throat
Splinters
Sprains
Stomach disorders
Tapeworms (suppository)
Tuberculosis
Ulcers
Uterine bleeding
Warts
Wounds

ALFALFA   (Medicago sativa)
A.K.A.,: Buffalo herb, Lucerne.

BODILY INFLUENCE: Alterative, Anodyne, Antipyretic, Anti-rheumatic, Anti-scorbutic, Aperitive, Depurative, Diuretic, Galactagogue, Nutritive, Stomachic, Tonic.
PART USED: Herb, Seed, Sprout.

Alfalfa is a member of the legume family. As early as 1597, English herbalist John Gerard, recommended Alfalfa for upset stomachs. Frank Bouer, noted author and biologist discovered that the leaves of Alfalfa, had eight essential amino acids.

In the America's, Alfalfa has been used by the Colombians for coughs, while the Costanoan Indians applied it as a poultice for earaches. On the Asian Continent, the Chinese treat all five viscera with Alfalfa, especially intestinal and kidney disorders. In the Middle East, the Arabs called Alfalfa, the "father of all herbs." In fact, the origin of the term alfalfa has been traced to the Persian word "asparti" meaning horse fodder. Alfalfa has been cultivated by man for thousands of years probably originating in Armenia.

Spanish explorers brought Alfalfa to the New World and gold prospectors carried it from South America into California. It was imported into the eastern and central U.S. directly from Europe. In comparison with other choices for vitamin C, the fresh plant has four times the amount, than contained in citrus juice. It is rich in vitamin K, which is a friend to women suffering from morning sickness.

The leaves contain lots of beta-carotene for a healthy immune system, skin, and internal mucous membranes. As for vitamin E, it is considered one of the most reliable sources for animals. There is also a "vitamin U" factor, so-called because it prevents ulcers in test animals. Calcium is so high in this plant that it almost goes off the charts.

The reason human beings do not use Alfalfa at the kitchen table, is that it is one of the highest fibrous herbs in existence and human beings do not have the capability of breaking it down as animals do.

Alfalfa is the basis for liquid Chlorophyll, with a balance of chemical and mineral constituents almost identical to human hemoglobin. It is used therapeutically for arthritis, a wide range of intestinal and skin disorders, liver problems, breath and body odor and even cancer. In essence, eating any of the green super foods is like giving yourself a little transfusion to help treat illness, enhance immunity and sustain well-being.

• Alfalfa contains all the known vitamins and minerals for life. Some of these are in trace amounts so Alfalfa is not a perfect food, because it does not contain enough of these nutrients or carbohydrates in high enough amounts to sustain life by just eating Alfalfa.

- Alfalfa neutralizes acids and poisons.
- Alfalfa has roots that extend deep into the soil where it reaches mineral rich soil which gives it a high nutrient value. Alfalfa roots have even been found to come through the tops of coal miner's tunnels. Alfalfa is one the highest Chlorophyll bearing plants known to man. Certain religious groups have used Chlorophyll in place of blood transfusions before, during and after operations.
- Alfalfa has a natural ability to stimulant and feed the Pituitary gland.
- Many vegetarians have trouble in this day and age maintaining B-12, for them Alfalfa is a rich source of B-12.
- Green plants contain natural Fluoride; Alfalfa is no exception, as it helps to prevent tooth decay and harden bones naturally.
- Fluoride in Alfalfa is not the artificially made sodium fluoride, which is an aluminum manufacturing by-product, that is poisonous to the system.
- Alfalfa is known to be a natural deodorizer mainly because of its high Chlorophyll content and is also a natural infection fighter due of its high natural source of vitamin A.
- Alfalfa, because of its high fiber content, has the ability to absorb and carry intestinal waste out of the body.
- The high enzymes content of fresh or freeze-dried Alfalfa helps the body to balance its systems, enabling it to ward off infectious diseases and even helps to restore the body's immune system to defeat many degenerative diseases such as cancer and arthritis.
- Alfalfa is a panacea for almost everything and if you're taking it for one major problem, it may well be helpful for a dozen other minor problems.

ACIDITY
Alcoholism (liver)
ALLERGIES
ANEMIA (supplies iron)
APPETITE STIMULANT
ARTHRITIS
ASTHMA
Atherosclerosis
BELL'S PALSY
Bladder
BLOOD NORMALIZER, clotting
    (hemorrhaging) or not clotting
Blood pressure, high
BLOOD PURIFIER
Body building
Boils

Bowels (sluggish)
Breath odor
BURSITIS
CANCER (COLON
    PREVENTION)
Colds
Constipation
Cramps (muscle spasms)
DIABETES
DIGESTIVE DISORDERS
Dysuria (painful urination)
FATIGUE (MENTAL &
    PHYSICAL)
Fever (reduces)
Flu
Fungal/yeast infections

GOUT
Gravel
Heart disease
HEMORRHAGES
Hormone imbalance
Hypertension
Hypoglycemia
Infections (bacterial)
Inflammation
Insomnia
Jaundice
Joint inflammation/swelling
Kidney cleanser
LACTATION (increases both quality & quantity of Mother's milk)
Liver conditions
Lupus (systemic)
MORNING SICKNESS
Muscle tone
NAUSEA
Nervousness
Nosebleeds
Pain, minor
PITUITARY GLAND (Cushing's disease)
RHEUMATISM
Scurvy
Stomach inflammation
Strokes
TOOTH DECAY
Toxemia
Tumor regression
Uric acid retention
ULCERS (PEPTIC)
Weakness (chronic)
Weight gain/loss (normalizes)
Whooping Cough

ALOE (Aloe vera)
A.K.A.,: Barbados Aloe, Medicine Plant, Lily of the Desert.

BODILY INFLUENCE: Abortifacient, Alterative, Anthelmintic, Antibacterial, Antibiotic, Anti-inflammatory, Antiseptic, Bitter, Cathartic, Cell proliferant, Cholagogue, Decoagulant, Demulcent, Depurative, Emmenagogue, Emollient, Insecticide, Laxative, Purgative, Stimulant, Stomachic, Tonic, Vemifuge, Vulnerary.
PART USED: Leaf.

Worldwide, Aloe Vera carries the idea of its being a plant that heals. Its inner mucus-like sap, called gel, is rich in over 200 hundred nutrients known to be beneficial to mankind. It will be commonly found in the better cosmetics, because it naturally balances the pH of skin. The plants. enzymes soften skin by removing dead cells and increases moisture which fight the effects of aging.

Aloe vera is one of the oldest known therapeutic herbs. All Aloe plants exhibit more or less the same properties; however, the Aloe vera variety is easiest to use medicinally because of its size and softness of the leaf. The Greek Historian Dioscorides wrote 2,000 years ago, that Aloe vera was an effective treatment for everything from constipation to burns to kidney ailments. The Egyptians secret of embalming was believed to have incorporated the Aloe plant in its process.

Aloe's are a member of the Lily family. The term "Aloe" is from the Arabic "alloeh" or the Hebrew "halal", which means a shining and bitter substance. "Vera" is from the Latin root "verus", which means "true".

The inner chamber of the Aloe vera leaf is made up of the clear pulp, which resembles slightly-melted lemon Jell-O. The pulp is believed to contain the wound-healing agents. The Russians call these "biogenic stimulators." They now have developed a process by where they can use the leaf of the plant, which is also the strongest part of the plant, for nutrients. It was not used as food before because of its strong purgative qualities. It caused uncontrollable bowel spasms in its raw form. This new processing has enabled the leaf to now be used nutritionally, but without the accompanying strong laxative effect. This is now called Whole Leaf Aloe. Whole Leaf Aloe is many times stronger in nutrients than the gel. This product can be used very effectively for people in debilitated conditions. It is very high in nutritive properties that are easily absorbed.

Aloe has a natural antidotal effect, neutralizing body toxins thus, reducing arthritic pain caused by tissue toxicity.

• Aloe Vera has been used widely in Holistic medicine in the treatment of the HIV virus which is related to AIDS. It buffers the HIV virus from entering one cell to the next, inhibiting the virus from moving throughout the body. The effect is to stabilize the life force; thereby, contributing to balancing the blood. It is believed to boost the immune system by balancing the pH of the blood and also increases digestion and absorption.

• As early as 1935, Aloe Vera juice was recommended in treating certain types of burns, such as third degree x-ray burns and more recently, it has been advocated in treating atomic radiation burns.

• Aloe Vera has properties for promoting the removal of dead skin and stimulating the normal growth of living cells.

• During the healing process, it can stop pain and reduce the chance of infection and scarring and is especially beneficial for first and second degree thermal burns.

• Aloe Vera is excellent for absorbing toxins and promoting growth of friendly colon bacteria.

Abrasions
ACNE
AIDS (whole leaf)
ALLERGIES
Amenorrhea
Anemia
Asthma
Athlete's foot
BED SORES
BLEEDING
Blood cleansing

Bowels (regulates)
Bruises
BURNS or SCALDS
CANKER SORES
CHICKEN POX ITCH
COLITIS
Constipation
DENTURE SORES
DEODORANT
DIGESTION or INDIGESTION
ECZEMA

Fever blisters	RADIATION BURNS
FLU	RINGWORM
Hair growth (promotes)	SCALDS
Headache	SCAR TISSUE
Heart (increase oxygen)	Shingles
HEARTBURN	SKIN ERUPTIONS
HEMORRHOIDS	STOMACH (SOOTHES)
HERPES	SORES (ULCERATED)
Inflammation	SUNBURN
INSECT BITES or STINGS	Tapeworm
Jaundice	THERMAL BURNS
Leg ulcers	Tinnitus
Liver disorders	Tuberculosis
PAIN	ULCERS (LEG)
Pink eye	Ulcers (peptic)
PIN WORMS	Varicose veins
Pimples	Weaning
POISON IVY or OAK	WOUNDS
PSORIASIS	Wrinkling of skin

ALTHEA   (SEE MARSHMALLOW ROOT)

AMARANTH   (Amaranthus spp.,)
A.K.A.,: Lovely Bleeding, Love lies bleeding, Prince's feather.

BODILY INFLUENCE: Alterative, Astringent, Demulcent, Diuretic, Nutritive, Styptic-mild, Tonic.
PART USED: Leaves and Flowers.

Amaranth is named from a Greek word meaning "unfading". Amaranth is a grain-like seed, which contains a rich variety of life-sustaining nutrients making it an excellent food. In the past, this Native American plant was harvested and was used as a survival food by the Indians of Central and North America, most notably among the Aztec or Meztec Indians. Today, it is popped to be eaten as a form of pop-corn garnished with honey.

Amaranth gained its folk name "love lies bleeding" from its use in treating excessive menstruation. Another historical use of Amaranth was by early herbalists in the treatment of diarrhea and dysentery.

Amaranth is currently being rediscovered in America due to its content of very high quality protein. It has a high concentration of the amino acid L-Lysine, which is not normally found in plants.

• L-Lysine has been found to be an excellent herbal cure for Herpes, which according to some statistics, 70% of all the people in the United States have had already in some form, such as

Herpes (Simplex I & II). This problem greatly weakens the immune system. Even "The Saturday Evening Post" magazine is now promoting a corn that produces high amounts of Lysine. L-Lysine deficiencies seem to be world-wide in humans and animals. They have proven that L-Lysine in the diet greatly boosts the immune system.
• Amaranth has been found to be an excellent food to help control the spread of Candida Albicans. This grain-like seed has been found compatible with the curtailment of the rapid growth of CANDIDA ALBICANS and can be used in place of grain in grain-free breads and desserts.
• Amaranth leaves are eaten as a pot herb in place of spinach in France.

Blood (spitting up)
CANDIDA ALBICANS
Canker sores
Convalescence (as nutritive)
DIARRHEA
DYSENTERY
Gastroenteritis
Gums (bleeding)
Hemorrhage
HERPES
Kidneys
MENSTRUATION (EXCESSIVE)
Nosebleeds
Spleen
Stomach flu
Swelling
Ulcers (mouth & stomach)
VIRUSES
Worms
Wounds

ANGELICA   (A. atropurpurea)
A.K.A.,: Wild Archangel, Masterwort.

BODILY INFLUENCE: Aromatic, Bitter, Carminative, Diaphoretic, Diuretic, Emmenagogue, Expectorant, Stimulant, Stomachic, Tonic.
PART USED: Root, leaves, seeds.

This plant had historical use during the great plague of Europe. It is reported that a monk said he was told by an angel in his dreams that Angelica would cure the plague. Appropriately, Angelica water became an ingredient in an official remedy published by the College of Physicians in London called "The King's Majesty's Excellent Recipe for the Plague." Angelica water was mixed with nutmeg and other herbs, made into a tea and then drunk twice a day for the plague.
• Today, Angelica is mainly valued for its stimulating effects on the digestive system.
• People have chewed on the root of Angelica prior to World War I in the hopes that they would be protected from the influenza epidemic.
• Angelica is used for digestive, heartburn, gas and bronchial

problems.
- Angelica is invigorating and strengthening to the body and can be used as a tonic to improve vitality and mental well being.
- Angelica is used to clean wounds aiding in the healing process.
- Angelica has been used for treating hypertension of the heart.

CAUTION: NOT TO BE TAKEN IN LARGE AMOUNTS DURING PREGNANCY, AS IT IS AN EMMENAGOGUE THAT CAUSES UTERINE CONTRACTIONS AND ALSO SHOULD NOT BE TAKEN WHEN YOU'RE HAVING EXCESSIVE BLEEDING.

APPETITE STIMULANT
Arthritis
Asthma
Backaches
Blood pressure (lowers)
BRONCHIAL PROBLEMS
COLDS
COLIC
Coughs
Digestive problems
Ears (drops for deafness)
Epilepsy
EXHAUSTION
Fever (intermittent)
Flu
GAS
Gout
Headaches
Heart (strengthens)
HEARTBURN
Hemorrhoids
Inflammation
Intestinal problems
Liver
Lungs
Menstruation (promotes)
Prostate problems
RHEUMATISM
Spleen
Stomach troubles
TONIC
Toothaches
Ulcers
Urination (increases)
Vomiting

ANISE   (Pimpinella anisum)
A.K.A.,: Aniseed.

BODILY INFLUENCE: Abortifacient, Anodyne, Antiseptic, Antispasmodic, Aromatic, Carminative, Diaphoretic, Diuretic, Expectorant, Galactagogue, Pectoral, Stimulant, Stomachic.
PART USED: Oil and Seeds.

Anise was used by the Romans, primarily as a flavoring. It is noted that they served cake heavily flavored with Anise which worked to provide a delightful palette and to help prevent indigestion from overeating. It is believed that wedding cakes were treated as such and that this ultimately resulted in the traditional wedding cake.
In modern times, Anise is found in both culinary and

medicinal products, including such products as cough medicine, candies and bakery goods.

Hypocrites used the herb for coughs. Later in history, a Roman scholar stated that by chewing Anise in the morning, all bad odors in the mouth would be removed. It is still recommended for this purpose today.

* Anise is very similar to Fennel and is used to improve the flavor of herbal formulas.
* Anise stimulates the female glands by helping to control estrogen levels. In the blood, it stimulates most of the other glands as well.
* Anise effects the digestive system and breaks up mucus blockage. It helps to prevent fermentation and gas in the digestive tract.
* Anise is a cell stimulator for the heart, liver, brain and lungs.
* The volatile oil of Anise can be helpful for treating bronchitis and spasmodic asthma.
* Anise oil can help relieve those suffering from emphysema.

Appetite stimulant	Epilepsy
Asthma	Gallbladder
Breath sweetener/Halitosis	GAS
Bronchitis	INDIGESTION
Cholera	Insomnia
COLDS (HARD AND DRY)	MUCUS
COLIC	NERVOUSNESS
Convulsions (spasms)	Pneumonia
COUGHS (EXPECTORANT)	Postpartum
Dysmenorrhea	Whooping cough
Emphysema	

ANTLER (Deer and Elk)
A.K.A.,: Dragons tooth, Dragon bone.

BODILY INFLUENCE: Adaptogen, Antipyretic, Antispasmodic, Aphrodisiac.
PART USED: Entire Antler.

The use of Antler dates back over two thousand years. Powders made of antler are fundamental in Oriental medicine. The first documented evidence of the use of Antler was during the Han dynasty in the Hunan province of China. It is usually found in combination with herbs.

Antlers are unique in that no other living animal produces a growth that reproduces itself once each year. Of these, the Elk and the Deer, are considered by the Chinese to be some of their most important animals, where medicine is concerned.

To the Asians, the prized part of the Deer or Elk is its antler rack. The velvet taken from the rack of a young buck is used as an elixir for strength and vitality to maintain good health. It is also used in the treating of sickness to restore a weakened condition. The deer antler velvet is a medical tool for increasing blood volume. It works on the basis that, with the increase of the blood, energy will be increased and better health will result.

The ground products are rich in Calcium and trace elements, dependent upon the diet of the animal providing the rack. This is considered of particular benefit to older folks needing Calcium. The elixir of antler velvet, according to Chinese Medicine, will provide vital energy, increasing strength, memory and will.

AGING
Anemia
Arthritis
Back (soreness, aching)
Blood deficiency
Blood pressure (low)
Carbuncles
Childbirth (easier)
Cholesterol (high)
Consumption
EJACULATION (PREMATURE)
ENERGY DEFICIENCY
Epilepsy
Fevers
Flu
Frigidity
Gastro-intestinal disorders
HORMONAL DEFICIENCY
IMPOTENCY
INFERTILITY
Kidney deficiency
Learning disabilities (child)
Leukorrhea (discharge from vagina)
Liver problems

Lochia (discharge following childbirth)
Longevity
Lumbago
Memory
Menopause
Menstrual disorders
Metabolism (raises)
Miscarriage (prevents)
Osteomyelitis
Rheumatism
Sinuses
Skeletal deformities (children)
Skin growth (promotes)
Sores
Stamina
Stress
Teeth (generating)
Tonic (for children)
Urination (frequent)
Vaginal (blood discharges)
WEAKNESS (GENERAL)
Weight (excessive loss of)

ASTRAGALUS (A. membranaceus)
A.K.A.,: Huang qi, Astragali.

BODILY INFLUENCE: Adaptogen, Antibacterial, Anhydrotic(stops sweating), Anti-hypertensive, Anti-inflammatory, Antiviral, Cardio-tonic, Diuretic, Immuno-stimulant, Pectoral, Tonic.
PART USED: The Root.

Astragalus is rich in polysaccharides which are basically the main nutrient that feeds our bodies.   Astragalus is known for its supporting of T-cell function and overall immune strength at a very deep level (bone marrow reserves) and is highly acclaimed as probably the most important of all deep immune tonics.
The use of Astragalus increases the level of interferon and antibodies.   It is known to increase strength, and vitality. Astragalus helps in the elimination of toxins thus promoting the healing of damaged tissue.   It supports liver and spleen function and in supporting the liver protects it against chemical damage caused by chemotherapy and also helps to normalize blood pressure.   When added to the program, Astragalus actually doubled the life of cancer patients who opted to be treated by chemotherapy and radiotherapy.
• Astragalus is primarily used in traditional Chinese Medicine in compounds with other herbs.
• Astragalus is a strong immune-enhancing herb and superior tonic, thus aids in recovery from illness and surgery. It combats fatigue by nourishing exhausted adrenals.
• Astragalus is an adaptogen herb which has been credited with long life of the cell. Research has been done to show that Astragalus increases the strength of T-cells. T-cells are the white blood cells of the body that attack the invaders that cause disease in the body. The T-cells are also called "killer cells" because of their ability to destroy foreign invaders in the body. It seems to protect the healthy cells even when chemotherapy is used.
• Urine flow is improved by Astragalus by reducing the potential of infection predominantly in the bladder.
• Astragalus is an anti-clotting agent and has vaso-dilating properties, helping prevent coronary heart disease and improving circulation.
• Astragalus has been demonstrated to increase energy, by the reduction of toxicity in the liver. As such, it acts as a heart tonic, which lowers blood pressure, dilates blood vessels and increases endurance to fatigued hearts.
• Astragalus increases the flow of bile and digestive fluids.

Adrenals
AIDS
Allergies
Arthritis
Blood pressure (lowers)
Cachexia (malnutrition)
Cancer (uterus)
Candida Albicans
COLDS
Debility
Degenerative conditions
Diabetes
DIGESTION (strengthens)
Edema
Epstein-Barr virus
Fatigue
Flu
Heart disease
Hepatitis
Hypertension
Immune system function
Infections (chronic)

Injuries (healing of)
Kidneys
Lesions (chronic)
Leukemia
LIVER CONDITIONS
Lungs (weak, short of breath)
Malaria
Metabolism (raises)
Muscle spasms
NEPHRITIS
Night sweats
PROLAPSED ORGANS
Spleen
Stress
Sweating (spontaneous)
Thymus (T-cells)
Ulcers
Urination (increases)
Vaginitis
Weakness (long term)
Wounds

BARBERRY   (Berberis vulgaris)
A.K.A.,: Jaundice Berry, Pepperidge Bush.

BODILY INFLUENCE: Alterative, Anthelmintic, Anti-bacterial, Antiseptic, Aperitive, Aromatic, Astringent, Bitter, Blood Purifier, Cholagogue, Diuretic, Hepatic, Hypotensive, Laxative, Refrigerant-Berries, Stomachic, Tonic-liver, Tonic.
PART USED: Bark, Root, Berries.

Historically, Barberry was found to be used by the North American Indians for treating the liver. It was found to be effective in cases of jaundice. Physicians have found that Barberry increases the secretion of bile, eliminating the stress of the liver that is contaminated by impure blood.

Barberry has a long history of use that goes back to ancient Egypt. They mixed it with Fennel seed to prevent the plague.

Barberry contains an alkaloid called Berberine which dilates blood vessels, thereby lowering blood pressure. Berberine is a strong antiseptic that is also found in Golden Seal. It is a stimulant on the myocardium and intestinal smooth muscle. If taken excessively, it may cause depression. It is also known to exhibit effects on respiration. Berberine reduces bronchial constriction, while it also is a mild anesthetic. It also works to care for the mucous membranes.

- Barberry is one of the best medicinal herb plants in the America's.
- Barberry helps to strengthen the body and is a system Invigorator.
- Barberry works to increase bowel functions thus stimulating appetite and promoting bile secretion. It is claimed to have no equal in normalizing liver secretions.
- Barberry exhibits superior stimulatory effects when used with Cayenne, which is a frequently used compound in mixtures.
- Barberry soothes and works to heal sore throats when used as a gargle and mouthwash. This is due to its astringent and antibacterial properties.
- Barberry alleviates anemia and general malnutrition.
- Barberry will reduce inflammation of the spleen caused by irritations due to contaminated blood and is effective at loosening obstructions in the intestinal tract.

Anemia
APPETITE (lack of)
Arthritis
Bladder
Blood cleanser
BLOOD PRESSURE (HIGH)
BLOOD PURIFIER
Boils
Breath odor
Bright's disease
Bronchials (constriction)
Cholera
CONSTIPATION (LIVER RELATED)
Debility (general)
DIARRHEA
Digestive disorders
DYSENTERY
Dyspepsia
FEVERS
GALLBLADDER (sluggish)
Gallstones
Gum diseases
Heart
Heartburn
Hemorrhaging
INDIGESTION
INFECTIONS
Itching
JAUNDICE
Kidneys
LIVER CONDITIONS
Migraine headaches
MOUTH ULCERS
PYORRHEA
Rheumatism
Ringworm
Skin disorders
SORE THROAT
Spleen
SYPHILIS
TYPHOID FEVER

BARLEY JUICE POWDER

BODILY INFLUENCE: Adaptogenic, Anti-inflammatory, Demulcent, Emollient, Immuno-stimulant, Nutritive, Stomachic, Tonic.
PART USED: Young leaves. young grass

Barley was one of the first crops planted in the Virginia Colony in 1611. It was known as a sacred grain to the Egyptians and Greeks. It is one of the most ancient of cultivated grains. In the grain form, it is known for its soothing and strengthening properties. It is easy to assimilate into the system. An entire book on the benefits of gruel made from Barley was written by Hypocrites.

In this section, however we will deal with the young grass of the Barley and relate to the benefits of young Barley Grass Juice.

Barley Grass Powder provide SOD (super oxide dismutase), a free radical scavenger, in greater amounts than most any other food source available. It is an excellent blood and immune builder.

Comparison tests have shown Barley Grass Juice Powder to have as much as thirty times more vitamin B-1 than cow,s milk and eleven times the amount of Calcium. Barley Grass Juice Powder holds about six times the amount of carotene than does spinach. It has seven times the amount of vitamin C, than an equal amount of oranges. Barley also has B-12, a vitamin that works to overcome fatigue and anemia, an important factor for many vegetarians.

Barley Grass Juice Powder is made by separating the juice in the Barley Grass from the grass solids, and then by a specially freeze dry process, evaporates the water off the juice leaving the Barley grass juice powder. This process further concentrates the food elements which are in the whole Barley Grass. The process itself must be done carefully at low temperatures, to protect the vital and sensitive nutritious components found in Barley.

Barley grass promotes natural tissue repair and nourishes anti-aging mechanisms of the body. Barley Grass Juice Powder was determined to be an anti-inflammatory agent, therefore it will be found effective in the healing of stomach and duodenal ulcers. It will help chronically inflamed hemorrhoids and should work to reduce pancreas infections.

• Barley juice powder is a great cleanser and booster for the immune system.
• Barley juice powder detoxifies cells and normalizes the metabolism. It assists in balancing the body chemistry and acts as a cell detoxifier.

- Barley juice powder neutralizes heavy metals such as lead and mercury.
- Barley juice powder is a cholesterol reducer along with being a blood purifier.

Acne
AGING (anti-)
AIDS
Allergies
ANEMIA
APPETITE (EXCESSIVE)
ARTHRITIS
Asthma
Blood pressure (high)
BLOOD PURIFIER
Body odor
BOILS
Bronchitis
CANCER
CATARRH
Cholesterol
Constipation
Diabetes
Digestion
Eczema
FEVERS
Gastritis
Hay Fever
Heart disease
Heavy metals

Hepatitis
Herpes
ILLNESS (general)
Impotence
Infections
Inflammation
Kidney problems
Leprosy
LIVER SPOTS
Lumbago
Lung problems
METAL POISONING
MUSCULAR DYSTROPHY
Obesity
Pancreatitis
POLYPS
Psoriasis
Skin problems
Smoking
Syphilis
Toxic conditions
Tuberculosis
Ulcers
Virus attack

BASIL (Ocimum basilicum)
A.K.A.,: Common Basil, Sweet Basil.

BODILY INFLUENCE: Antibacterial, Antispasmodic, Demulcent, Diaphoretic, Diuretic, Febrifuge, Galactagogue, Pectoral, Refrigerant, Stimulant, Stomachic, Vermifuge.
PART USED: Herb, Leaves.

In the Far East, it has been used as a cough medicine and in Africa, it has been used to expel worms. Basil was looked upon highly in India where it was worshipped as a sacred herb and was considered more valuable than the kings and queens of ancient times.

* In case of complete exhaustion, Basil has been used very effectively as a stimulant.
* Basil has positive antispasmodic and antibacterial properties. It is therefore useful for drawing out poisons when applied to wasp and hornet stings or venomous bites.

Bladder problems
Catarrh (intestinal)
COLDS
Colon
Constipation
CROUP
DYSENTERY
EARACHES
Enteritis
FEVERS
Flu
HEADACHES
INDIGESTION
INSECT BITES
Kidney problems
Liver
Menstruation (suppressed)
Nausea
Nervous conditions
Parasites
Respiratory infections
Rheumatism
SNAKE BITES
SORES
SPASMS
Spleen
Stomach cramps
Vomiting (excessive)
WHOOPING COUGH
Worms

BAYBERRY (Myrica cerifera)
A.K.A.,: Candle Berry, Wax Myrtle.

BODILY INFLUENCE: Antibacterial, Antiseptic, Astringent, Deobstruent, Emetic, Febrifuge, Insecticide, Stimulant, Tonic.
PART USED: Dried root bark and sometimes the leaves.

It is believed that Bayberry powder may be sniffed up the nose for relief of sinus congestion and has been used to alleviate nasal polyps. However, be warned that Bayberry snuff may cause sneezing and headaches. Bayberry is more effectively used as a tea for douches for treatment of excessive vaginal bleeding.

- Bayberry is a stimulant which invigorates and strengthens the body.
- Bayberry is very desirable in treating any problem associated with the female organs as such and has been found useful to check menstruation.
- Bayberry can be applied on the skin for cancerous and ulcerated sores. It is a strong cleanser and healer.
- When taken along with Capsicum, Bayberry can be helpful in warding off colds, fevers and chills at their onset.
- Bayberry's major effect is said to be on the mucous accumulation in the respiratory and alimentary tracts. It is also used as a gargle for tonsillitis and sore throats.
- In India, Bayberry and Ginger when combined together has reportedly been able to combat even the effects of cholera.
- Bayberry is used as a tonic, which stimulates the body, helping to raise vitality.
- Used as a tonic, Bayberry creates a resistance to disease and helps to aid digestion, nutrition and blood building.
- Bayberry also is reported to soothe the mucous membranes and to stimulate blood circulation.
- Poultices made with the root bark are said to help heal ulcers, cuts, bruises, and insect bites.
- Bayberry inhibits bacteria and therefore is a useful agent in fighting infection.

ADRENAL
    WEAKNESS
Asthma
BLEEDING
    (external)
Bronchitis
CANKER SORES
Catarrh (intestinal)
Chills
COLDS (breaks up
    mucus)
CHOLERA
Colon
CONGESTION
    (general)
Cramps
CUTS
DIARRHEA
    (chronic)
Digestive disorders
DYSENTERY
Dyspepsia
ENDOMETRIOSIS

Eyes
FEVERS
FEMALE
    PROBLEMS
FLU
Gangrenous sores
Gargle
GLANDS
GOITER
GUMS (BLEEDING,
    SPONGY)
Headache (sinus)
HEMORRHAGE
HEPATITIS
INDIGESTION
Infection
JAUNDICE
Liver problems
Lungs
MENSTRUAL
    BLEEDING
    (EXCESSIVE)

MENSTRUAL
    DISORDERS
MISCARRIAGE
    (STOPS
    BLEEDING)
Mucus membranes
Nasal congestion
Scarlet fever
SCOFULA
Scurvy
SINUSITIS
Sore throat
Stomach
Thyroid
Ulcers
UTERINE
    HEMORRHAGE
Uterus (prolapsed)
Vaginal discharge
Varicose veins

BEE POLLEN

BODILY INFLUENCE: Corrects polarity, Hormonal, Nutritive, Stimulant, Tonic-General.
PART USED: Bee Pollen

Pollen is created from the male parts of flowering plants and is provided in nature to fertilize the female flowers that produce seeds.

The bees store their pollen, upon returning to their home. It remains stored until used for food and other things in the hive.

• Bee Pollen is completely balanced for vitamins, minerals, proteins, carbohydrates, fats, enzyme precursors and all essential amino acids.

• Bee Pollen is a complete blood building food that rejuvenates and is especially beneficial for the extra nutritional needs of athletes and patients rebuilding the body from illness.

• Bee Pollen is often used as a antidote during allergy season. Bee Pollen also relieves other respiratory problems such as bronchitis, sinusitis and colds. U.S. Senator Harkin said that taking large doses of Bee Pollen cured his asthma which had plagued him most of his life. He also said he had taken everything that modern medical science ever had and none of it worked until he took Bee Pollen.

• As with Royal Jelly, Bee Pollen helps balance the endocrine system, showing especially beneficial results in menstrual and prostate problems.

• The enzyme support in Bee Pollen normalizes chronic colitis and constipation/diarrhea symptoms.

• Recent research has shown that Bee Pollen helps counteract the effects of aging, increases both mental and physical capability and and fortifies the body against illnesses.

• When taking Bee Pollen as part of a health program, always start out with small doses as some have reported allergy symptoms connected with its use.

ALLERGIES
APPETITE STIMULANT
Asthma
Blood pressure (lowers)
Cancer
CAPILLARY WEAKNESS
CONVALESCENCE
Depression
ENDURANCE (lack of)
ENERGY (lack of)
EXHAUSTION
FATIGUE (builds energy)

HAYFEVER
Hypoglycemia
IMMUNE DEFICIENCY
Indigestion
Liver diseases
LONGEVITY
MULTIPLE SCLEROSIS
PREGNANCY
Prostate disorders
Radiation
Vitality

BEE PROPOLIS

BODILY INFLUENCE: Antibacterial, Antibiotic, Anti-fungal, Anti-inflammatory, Anti-viral, Bacteriocide, Cell proliferant, Immuno-stimulant.
PART USED: Tree Bud Resin.

Bees use Propolis as a building material together with beeswax in the construction of hives. Propolis has a pleasant sweet-smelling odor with the texture resembling resin collected by the bees from the bark of leaf buds of trees, especially the popular tree.

Recorded history shows that Bee Propolis has been used in medicine, perhaps as far back as the first century A.D. The medicinal value of Bee Propolis was known by the Roman philosopher, Celsus, when he wrote in the first century A.D. giving instructions on preparing resin poultices containing Bee Propolis.

Bee Propolis was mentioned in the Islamic book of the Koran in manuscripts from the 6th and 8th centuries. There it is cited as an effective remedy for blood purification, skin disorders and bronchial catarrhs.

Bee Propolis is a strong source of trace minerals such as copper, magnesium, silicon, iron, manganese and zinc. It is also rich in amino acids. As with all bee products, Bee Propolis has strong antibiotic properties. It is also a powerful anti-viral which is effective against pneumonia and similar viral infections. It is used to treat stomach and intestinal ulcers. It aids the healing of broken bones, by accelerating new cell growth and has a part in the natural treatment of gum, mouth and throat disorders.

Research has confirmed its traditional reputation for lowering high blood pressure, reducing arteriosclerosis and lessening the risks of coronary heart disease. New research is currently being done on Propolis and its healing effects on certain skin cancers and melanomas. In Russia, scientists have reported that Bee Propolis induces phagocytosis, that works to destroy bacteria by improving white blood cells. In addition, surgeons in Russia now use honey as a proactive remedy to combat infection resulting from surgery.

• As the first line of defense against beehive micro-organisms, Bee Propolis is a natural antibiotic, antibacterial, anti-viral and anti-fungal substance. In humans, it stimulates the thymus gland and thus boosts the thyroid gland for improved immunity and resistance to infections.

Abscesses
ACNE
ARTERIOSCLEROSIS
BLOOD PRESSURE (HIGH)
Bruises
Burns
CORNS
Cystitis
DUODENAL ULCERS
ECZEMA (DRY)
GASTRIC ULCERS
Gum disorders
Halitosis
HERPES LESIONS
IMMUNE SYSTEM STIMULANT

INFECTIONS (MOUTH & THROAT)
Migraine headaches
MOUTH ULCERS
PNEUMONIA
Prostate trouble
Psoriasis
RESPIRATORY AILMENTS
SHINGLES
SKIN PROBLEMS
STOMACH ULCERS
Throat
Tonsillitis
Ulcers
WARTS

BEE'S ROYAL JELLY

BODILY INFLUENCE: Adaptogen, Antibacterial, Antibiotic.
PART USED: Royal Jelly.

Royal Jelly is the thick, sweet, milky substance secreted from the pharyngeal glands of a special group of young nurse bees who ingest honey and pollen. These young nurse bees are active between their 6th and 12th days of life when they produce what is called Royal Jelly.

It is Royal Jelly which is fed to an ordinary female bee who then becomes a Queen Bee. Those chosen to be queens are fed this Royal Jelly and then amazing things begin to happen. The bee transforms into a Queen Bee, which grows far larger than the other bees. In the process, she develops great energy and stamina. The Queen Bee will be able to produce the raw materials to lay as many as 2,000 eggs daily and live 60 times as long as other bees.

• Royal Jelly revitalizes the endocrine glands in the manner of live cells, reviving endocrine glands, boosting the immune system, reviving a weak constitution, improving poor skin and extending youthfulness.

• Argentinian researchers found that Royal Jelly contains globulinic acid (gamma globulin), which increases resistance to bacteria and viruses. It also contains a gelatinous amino acid, a basic ingredient in collagen, which is a fibrous protein important for connective tissue, essential to youthful, firm skin.

• It increases resistance to infection and helps to relieve gastro-duodenal ulcers.

• Royal Jelly fights the aging process by means of its inositol (related to the B complex) content, which Canadian researchers have found reduces cholesterol. They also contend that it blocks the deposition of cholesterol on the walls of the blood vessels. Further, with the inositol, it was reported that blood vessels remained youthful and free of hazardous plaque.

- It is a powerhouse of vitamins being high in B-5 & B-6, and has all the B vitamins, minerals, enzyme precursors and 8 essential amino acids required by the body.
- Royal Jelly contains every nutrient necessary to support life. It is one of the world's richest sources of pantothenic acid which is needed for the adrenal glands.
- It has the necessary nutrient for proper digestion and healthy skin and hair.
- Royal Jelly is a natural antibiotic, and promotes deep cellular health. It has been found effective for gland and hormone imbalances that may be experienced in menstrual and prostate problems.

Anxiety
ASTHMA
Bone fractures
Bronchials
Cholesterol (reduces)
Depression
Digestive disorders
Eczema
ENERGY/STAMINA
Flu
Gallbladder troubles
Herpes
Hormone imbalances
IMMUNE SYSTEM
Impetigo
INSOMNIA
Kidney disease
Liver disease
LONGEVITY
MENTAL ALERTNESS
MENSTRUAL PROBLEMS
Migraine headaches
Pancreatitis
PROSTATE PROBLEMS
Senility
Sexual dysfunction
Shock
Skin disorders
Stomach ulcers

BILBERRY (Vaccinium myrtillus)
A.K.A.,: BLUEBERRY, HUCKLEBERRY.

BODILY INFLUENCE: Antiseptic, Astringent, Diuretic, Nutritive.
PART USED: Leaves and berries.

Bilberry is native to northern Europe and Asia and one can eat the berries or make them into jams and jellies with honey.

One of the most recent advances in the use of Bilberry was found during World War II. The story goes that British RAF pilots were using Bilberry jam on their bread. It was noted that these pilots seemed to be far more successful at hitting their targets. After research was done on the use of Bilberry in the use of eye disorders, it was found to help against fatigue, reduce eye irritation, nearsightedness and nightblindness, extend the range and sharpness of vision, aid in the adaptation to darkness by accelerating regeneration of the retina and help to restrain the development of conditions such as glaucoma cataracts.

The berries of the plant contain anthocyanins associated with P-vitamin (bioflavonoid) functions. Anthocyanins are distributed generously in the plants and the P-vitamin effect is noted even stronger in Bilberry than in other combinations, particularly citrus fruits. This works well in the strengthening of capillaries in the peripheral circulation, lessening the permeability of the capillary membranes.

• The dried berries of Bilberry are primarily used for their astringent qualities in the treatment of dysentery and diarrhea.

• Bilberry improves blood circulation by increasing the ability of fluids and nourishment to pass through veins and to capillaries.

THIS IS A BENEFICIAL HERB TO USE DURING PREGNANCY: IT CAN BE A STRONG BUT GENTLE ASTRINGENT AND WILL FORTIFY VEIN AND CAPILLARY SUPPORT, AIDS IN KIDNEY FUNCTION AND IS A MILD DIURETIC FOR BLOATING.

BLADDER STONES	INFECTIONS
Blood thinner	Kidney problems
BLOOD VESSELS	Light sensitive
COLD HANDS & FEET	NIGHT BLINDNESS
DIABETES	Raynaud's disease
DIARRHEA (INFANT)	Scurvy
Dropsy	Skin (ulcerative)
DYSENTERY	Typhoid epidemics
Eye problems	URINARY PROBLEMS
HEMORRHOIDS	VARICOSE VEINS
Immune system	Water retention

BIRCH (Betula alba, B. lenta)
A.K.A.,: White birch, Black birch, Mountain Mahogany.

BODILY INFLUENCE: Anthelmintic, Anti-rheumatic, Astringent, Depurative, Diuretic, Stimulant, Sudorific.
PART USED: Bark and Leaves.

The American Indians used Birch bark to make a tea to help relieve headaches. Some tribes brewed a tea from the leaves and dried bark for fevers, kidney stones, and abdominal cramps caused by gas in the digestive system.

• Poultices of boiled bark were used to aid in the healing of burns, wounds, and bruises.

- The natural properties of Birch are used for blood cleansing.
- The bark produces, "birch oil", by a dry distillation process. The oil is used in cases of certain skin conditions.
- Glycoside in Birch decomposes to produce methyl salicylate (aspirin) which is used as a remedy for rheumatism in North America.
- It has a mild sedative effect and can be taken for insomnia.

ARTHRITIS
BLADDER
Bleeding gums
BLOOD CLEANSER
Boils
Cancer
Canker sores
Cholera
Diarrhea
Dysentery
Dropsy
ECZEMA (EXTERNAL)
Fevers
Gas
Gonorrhea
Gout
Insomnia
Kidney problems
Kidney stones
PAIN
Pyorrhea
RHEUMATISM
Urinary tract problems
Worms (expels)

BISTORT   (Polygonum bistorta)
A.K.A.,: Dragonwort, Patience dock.

BODILY INFLUENCE: Antiseptic, Astringent, Diuretic, Expectorant, Hemostatic, Tonic.
PART USED: Root and leaves.

The name Bistort comes from Latin word elements meaning "twice-twisted.. This refers to the gnarled appearance of Bistort's dark brown rhizome or underground stem.

Bistort is one of the strongest astringents in the herb kingdom and has been used as a gargle for spongy gums. It is known to contains 20% tannins, therefore it is not for excessive use.

- Powdered Bistort has antiseptic properties when applied to wounds and is good for infectious diseases, driving them out by sweating.
- Externally, it is used as a wash for sores and hemorrhages.
- Bistort is a member of the buckwheat family and contains starch which in times of famine was dried and ground up for use as flour.
- Bistort is useful in all bleeding internally and externally.
- Although Bistort cleanses the entire body, it primarily purifies the alimentary canal.

Bedwetting
BLEEDING (EXTERNAL &
  INTERNAL)
Bowels
Canker sores
CHOLERA
CUTS
Diabetes
DIARRHEA
DYSENTERY
FEVERS
GUMS (SPONGY)
Hemorrhage
HEMORRHOIDS

Insect stings
Jaundice
Measles
Menstruation (regulates)
MOUTH WASH
Mucus
Plague
Skin eruptions
Smallpox
Tonic (spring)
Tumors
Vaginal discharge
Worms (expels)
Wounds

BLACKBERRY   (Rubus fructicosus and spp.,)
A.K.A.,: Bramble Berry, Dewberry.

BODILY INFLUENCE: Antipyretic, Astringent, Bitter, Hemostatic- Topical, Tonic.
PART USED: Roots , Leaves, Fruit.

In the Middle East, the mastication of leaves has been a remedy for bleeding gums since the time of Jesus.

A tonic made from the root of the Blackberry plant works effectively as an astringent and is mild enough to use for watery diarrhea in children.

Historically, Blackberry was used to treat diarrhea and also effectively used for the elimination of water from the system.

In Chinese herbal medicine, herbs are noted for either Yin or Yang application. The fruit is believed to apply to the Yin principle; therefore, it is the female functions of the body that would be affected. This means stamina and vigor for most.

Anemia
BLEEDING
Boils
CHOLERA
DIARRHEA (CHILDREN)
DYSENTERY
Female problems
Fevers
Vaginal irritations

Gums (bleeding)
Menstruation (excessive)
Rheumatism
Peristalsis, weak
SINUS DRAINAGE
Snakebite
Stomach (irritable)
VOMITING
Wounds

BLACK COHOSH (Cimicifuga racemosa)
A.K.A.,: Black Snakeroot, Bugbane.

BODILY INFLUENCE: Alterative, Analgesic, Anti-rheumatic, Antispasmodic, Antivenomous, Astringent, Bitter, Diaphoretic, Diuretic, Emmenagogue, Expectorant, Hormonal-female, Nervine, Oxytocic, Parturient, Sedative, Stomachic, Tonic-Glandular.
PART USED: Root.

Black Cohosh when flowering, exhibits a strong aroma that makes it effective as an insect repellent. The botanical name Cimicifuga is Latin for "bug repellent." Black Cohosh is called Snakeroot by the American Indians because of its use for snake bites. Also, it has proven its worth for those allergic to bee stings.

Black Cohosh was used by the early American Colonists for yellow fever, malaria, fevers, bronchitis, dropsy, uterine problems, and nervous disorders.

Black Cohosh was made famous by Lydia Pinkham who was credited with about 1/3 of the population of the United States. The label on the bottle said vegetable herbal compound, but everybody knew it as a "baby in every bottle."

Black Cohosh is used very effectively for spinal meningitis.

• Black Cohosh works directly on and calms the nervous system. It promotes menstruation, relieves menstrual cramps and has been employed for the after-pains of delivery.

• Black Cohosh breaks up mucus and phlegm deposits. It also soothes local pain and is used for headaches.

• Black Cohosh is used as a tonic for the central nervous system and is regarded as a nervine. It is an excellent, safe sedative. It is reported to be good for medulla oblongata damage, caused by hallucinogenic drugs.

• Black Cohosh relieves or prevents spasms, is used for epilepsy and causes perspiration.

• Black Cohosh contains natural estrogen, the female hormone and is a specific for female problems. Black Cohosh is also used many times in nervine combinations and for nervous conditions in the male also.

• Black Cohosh helps in hot flashes, it contracts the uterus and increases menstruation when its sluggish.

• Black Cohosh loosens and expels mucus from the bronchial tubes and stimulates the secretions of the liver, kidneys and lymph system and has a stimulating effect on the secretion of the spleen, liver and lymphatic system.

• A Black Cohosh poultice can be used for all kinds of inflammation.

- Black Cohosh equalizes blood circulation.
- Black Cohosh acts directly on the lungs, heart, stomach, kidneys and the reproductive organs. It is a mild cardiac tonic, especially on fatty hearts.
- Black Cohosh slightly lowers the heart rate, while increasing the force of the pulse.
- Black Cohosh, if taken in larger amounts than needed, can cause a headache at the base of the skull.

CAUTION: NOT TO BE TAKEN DURING EARLY PREGNANCY, EXCEPT IN COMBINATION WITH OTHER HERBS. IT CAN BE USED FOR FINAL WEEKS OF PREGNANCY, BUT ONLY TO EASE/ AND OR INDUCE LABOR.

Angina
Aphrodisiac (female)
Arthritis
ASTHMA
Bedbugs
BEE STINGS
BLOOD CLEANSER
BLOOD PRESSURE (HIGH)
Bowels
BRONCHITIS (CHRONIC)
CHILDBIRTH
Cholera
Chorea
Convulsions
Coughs
Diabetes
DIARRHEA
Digestive disorders
DROPSY
DYSMENORRHEA
EPILEPSY
ESTROGEN DEFICIENCY
FEVERS
Gallstones
Headaches
Heart palpitations
HORMONE BALANCER
HOT FLASHES
HYSTERIA
INSECT BITES
Kidney ailments

Inflammations (of all kinds)
Insomnia
Liver
Lumbago
LUNGS
MALARIA
MEASLES
MENOPAUSE
MENSTRUAL PROBLEMS
Nervous disorders
NEURALGIA
Pain
Paralysis
Pelvic disorders
POISON ANTIDOTE
POISONOUS BITES
RHEUMATISM
Skin disorders
Smallpox
SNAKE BITES
SORES
Sore throat
SPASMS
SPINAL MENINGITIS
ST. VITUS DANCE
Syphilis
TUBERCULOSIS
Typhoid fever
Uterine problems
WHOOPING COUGH
Worms

BLACK WALNUT   (Juglans nigra)
A.K.A.,: English Walnut.

BODILY INFLUENCE: Anthelmintic, Antifungal, Antiparasitic, Antiseptic, Astringent, Bitter, Insecticide, Laxative, Parasiticide, Vermifuge.
PART USED: Bark, Leaves, Nut.

Herbalists have traditionally used the husks of Black Walnut as a nutritional aid for the intestinal system. American Indian tribes have been known to use Black Walnut as a laxative. For many centuries in Europe, Black Walnut was used as a laxative and for skin aliments, especially herpes and eczema.

Black Walnut has been used on patients suffering from electrical shock.

• Black Walnut oxygenates the blood which helps to kill parasites. Black Walnut aids in expelling tapeworms, pinworms and ringworms and has been shown to be specific for treatment of Candida Albicans.

• Black Walnut is able to burn up excessive toxins and fatty materials, while it helps balance sugar levels.

• The green husk of Black Walnut produces a brown stain resulting from the high organic iodine content. This makes it antiseptic and useful in healing. It properties are useful in all sorts of cleansing programs, especially in expelling parasites.

• Black Walnut has been very successful in the treatment of Valley fever. There has been a massive increase in these cases since recent earthquakes and major excavations have occurred.

• Black Walnut has been highly thought of as a dependable remedy for "bad blood" diseases such as scrofulous, syphilis and Diptheria.

Abscesses	Diarrhea
Acne	Diptheria
Antiperspirant	Dysentery
ANTISEPTIC (EXTERNAL)	ECZEMA
Asthma	Eye diseases
ATHLETE'S FOOT	Fevers
BOILS (EXTERNAL	FUNGUS
APPLICATION)	Gargle
Cancer	GOITER
CANDIDA ALBICANS	GUM DISEASE
CANKER SORES	Hemorrhoids
Carbuncles	HERPES
COLD SORES (TOPICALLY	IMPETIGO
APPLIED)	INFECTIONS (INTERNAL)
Colitis	LACTATION (STOPS)
DANDRUFF	Liver congestion

LUPUS
MALARIA
Mouth sores
OXYGEN (DEFICIENCY IN
   BLOOD)
PARASITES (INTERNAL)
PINWORMS
POISON IVY/OAK
PROLAPSUS
RASHES (SKIN)
RINGWORM
Scrofula
Skin diseases

Syphilis
TAPEWORM
Teeth
Throat
Thyroid (low)
Tonsillitis
TUBERCULOSIS
Ulcers (internal)
Urinary bladder
Uterus (prolapsus)
Vaginal discharge
VALLEY FEVER
WORMS

BLESSED THISTLE (Cnicus benedictus)
A.K.A.,: St. Benedict Thistle, Holy Thistle, Spotted Thistle.

BODILY INFLUENCE: Alterative, Anthelmintic, Anti-pyretic, Aperitive, Carminative, Cholagogue, Diaphoretic-Stimulating, Diuretic, Emetic (in large doses), Emmenagogue, Galactagogue, Hormonal, Intoxicant, Nervine, Stimulant Tonic, Tonic-liver, Vermifuge.
PART USED: Leaves, flowers, seeds.

In 17th century England, the herbalist Culpepper lists Blessed Thistle for use in headaches, female complaints and for fevers.

In America, the Quinault Indians used the whole plant to create a birth-control medicinal.

In Europe, monks grew Blessed Thistle as a cure for smallpox, which is believed where this plant derived it name.

• Blessed Thistle acts to strengthen the heart, lungs, increases circulation to the brain by bringing oxygen to it which strengthens the memory and also aids in all liver disorders.

• Blessed Thistle stimulates milk production in nursing mothers, more so when taken in combination with Red Raspberry.

• Blessed Thistle has a long history as a digestive and general tonic.

• Blessed Thistle is useful for headaches in menopausal problems.

• Blessed Thistle helps to reduce and control fevers.

• Blessed Thistle helps with cramps, painful menstruation, headaches associated with female problems and also is a female hormone balancer.

• Blessed Thistle has been used for treating internal cancer.

ANGINA
Arthritis
Birth control
BLOOD CIRCULATION
BLOOD PURIFIER
BRAIN (circulation to)
BREAST MILK (TO ENRICH)
CALCIUM DEPOSITS
CANCER
CONSTIPATION
Cramps
DEPRESSION
DIGESTIVE DISORDERS
Dropsy
FEMALE PROBLEMS
FEVERS
GALLBLADDER
GAS
HEADACHES

HEART (STRENGTHENS)
HORMONE BALANCER
HYSTERIA
Inability to concentrate
Jaundice
Kidneys
LACTATION
Leucorrhea
LIVER CONDITIONS
LUNGS (strengthens)
MEMORY PROBLEMS
MENSTRUATION (PAINFUL)
Migraine headaches
PREGNANCY
Respiratory infection
Senility
Spleen
Vaginal discharge
Worms

BLUE COHOSH (Caulophyllum thalictroides)
A.K.A.,: Papoose root, Blue Ginseng, Squawroot.

BODILY INFLUENCE: Anthelmintic, Antispasmodic, Bitter, Diaphoretic, Diuretic, Emmenagogue, Nervine, Oxytocic, Sedative, Stimulant.
PART USED: Root.

Blue Cohosh was used by the North American Indians for cramps and menstrual problems. Cherokee, Chippewa, Iroquois, and other native North American Indians used Blue Cohosh herb for delayed delivery and to promote menstruation.

In recent times, Blue Cohosh has been shown to be useful in the regulation of menstrual cycles in women and is helpful in relieving painful menstruation. It is effective as an inhibiting agent to stop false labor pains in childbirth.

Blue Cohosh acts to stimulate the uterine muscle thereby advancing a delayed delivery. Because Blue Cohosh has a well deserved reputation for helping in cases of prolonged labor, it has been nick-named "a woman's best friend." It helps to relax the uterus so that delivery is easier, thus preventing pain and exhaustion. It is also useful to reduce inflammation of the uterus. If Blue Cohosh is given hours previous to delivery, it is said to be reliable and less dangerous where cases of labor are slow and painful.

• Blue Cohosh increases the flow of urine, and causes profuse perspiration.
• Blue Cohosh has a strong antispasmodic effect on the whole

system; thereby, has an effect on the nervous system and it can relieve muscle cramps and spasms.
• Blue Cohosh should be used in combination with other herbs, such as Black Cohosh.
• A Blue Cohosh poultice has been used as an emergency remedy for allergic reactions to bee stings.
Blue Cohosh has the ability to stop false labor pains.

AMENORRHEA
Bladder infection
Blood cleanser
Blood pressure (high)
Bronchitis
CHILDBIRTH PAIN
Colic
CRAMPS
DIABETES
Dropsy
Edema
EPILEPSY
ESTROGEN (LOW)
FEMALE PROBLEMS
Fits
Heart palpitations

Hysteria
Insect bites
Kidneys
LABOR (INDUCES)
Leucorrhea
MENSTRUAL DISORDERS
MENSES (REGULATES)
Mucus
NERVOUS DISORDERS
PALPITATIONS
RHEUMATISM
Spasms
URINARY TRACT INFECTIONS
UTERINE INFLAMMATION
VAGINITIS
Whooping cough

BLUE VERVAIN (Verbena hastata)
A.K.A.,: Indian Hyssop, Simpler's Joy.

BODILY INFLUENCE: Alterative, Analgesic, Anti-inflammatory, Anti-periodic, Anti-pyretic, Anti-spasmodic, Astringent, Diaphoretic, Diuretic, Emmenagogue, Expectorant, Galactagogue, Nervine, Parasiticide, Relaxant, Tonic. Blue Vervain is an alternative to Lobelia. Large doses may induce vomiting.
PART USED: Whole plant.

Blue Vervain, as with so many other of the herbal remedies dates back in time of use to ancient times. The root was used for malaria and dysentery in China, they used the stalk and leaves for blood conditions and for relieving congestion and helping to cleanse out body toxins. Blue Vervain was used as a cure all and by some as being a sacred plant. It was used to save lives during the Medieval plagues.

The leaves of the Blue Vervain were used to make a tea by the American Indians as a female tonic. They also used it for colds fevers and complaints of bowel problems. In liquid form, Blue Vervain is given to small children to help relieve colds, fevers and minor ailments. Blue Vervain has a calming, relaxing effect on the system which aids in breaking down obstructions and with a stimulating effect helps to expel waste from the system.
• Blue Vervain can be helpful as part of a liver cleanse when there is inflammation and jaundice.

- Blue Vervain is a quieting herb that helps calm coughing and is a natural tranquilizer.
- Blue Vervain is a mild laxative, causes perspiration and has the over-all effect of inducing relaxation.
- Blue Vervain has the ability to alleviate fevers, settle stomachs and produce an overall feeling of well being.
- Blue Vervain is one of the best herbs to use to help alleviate the onset of a cold, especially with upper respiratory inflammation of the lungs.
- Blue Vervain will aid in expelling phlegm from the throat and chest.
- Blue Vervain is helpful at expelling worms and often works where other remedies fail.

ADENOIDS (NOSE DROPS)
Ague (malaria)
ASTHMA
BLADDER
BOWELS
BRONCHITIS
Catarrh
CIRCULATION (POOR)
COLDS (CHILDREN)
COLON
CONGESTION (GENERAL)
Constipation
CONSUMPTION
CONVULSIONS
COUGHS
CROUP
CYSTIC FIBROSIS
DIARRHEA
Dysentery
Earaches
Epilepsy
Eyes (tonic)
FATIGUE
FEVERS
Female troubles
FLU
Gallstones

Headache (nervous)
Hysteria
INDIGESTION
INSOMNIA
Kidneys
Laxative
LIVER (TOXIC)
LUNG CONGESTION
Measles
Menstruation (painful/irregular)
Mucus
NERVOUS DISORDERS
Pain
Paralysis
PLAGUE
Pneumonia
SEIZURES
Skin diseases
Smoking
Sores
SORE THROATS (CHILDREN)
Spleen
Stomach troubles (settles)
SWELLINGS
WHOOPING COUGH
WORMS

BONESET   (Eupatorium perfoliatum)
A.K.A.,: Agueweed, Indian Sage, Feverwort.

BODILY INFLUENCE: Analgesic, Antipyretic, Aperitive, Bitter, Diaphoretic, Emetic, Febrifuge, Stimulant.
PART USED: Flower, leaf.

Research done in Western Germany suggests that one of the constituents of Boneset is that it stimulates white blood cells to consume more foreign agents. Thus, Boneset's traditional use as a remedy for infectious diseases has some scientific merit.

From the name of this herb, you might think its powers

included, the ability to mend broken bones; however, Boneset traditionally is used as a cough and fever remedy. It perhaps gets its name because of its usefulness in treating the flu. A flu that caused severe body aches, right to the bone was treated with Boneset and its application was called a "breakbone fever".

It had no equal as a cough, cold, and fever remedy during the eighteenth and nineteenth centuries. Civil War troops received Boneset infusions not only as remedies when they fell victim to fevers, but also as tonics to keep them healthy.
• It is a used as a mild tonic and useful in the indigestion of older folks.
• Boneset is a slow but continuous stimulant and tonic for the stomach, liver, bowel and uterus.
• Before the wide use of Aspirin, Boneset tea was one of the most popular home remedies for treating fever and colds.

Bronchitis
Catarrh
CHILLS
COLDS (WITH FEVER)
COUGHS
ENCEPHALITIS (BRAIN FEVER)
FEVERS (ALL KINDS)
FEVERS (TO BREAK)
FLU
Jaundice
Liver disorders
MALARIA

MEASLES
Mumps
Muscle aches
PAIN
Rheumatism (muscular)
Rocky Mountain Spotted Fever
Scarlet Fever
Sore throat
Tonic
TYPHOID FEVER
Worms
YELLOW FEVER

BORAGE (Borago officinalis)
A.K.A.,: Common Bugloss, Starflower.

BODILY INFLUENCE: Bitter, Depurative, Diaphoretic, Emollient, Febrifuge, Galactagogue, Laxative, Pectoral, Sudorific, Tonic.
PART USED: The Herb, Flowers, Leaves.

• Borage is used to treat bronchitis because it is soothing and reduces inflammation. It has been recommended for treatments involving the digestive system.
• Borage is helpful in treating the kidneys to dispose of mucous generated from a fever.
• Borage stimulates the adrenal glands, which helps restores vitality when recovering from illness.
• Borage has been used to soothe the mucous membranes of the mouth and throat.
• As a tonic, Borage tea is good as an eyewash for sore or irritated eyes.

- Borage has been used to increase the quantity of mother's milk.

Bladder	HEART (STRENGTHENS)
Blood purifier	Insomnia
BRONCHITIS	Jaundice
CATARRH (CHRONIC)	LACTATION
Colds	Lungs (decongestant)
Congestion (lung phlegm)	Nerves (calms)
Corns	Pleurisy
Digestion	RASHES
EYES (INFLAMMATION OF)	RINGWORM
FEVERS	Spasms

BRIGHAM TEA (AKA - MORMON TEA)
(SEE MA HUANG)

BRINDALL BERRIES (SEE GARCINIA)

BROAD BEAN (Vicia faba)
A.K.A.,: Horse Bean, Fava Bean, Windsor Bean.

BODILY INFLUENCE: Antispasmodic, Diuretic, Tonic.
PART USED: The Bean.

A general description of this plant is that it is sweet to the taste. It has been used as a tonic to strengthen the spleen. It is used to improve appetite and is nutritional, as well. As a food, it is effective to feed those who suffer from hypertension.

Broad bean is effective at eliminating water retention. Broad beans can remove water from the body because the lymphatics of the body are toned and nourished to strike a balance with the internal organs.

Broad beans can increase body energy, control seminal emission in men and make the intestines stronger.

- It contains L-lysine which is good for treatment of canker sores, fever blisters and Herpes.
- It contains L-dopamine, an essential ingredient in the treatment of Parkinson's disease and other disorders related to spasmodic reaction between nerves and muscle.

CANKER SORES	Kidneys
Ejaculation (premature)	Lymphatics
FEVER BLISTERS	PARKINSON'S DISEASE
HERPES	Spasms

BUCHU   (Barosma betulina)
A.K.A.,: Bookoo, Bucku.

BODILY INFLUENCE: Antilithic, Antiseptic, Aromatic, Astringent, Carminative, Diaphoretic, Diuretic, Lithotriptic, Stimulant, Stomachic, Sudorific, Tonic.
PART USED: Leaves.

Buchu is found in the southwest region of Cape Colony in South Africa where it was discovered being used by the indigenous people. The Hottentot people used it as a stimulant-tonic and stomach remedy because it soothed.

Buchu is an excellent plant to use in the treatment of chronic kidney inflammations from high acidity of the urine and mucus formation. Treatment in such conditions will result in increased frequency of urination, thus a cleaner system.

In the pelvic area, when combined with Squaw Vine and Unicorn, Buchu helps alleviate lower back and loin pains by soothing the pelvic nerve.

• Buchu finds it primary application in urinary disorders and is considered one of the best herbs for the urinary organs and is especially soothing when there is pain while urinating. It is also one of the best herbs for the prostate gland.

• Buchu absorbs excessive uric acid, thus reducing bladder irritations.

• Buchu increases the quantity of urine fluids and fecal solids and at the same time it acts as a tonic, astringent and disinfectant to the mucous membranes.

• Buchu may find use in treating the first stages of diabetes.

• Combined with Uva Ursi, Buchu has been used for treatment of water retention and urinary tract infections.

Bedwetting	Liver
BLADDER CATARRH	Lungs
Bladder (weak)	NEPHRITIS
Blood pressure (high)	Pancreas
Catarrh	PMS (bloating)
Cystitis	PROSTATE PROBLEMS
Diabetes (first stages)	Rheumatism
Dropsy	Spleen
Fluid retention	Stomach (mucous membrane)
Gallstones	URETHRITIS
Glands	Urinary antiseptic
Gravel (stones)	URINARY TRACT
Hypoglycemia	Vaginal problems
Indigestion	Venereal disease
KIDNEY PROBLEMS	Water retention
Kidney stones	Yeast infection

BUCKTHORN   (Rhamnus frangula)
A.K.A.,: Alder dogwood.

BODILY INFLUENCE: Alterative, Anthelmintic, Bitter, Cathartic, Depurative, Diuretic, Emetic, Laxative, Purgative.
PART USED: Bark, Berries, Root.

Buckthorn is a purgative and acts similar to Rhubarb root.

Nicholas Culpepper, the 17th-century herbalist, said that a poultice of the bruised leaves of Buckthorn would help stop the bleeding from a wound. He also said that an application of the bruised leaves would get rid of warts.

Buckthorn was historically used in the Americas. The Cherokee Indians used Buckthorn as a cathartic and as a solution for skin problems.

* Buckthorn is a close relative of Cascara Sagrada.
* Buckthorn helps the bowels evacuate normally, by stimulating the flow of bile from the liver to the gall bladder.
* Buckthorn is a bitter herb which expels impurities.
* Buckthorn does not gripe and it has a calming effect on the gastrointestinal tract, without being habit forming, when used as directed. If used in excessive amounts, it can cause griping and excessive catharsis.
* Buckthorn taken hot, will produce perspiration and lower fevers.

APPENDICITIS (ACUTE)	Gout
BLEEDING	Hemorrhoids
BOWELS	ITCHING
CANCER	LEAD POISONING
Colic	LIVER CONGESTION
CONSTIPATION (CHRONIC)	Parasites
Dropsy	Rheumatism
FEVERS	Skin disorders
GALLBLADDER (SLUGGISH)	WARTS
GALLSTONES	Worms

BUGLEWEED   (Lycopus virginicus)
A.K.A.,: Water Horehound.

BODILY INFLUENCE: Antithyroid, Astringent, Bitter, Cardiac, Diuretic, Emmenagogue, Hemostatic, Sedative (effective for sedating hyper-thyroid), Tonic.
PART USED: The whole plant.

Bugleweed has been used successfully in hemorrhages from the lungs and bowels.

This plant has the characteristic of regulating the body by relaxing some systems while working to tighten others. It has the ability to improve the tone of the heart and also improve blood circulation through the capillaries. It is a nutritional aid to balance and strengthen circulatory system function. It is used to support a weak heart in cases of extreme edema.

Bugleweed makes an effective cardiac tonic, stabilizing rapid, or irregular heartbeat due to a nervous condition. It is reported to be effective at arresting internal bleeding. For women, it has been successful in working to control excessive menstruation.

Bugleweed has a similar body function to that of digitalis as it acts to lower and regulate the heart rate. Bugleweed is milder than digitalis but is non- toxic and does not accumulate. It is also useful when there is an enlargement of the thyroid gland.

Currently the United States Federal Drug Administration (FDA) is in denial of the qualities given to be inherent to Bugleweed.

- Bugleweed is effective in arresting irritations resulting from coughs.
- Bugleweed is useful in treating some pain; however, the source or reason for pain should be determined before arbitrary use as a pain killer.
- Bugleweed contains ingredients that work as compounds which contract tissues of the mucous membrane and reduce fluid discharges.

Asthma
Bleeding (internal-lungs)
Bronchitis
Bruises (traumatic)
Cardiac problems
COUGHS
Colds
Diabetes
DIARRHEA
FEVERS
Goiter
HEART (CALMS)
Hemorrhages (pulmonary)

HYPOTHYROIDISM
INDIGESTION (NERVOUS)
Lungs (fluid in)
MENSTRUATION (EXCESSIVE)
NERVES
Nosebleeds
PAIN
Pneumonia
Sores
THYROID (OVERACTIVE)
Tuberculosis
Ulcers
Urinary problems

BURDOCK   (Arctium lappa)
A.K.A.,: Turkey burrseed, Hurr-bur

BODILY INFLUENCE: Alterative, Antidote, Anti-phlogistic, Anti-tumor, Aperient, Bitter, Bacteriocide, Blood purifier, Carminative, Cholagogue, Demulcent, Depurative, Diaphoretic, Diuretic, Hepatic, Laxative, Lithotriptic, Stomachic, Tonic.
PART USED: Root, seeds and sometimes leaves.

Burdock has the historical reputation of being an "alterative," meaning herbalists have considered it as a good source of nutrients to help build the body. Our great-grandparents called plants like Dandelion and Burdock "blood purifiers." Menominee and Micmac Indians used Burdock for skin sores, while the Cherokees used it for a broader base of ailments.

Burdock is an herb to use during pregnancy. It is a mineral-rich, hormone which can help in balancing all systems. It helps prevent water retention and jaundice in the baby.

Burdock is a strong liver purifying and hormone balancing herb with particular value for skin, arthritic, and glandular problems. It is a specific in all blood cleansing and detoxification problems.

Burdock is an excellent blood purifier and cleanser and eliminates long-term impurities from the blood very rapidly. It is also an antidote for acute poisoning. Burdock can reduce swelling around the joints by promoting kidney function, thus increasing the flow of urine. It helps to clear the blood of harmful acids due to calcification deposits.

• Used as a poultice, Burdock was found to be an effective remedy when applied to sores and bug bites.
• Inulin, the source of most of Burdock's curative powers, consists of 27% to 45% inulin which is a form of starch important in the metabolism of carbohydrates.
• Burdock has been used extensively by some for cancer cases, as it is an alterative. When used as a poultice on skin cancer, it has manifested its greatest success.
• In Europe, it has been used as a remedy where there is a prolapsed and displaced uterus.
• Burdock works on the pituitary gland helping it to release protein in proper amounts, thus maintaining hormonal balance for a healthy body.
• Burdock is a good source of iron making it an excellent choice for treating iron deficiencies.
• The Chinese have used Burdock for coughs, colds, sore throats, tonsillitis, measles, sores and abscesses.
• Burdock has the ability to neutralize most poisons, relieving both the kidney and lymphatic system.

• Burdock has been used as a replacement for Chaparral very effectively.

HERB BENEFICIAL DURING PREGNANCY: AIDS IN BALANCING HORMONES AND HELPS PREVENT WATER RETENTION AND JAUNDICE IN BABIES.

ABSCESSES (INTERNALLY)
ACNE (blood cleansing)
ALLERGIES
ARTHRITIS
Bladder infections
BLOOD CLEANSER
Blood poisoning
BLOOD PURIFIER
BOILS
Bronchitis
BRUISES
BURNS/SCALDS
BURSITIS
CANCER
CANKER SORES
Carbuncles
CATARRH
CHICKEN POX
COLDS
CONSTIPATION
Coughs
Cystitis
Dandruff
Degenerative conditions
ECZEMA
FEVERS
FLUID RETENTION
Gall bladder
Gallstones
GOUT
Hair growth
Hair loss
Hayfever
HEMORRHOIDS
HERPES
HYPERGLYCEMIA

HYPOGLYCEMIA
Infection
Inflammation
ITCHING
KIDNEY PROBLEMS
LEPROSY
LIVER PROBLEMS
Lungs
LYMPHATIC CONGESTION
MEASLES
Nervous conditions
Obesity
Pimples
Pneumonia
POISON IVY/OAK
Poisons
PSORIASIS
RASHES
RHEUMATISM
SCIATICA
Scrofula
SKIN DISORDERS
Skin eruptions
Sore throats
SORES
Sties
Stomach disorders
SWELLING
SYPHILIS
TONSILLITIS
Tuberculosis
TUMORS (GLAND, SPLEEN)
Ulcers
Uterus (prolapsed)
Venereal diseases
Wounds

BUTCHERS'S BROOM   (Ruscus aculeatus)
A.K.A.,: Asparagaceae.

BODILY INFLUENCE: Anti-inflammatory, Aperient, Astringent, Deobstruent, Diaphoretic, Diuretic, Emmenagogue, Laxative, Prevents Blood Clots, Vasoconstrictive.
PART USED: Root.

Butcher's Broom acts on the blood vessels by stimulating the release of norepinephrine, which then produces a vasoconstricting effect. The production of norepineprine lengthens the time required to clot the blood and thus explains its use in preventing post-operative thrombosis. Butcher's Broom inhibits the formation of blood clots and will also help dispel them.

Butcher's Broom is also useful in pregnancy and for people who stand for lengthy periods of time.

20 - 30% of the people that go on the operating table in the U.S. either die in the operating room or die in recovery afterwards. The major cause is thrombosis (blood clots). In Europe, where Butchers Broom is used extensively, thrombosis in those operating rooms is a rare and unusual incident. Butchers Broom has been very beneficial for hemorrhoids also.

People who have complained of heavy legs have found great benefits taking Butchers Broom.

• Butcher's Broom contains anti-inflammatory properties, as well as having the characteristic of strengthening the walls of the blood vessels.

• On patients with post-operative tendencies toward circulatory problems like thrombosis, Butcher's Broom exhibits a constricting action on the veins, making it most effective.

• Butcher's Broom has been beneficial for improving peripheral circulation, while also increasing circulation to the brain, legs and arms.

• It has a diuretic effect, causing the constriction of blood vessels while also lowering cholesterol.

• Butcher's Broom may be a wise choice when we consider the fact that circulatory problems are the #1 killer in the United States.

ANEURYSM
ARTERIOSCLEROSIS
BLOOD CLOTS (TO PREVENT)
Brain circulation
Bruises
CAPILLARY WEAKNESS
Dropsy
Edema (legs)

GRAVEL
Headaches
HEMORRHOIDS
INFLAMMATION (GENERAL)
JAUNDICE
Leg cramps
Menstrual problems
PHLEBITIS (VEIN

INFLAMMATION)
STROKE PREVENTION
SURGERY (PREPARATION FOR)
THROMBOSIS (BLOOD
   CLOTTING)

Tumor (prostate)
URINATION (SCANT)
VARICOSE VEINS

CALENDULA   (Calendula officinalis)
A.K.A.,: Garden Marigold.

BODILY INFLUENCE: Alterative, Analgesic, Anti-inflammatory, Antiseptic, Astringent, Bitter, Cholagogue, Depurative, Diaphoretic, Diuretic, Emmenagogue, Hemostatic, Stimulant, Styptic, Vermifuge, Vulnerary.
PART USED: Leaves, Flowers, Petals.

    The Calendula plant received its name from the ancient Romans. They noted that the plants bloomed on the first day or "calends" of every month and named them "*Calendula.*" The Romans used this herb to treat scorpion bites.
    Nutritionally, Calendula supports the skin and connective tissues. It can be used internally as well as applied topically.
• Calendula is said to be similar to Witch Hazel and is considered to be one of the best antiseptics, due to its content of natural iodine.
• Calendula is used as a local application for healing of all types of skin irritations and injuries.
• Many consider Calendula to be the best tissue healer for wounds and skin irritations.
• Old herbal doctors believed that constant applications of Calendula would help or even prevent gangrene or tetanus.
• Calendula in a tea can be used as a nasal wash or gargle as it is soothing to tender mucus membranes. According to one homeopathic text, Calendula helps to heal, because it causes a local irritation which draws numerous white blood cells which reduce infection and promotes healing.
• Calendula is effective for healing membranes inside the body aiding such conditions as the colon, stomach, liver, gum diseases and healing after operations.
• Calendula promotes mending and healing of cuts or wounds when a poultice is applied.
• Calendula is most commonly applied externally as an ointment or oil, usually for injuries, burns, bruises and varicose veins.

Abrasions
Acne
Athletes foot
Bee stings
Bleeding
Blood cleansing

BLOOD PURIFIER
BRUISES (EXTERNAL)
Bug bites
Burns
Cancer
CHICKEN POX

CONNECTIVE TISSUES
(REBUILDS)
Cramps
CUTS (EXTERNAL)
Earaches
FEVERS
Flu
Frostbite
Gargle
Hemorrhoids
Indigestion
Injuries
Lupus
MEASLES

Menstruation (delayed)
Mouthwash
Mucous membranes
Nasal wash
Pyorrhea
SKIN IRRITATIONS
Skin ulcers
Sores
Sprains
TOOTHACHES
Ulcerations
Ulcers
Varicose veins
WOUNDS

CAPSICUM OR CAYENNE (Capsicum annum)
A.K.A.,: Red Pepper, Bird Pepper, African Bird Pepper.

BODILY INFLUENCE: Antibacterial, Antipyretic, Antiseptic, Antispasmodic, Aperitive, Aromatic, Astringent, Blood thinner, Cardiovascular tonic, Carminative, Condiment, Diaphoretic, Hemostatic, Hypertensive, Hypotensive, Rubefacient, Stimulant, Stomachic, Tonic-general, Vulnerary.
PART USED: The fruit.

The Capsicum fruit family has many herbs in its family. The activity of the herb in that family is measured by BTU ratings (British Thermal Units) in other words, how hot it is. In the following discussion, we will be using the names Cayenne or Capsicum, interchangeably being both of the same family.

The hot, biting taste of the fruit from the Cayenne pepper plant was first introduced to Europe with the return of Christopher Columbus from the New World. In fact, its name comes from the Greek word "to bite." Capsicum has been aptly described as the plant that *bites back*.

Although Cayenne was probably cultivated for hundreds, even thousands, of years in the tropical Americas, Africa, India, and other tropical areas of the world, Columbus seems to have been the first Westerner to take conscious note of food flavored with this pungent herb.

The North American Cherokee Indians used Cayenne for its stimulating properties, while the Navajo's used it as a means of weaning children. In 1943, the Dispensary of the United States of America reported that "Capsicum is a powerful local stimulant, producing when swallowed, a sense of heat in the stomach and a general glow over the body without narcotic effect." For many centuries, Cayenne has been used as an Ayurvedic herb.

Capsicum is used as a catalyst in almost every herbal

combination and thus aids the absorption and the effectiveness of the combination. It increases the body's ability to produce HCL which increases the body's ability to digest anything that's in the stomach. Because of this fact, Capsicum is used as a "carrier or catalyst" herb for almost any herb combination.

Those suffering from osteoarthritis and rheumatoid arthritis have been discovering relief using an experimental rub-on cream made with Capsaicin, an ingredient of Capsicum. Capsaicin is the most important and prominent compound in Capsicum.

- Capsicum promotes perspiration, which anyone who has eaten any "hot" food should know from experience. In tropical areas, many people eat goodly amounts of hot peppers every day. This may help to keep them "cool" since perspiration is the natural cooling mechanism of the body.

- Like many spices, Capsicum influences the flow of digestive secretions from salivary, gastric, and intestinal glands.

- Capsicum increases Thermogenesis for weight loss, especially when combined with caffeine type herbs or Ephedra. Capsicum gives the system a little cardiovascular lift by exciting the heart; thereby, effectively increasing circulation.

- Capsicum's red color is due in part to its high vitamin A content, which is essential for normal vision, growth, cellular activity, reproduction and healthy immunity.

- Capsicum is excellent for warding off diseases and equalizing blood circulation, which works to prevent strokes and heart attacks.

- It is useful to arrest hemorrhaging (external and internal) and it is cleansing and healing when used to purify external wounds.

- Capsicum helps heals ulcers in the cell structures of the arteries, veins, and capillaries.

- Capsicum is known as the best and purest stimulant in the herb kingdom and has been called by many as the purest and most effective stimulant in the herbal bag of medicine.

- Capsicum if taken internally, will work to heal an ulcerated stomach and may be used as poultice for any inflammation.

- Capsicum increases the heart action without increasing the blood pressure.

- Capsicum increases the power of all other herbs; it helps in digestion when taken with meals and promotes secretion of all of the organs.

- Capsicum is said to be unequaled for warding off diseases and equalizing blood circulation.

- Capsicum is a very useful herb when you want to quickly improve conditions caused by the flu or a cold.

- Capsicum can be useful to aid in the removal and cleaning of tissue in the stomach. The effect is to promote rebuilding of tissue which in effect heals the stomach and intestinal ulcers.

- Capsicum improves the ratio of (HDL) cholesterol which has a protective effect on (LDL) cholesterol which increases heart disease risk.

• It is reported that Capsicum significantly lowers serum cholesterol and serum triglycerides.

• Cayenne also increases the liver enzymes accountable for fat metabolism and decreases the fat deposits in the liver caused by a high fat diet. The natural conclusion might be that Cayenne peppers may reduce weight gain due to a high fat diet by increasing the speed of fat metabolism (Thermogenesis).

• Although Capsicum has an active, pungent principle, the irritant only has a strong effect upon the nerve endings of the sensory nerves and has very little action upon the capillary and other blood vessels. While the burning sensation may be severe, there is usually no reddening or blistering of the skin.

• Capsicum, by reducing blood vessel dilation, is able to help people stop their addiction to alcohol.

• Capsicum is useful for toothaches by rubbing the powder on the affected area.

• For use with arthritis, rub the extract of Capsicum over the affected joint then wrap with a cotton flannel cloth over night.

• By combining both Capsicum and Plantain and then applying this externally, it can draw out foreign items embedded in the skin, such as slivers and thorns.

• Place the powder or extract on or under the tongue for crisis situations such as shock, hemorrhage and heart attack.

• Sprinkle small amount of powder into socks to prevent frostbite.

• Capsicum has been used in tincture form along with a liquid nervine tincture with Valerian root and an Oriental oil which is then applied topically along the spine and on tense muscles. Keep the body warm, allowing the body to absorb these herbs into the effective areas to promote rapid healing. This is called an herbal adjustment.

SEE HERBAL ADJUSTMENT IN FIRST AID IN .DR. RITCHASON'S BOOK OF HERBAL THERAPIES' by Dr. Jack Ritchason.

Ague (malaria)
APPETITE STIMULANT
Arteriosclerosis
ARTHRITIS
Asthma
Backache (external)
BLEEDING (EXTERNAL &
    INTERNAL)
Blood cleanser
BLOOD PRESSURE EQUALIZER
BLOOD PRESSURE (HIGH)

BLOOD PRESSURE (LOW)
BRONCHITIS
Bruises
Burns
CHILLS
CIRCULATORY DISORDERS
COLDS
CONGESTION (GENERAL)
Contagious diseases
CONVULSIONS
Coughs

Cramps
Cuts
DIABETES
Digestive disorders
Eyes
FATIGUE
Fever
FROSTBITE (TO PREVENT)
Gas
HANGOVER
Hayfever
Headaches (cluster)
HEART
HEART ATTACKS
HEMORRHAGE
HYPOTENSION
INDIGESTION
INFECTION
Inflammation
Jaundice
Kidneys
LARYNGITIS (DRUNK AS A TEA)
Lethargy
Lock jaw
LUNGS (FLUID IN)
Male tonic
Mucus
NOSEBLEEDS

Pain (chronic)
Palsy
Pancreas
Paralysis
Parkinson's disease
PERSPIRATION (INCREASE)
Pleurisy
PHLEBITIS
Pyorrhea
RHEUMATISM
SENILITY
Shingles
SHOCK
Sinus problems
Skin problems
SORE THROAT (GARGLE)
Spasms
Spleen
Sprains
STOMACH (ULCERS)
STROKES
Sunburn
SURGERY (PREPARATION FOR)
SWEATING (PROMOTES)
TONSILLITIS
TUMORS
ULCERS
VARICOSE VEINS
WOUNDS (STOPS BLEEDING)

CARAWAY   (Carum carvi)
A.K.A.,: Caraway seed.

BODILY INFLUENCE: Antispasmodic, Carminative, Diuretic, Emmenagogue, Expectorant, Galactagogue, Laxative, Stimulant, Stomachic.
PART USED: Root, Seed.

One of the more popular uses of Caraway root and seeds is in relieving flatulence, even in the very young. It has been used for digestive problems for young and old.

Caraway is especially useful mixed with Cascara Sagrada and other herbal cathartics as a controlling factor, lessening the strong purgative effects making it less griping.

The oil of Caraway seed is used as an antiseptic as is the whole Caraway which relieves dental pain and discomfort. Caraway has been used to relieve menstrual cramps.

Caraway is very similar to Anise and is recommended for the same purposes.

APPETITE STIMULANT
Colds
COLIC
DIGESTION (ACIDS)
Female problems
GAS
INDIGESTION

Lactation
Lungs (mucus)
Menstruation (promotes)
SPASMS
Stomach (settles)
Toothaches
UTERINE CRAMPS

CASCARA SAGRADA   (Rhamnus purshiana)
A.K.A.,: Sacred Bark, California Buckthorn.

BODILY INFLUENCE: Alterative, Anthelmintic, Bitter tonic, Cathartic, Cholagogue, Emetic, Febrifuge, Hepatic, Laxative stimulant, Nervine, Stomachic, Tonic-colon.
PART USED: The aged, dried bark.

The name "sacred bark" dates back to the seventeenth century, when it was bestowed on this tree by Spanish and Mexican explorers. Apparently, they were intrigued by the American Indians use of the bark for a wide variety of medicinal purposes. Its most important use, however, was as a remedy for constipation for upset stomachs.
• Cascara Sagrada is an excellent remedy for chronic constipation.
• Cascara Sagrada is very invigorating to the body despite its bitter taste.
• Its bark is rich in hormone-like oils which promote peristaltic action in the intestinal canal.
• Cascara Sagrada is not considered to be habit-forming, as it cleanses and restores natural tone to the colon.
• Cascara Sagrada improves a sluggish colon that is chronically constipated, by improving the flow of secretions of the stomach, liver and pancreas.
• Cascara Sagrada is effective on the gall bladder ducts and helps the body rid itself of gallstones. Cascara Sagrada also increases the flow of bile. ↪ what is ?
• Cascara Sagrada has also been helpful for the treatment of hemorrhoids by being non-irritating and forming a soft stool allowing painless passage.
• Cascara Sagrada helps in cases where there is chronic hardening of the stool. It is believed that after prolonged use of Cascara Sagrada as a tonic, the bowels will operate naturally.
• Cascara Sagrada is reported to work because it excites the autonomic nervous system of the body. The stimulation of the

autonomic nervous system increases peristaltic action. The worm like movement of muscle in the large intestine is referred to as peristalsis.

• Many pharmaceutical companies use Cascara Sagrada along with other ingredients.

CAUTION; SHOULD NOT TO BE TAKEN EXCESSIVELY DURING PREGNANCY: TOO STRONG A LAXATIVE, CAN CAUSE CRAMPING AND STOMACH GRIPING.

Blood pressure (high)
BOWELS (TOXIC)
Catarrh
CONGESTION (GENERAL)
CONSTIPATION
CONSTIPATION (CHRONIC)
Colitis
COLON
Cough
Croup
Digestion
Diverticulitis
Dyspepsia
GALLBLADDER (SLUGGISH)
GALLSTONES
GAS
Gout
HEMORRHOIDS
Indigestion
Insomnia
INTESTINES
JAUNDICE
LIVER DISORDERS
Nervous disorders
PARASITES (INTERNAL)
Pituitary gland
Spleen
Stomach disorders
WORMS

CATNIP   (Nepeta cataria)
A.K.A.,: Catswort.

BODILY INFLUENCE: Analgesic, Antacid, Antispasmodic, Aperitive, Aromatic, Bitter, Carminative, Diaphoretic, Emmenagogue, Nervine, Refrigerant, Sedative, Stimulant, Stomachic, Tonic.
PART USED: Herb, Leaves.

In early Europe, Catnip was one of the most common teas in use, even before Chinese tea became popular. The North American Indians used Catnip for its sedative effect on the nervous system as well as for treating colic in infants. Culpepper mentions Catnip as a topical aid for hemorrhoids.

Catnip has been documented as normalizing blood pressure and it is said that putting several drops on the back of the tongue will decrease the desire for cigarettes.

• Catnip relieves pain, prevents spasms, and calms the nerves.

• Catnip is often used in colds and flu (especially children) since it produces "perspiration inducing sleep" without increasing body temperature. Catnip enemas will reduce a fever quickly for

adults and children.
- Catnip will work to quickly overcome convulsions in children. It also helps to control restlessness and colic by helping the body to rest. It is known to act as a pain killer because of its calming effect (especially for toddlers and infants).
- Catnip enemas cleanse the colon and reduce spasms. It is often used as a warm enema because of its relaxing action. Catnip relieves gas from the bowels, colic and is soothing and relaxing in general.
- Catnip reduces excess mucus from the body.
- Catnip improves circulation and it helps to reduce fatigue from muscle exhaustion.
- Take Catnip to reduce swellings, especially under the eyes.

ACHES
ACNE
ADDICTIONS
Anemia
BRONCHITIS
CHICKEN POX (to prevent)
Circulation (improves)
COLDS
COLIC
CONVULSIONS
Coughs
Cramps (menstrual)
Cramps (muscular)
CROUP
DIARRHEA
Drug withdrawal
Epilepsy
FEVERS
FEVERS (IN CHILDREN)
Fatigue
FLU
GAS (EXPELS)
Headaches (nervous)
Hemorrhoids
Hiccups
Hypoglycemia
Hysteria
Indigestion

Infertility
Inflammation
Insanity
INSOMNIA
Kidney stones
Liver
Lung congestion
MEASLES
Menstruation (stimulates)
Mental illness
Miscarriage (prevents)
Morning sickness
MUMPS
Nausea
NERVOUSNESS
Nicotine Withdrawal
PAIN RELIEVER
Restlessness
Shock
Skin problems
Sleeplessness
Sores (external)
SPASMS
Stress
Tension
Uterine problems
Vomiting
Worms (expels)

CAYENNE   (SEE CAPSICUM)

CEDAR BERRIES (SEE JUNIPER BERRIES)

CELERY   (Apium graveolens)
A.K.A.,: Garden celery, Wild celery.

BODILY INFLUENCE: Alterative, Anti-rheumatic, Antiseptic, Aperitive, Carminative, Diuretic, Emmenagogue, Nervine, Sedative, Stimulant, Stomachic, Tonic, Uterine stimulant.
PART USED: Root and Seeds.

Historically, Celery seed has been known to assist the process of digestion. Many believe that it lowers blood pressure, while being beneficial to aid kidney and liver function. Some believe that Celery seed will assist in controlling dizziness and headaches.

Celery produces perspiration and therefore, is good in helping those who are looking to lose weight. Medical use of Celery seed has found it to be effective for incontinence of urine. Celery seed has also been found to help regulate the nervous system by producing a calming effect.

• Celery helps in diseases of chemical imbalance and acts as an antioxidant.

• Both the stems and seeds of celery have been reported to help balance acidity in the body. It has been used to treat arthritis in cases of complete crippling and severe malformation. In some cases, where the patient was full of arthritic spurs, the spurs were dissolved from the body in about nine months to a year. In this research, Celery Juice was the primary ingredient being administered to the patients mixed with freshly squeezed carrot juice.

• Celery is a natural source of organic sodium which is needed for the lining of the stomach, joints and is a major mineral in the bloodstream.

• Celery stimulates sex drive and is helpful for the relief of headaches.

• Celery is a sedative, yet it has a stimulating effect on the kidneys and will produce an increased flow of urine.

ARTHRITIS
Bladder problems
Bright's disease
Cancer
Catarrh (post-nasal & pulmonary)
Diabetes
Dropsy
Frigidity
Gas
GOUT
Headache

Impotence
Insomnia
Liver problems
LUMBAGO
Menstruation (delayed)
NERVOUSNESS
Neuralgia
RHEUMATISM
Urine retention
Vomiting
Weight reduction

CENTAURY (Centaurium erythraea)
A.K.A.,: Bitter Herb.

BODILY INFLUENCE: Aromatic, Bitter, Blood Purifier, Cholagogue, Depurative, Digestive, Emmenagogue, Febrifuge, Stomachic, Tonic.
PART USED: The Herb.

In ancient times, Centaury was a primary treatment for intermittent fevers and for malaria, as well as a remedy for drawing out snake poison and infection from other animal bites.
• Centaury is used as an appetite promoter and digestive system strengthener in slow convalescence.
• Centaury works effectively in the treatment of muscular rheumatism.
• It also works to strengthen the bladders of elderly people or those with urinary control problems.
• Centaury has been used to treat bed-wetting.
• Centaury is a preventive in periodic febrile diseases, such as malaria.
• Centaury juice applied externally to the eyes can help clear the vision and promotes resolution of wounds.

Appetite (stimulates)	Jaundice
Bedwetting	KIDNEYS
BLOOD PURIFIER	LIVER
DIGESTION (PROMOTES)	MENSTRUATION (PROMOTES)
Dyspepsia	Rheumatism (muscular)
Eczema	Sores (external)
FEVERS	Tonic
Gall bladder	Ulcers
Gas	Worms
Heartburn	Wounds

CHAMOMILE (Anthemis nobilis-Roman)
A.K.A.,: Ground apple, Wild Chamomile.

BODILY INFLUENCE: Analgesic, Anodyne, Antibiotic, Anti-fungal, Anti-pholgistic, Antipyretic, Antiseptic, Antispasmodic, Aperitive, Aromatic, Bitter, Calmative, Carminative, Diaphoretic, Diuretic, Emmenagogue, Expectorant, Nervine, Sedative, Stimulant, Stomachic, Sudorific, Tonic, Vermifuge.
PART USED: The whole plant.

Greeks called it "ground apple." Chamomile comes from the Greek words kamai, meaning "on the ground" and melon, meaning "apple". Chamomile grows low to the ground everywhere the plant is found. Even though it is fragrant, the herb has a slightly bitter taste.

The only potential negative is that Chamomile may cause allergic reactions in persons sensitive to Ragweed, or the many varieties of Chrysanthemum.

It helps one to relaxes for quality sleep and aids digestive and bowel problems.

The Cherokee Indians used it in cases of colic, bowel complaints and vomiting.

• Chamomile, although a stimulant, is one of the finest nervine herbs that there is.

• Chamomile is invigorating and strengthening to the body.

• Chamomile is one of the best herbs that is both beneficial and trustworthy to keep on hand for emergencies.

• Chamomile is known as a soothing tonic which is sedative in nature and used for the nerves.

• It has been effectively used for menstrual cramps.

• In France and Spain, the orthodox medical profession recognizes Chamomile as a valuable tonic for the young on such problems as colic, upset stomachs and helps to induce sleep.

• Chamomile can be used as a diaphoretic to induce perspiration.

• Chamomile is also excellent for bilious fevers and colds.

• Chamomile is reportedly useful as a remedy for nightmares (especially in children).

• Chamomile is especially beneficial for a good night sleep.

HERB BENEFICIAL DURING PREGNANCY: RELAXES FOR SOUND SLEEP AND HELPS WITH DIGESTIVE AND BOWEL PROBLEMS.

ABSCESSES
Air pollution
ALCOHOLISM
Anxiety
APPETITE (STIMULANT))
Asthma
Bladder problems
Blood disorders
BRONCHITIS
Callouses
Catarrh
Childhood diseases
CIRCULATION (POOR)
Colds
COLIC
Colitis
Constipation

CORNS
Coughs
Cramps (menstrual)
CYSTS (BREAST)
Dandruff
Diarrhea
Diverticulitis
Dropsy
DRUG ADDICTION
Earache
Eyes (sore)
Eye wash
FEVER
Flu
Gallstones
Gangrenous sores
GAS (expels)

Headaches
Heartburn
Hemorrhoids
HYSTERIA
INDIGESTION
Inflammation
INSOMNIA
Jaundice
Kidneys
Liver (stimulates)
Lungs
Measles
Menstrual regulator
MENSTRUATION (PAINFUL)
MUSCLE PAIN
Nausea
NERVOUS DISORDERS

Pain
SLEEP
SMOKING (CALMS NERVES)
Sore throat
Spasms
Spleen
Stomach (cramps)
Stomach upset
Teething
Throat (gargle)
TOOTHACHE
Tumors
Typhoid
Ulcerations
Ulcers (peptic)
Worms (expels)

CHAPARRAL   (Larrea tridentata, L. divaricata)
A.K.A.,: Creosote bush, Greasewood, Gobernadora.

BODILY INFLUENCE: Alterative, Anodyne, Antibiotic, Anti-carcinogenic, Anti-inflammatory, Antioxidant, Antiseptic, Anti-tumor, Bitter, Blood Purifier, Diuretic, Expectorant, Parasiticide, Tonic.
PART USED: Leaves.

Chaparral is nicknamed "Creosote bush" which gets its name from the oil which is used to treat wood. The word *Chaparral* comes from the Spanish language, meaning a low growing shrub.

In Mexico, Chaparral has been used for centuries as an anti-cancer remedy. North American Indian tribes, the Kawaiisu, the Paiute and the Sho-shone, used the "Creosote bush" for ailments relating to sepsis (bacteria) and elimination.

The plant is known to act against free radicals and thus may be effective in preventing degenerative disease associated with aging. This plant is of particular interest to us in cleansing the lymph system, an important part of rejuvenation. It is anti-inflammatory and non-toxic. It is so powerful, however, that parasites will leave the system, while dangerous microbes will either leave or succumb to it.

• Many universities have tested Chaparral and found it an aid in dissolving tumors and in fighting cancer.

• It is a strong antioxidant, pain-killer and antiseptic.

• Chaparral has the ability to cleanse deep into the muscles and tissue walls.

• Chaparral tones the system, rebuilds tissues and is a very effective healer for the urethral tract, blood, liver and lymphatic system. Fluid intake may be helpful, as Chaparral is a strong cleansing herb for the kidneys.

- Chaparral works by constraining undesired rapid cellular growth, by way of the essential respiratory process present throughout the whole human system.
- Chaparral has been said to eliminate the residue of LSD from the body helping prevent the recurrences or flashbacks caused by LSD.
- The oil from Chaparral's resin has been shown to reduce inflammation of the intestinal and respiratory tracts. In plants this same oil stops aerobic combustion in plant cell mitochondria, thereby preventing competition from other plants growing near it.
- Chaparral is famous for its role in combating cancer, by virtue of its primary constituent, NDGA (nordihydroquaiaretic acid), a powerful antioxidant and anti-tumor agent.
- Chaparral also relieves pain, has increased ascorbic acid levels in the adrenals and has vasodepressant properties.
- After 2,000 years of recorded history, and after multiple universities have tested the plant, have found that it aids in dissolving tumors and fighting cancer. The FDA now wants to take Chaparral off the market.

Aches
Acne
Allergies
Antioxidant (potent)
ARTHRITIS
Backaches (chronic)
Blood cleanser
Blood poisoning
BLOOD PURIFIER
Boils
Bowels (lower)
Bruises
Bursitis
CANCER
Cataracts
Colds
Cramps
Cuts
Eczema
Eyes (strengthens)
Fibrositis
Glaucoma
Hair growth (promotes)

Hay fever
Kidney infection
Lungs
LEUKEMIA
Osteoarthritis
Pain
Parasites (intestinal)
Prostate problems
Psoriasis
Respiratory system
RHEUMATISM
SKIN DISEASES
Skin problems (blotches)
Sores
Stomach disorders
Swelling
TUMORS
Venereal diseases
Viral illnesses
Warts
Weight reduction
Wounds

CHICKWEED   (Stellaria media)
A.K.A.,: Starweed, Stitchwort.

BODILY INFLUENCE: Alterative, Breaks Down Fat, Demulcent, Discutient, Diuretic, Emollient, Expectorant, Mucilant, Nutritive, Pectoral, Refrigerant, Stomachic.
PART USED: The Herb.

The North American Chippewa and Iroquois Indians were known to have used Chickweed as an eyewash and wound poultice.
• Chickweed can be applied externally (as a poultice) to any skin problem including boils, burns, and sores in the mouth and throat. A Chickweed ointment would be an excellent treatment for diaper rash.
• Chickweed is also used for breast inflammation during lactation (both internally and externally).
• Chickweed poultices are good for sore eyes and has been used for swollen testes and hemorrhoids.
• Chickweed has been used on tumors.
• The mucilage content, known as a demulcent, help heal stomach ulcers, inflamed bowels, lungs and most any inflammation whether internal or external.
• Chickweed moistens phlegm and aids in its expectoration from the lungs, while relieving sore throats, lowering fevers and treating stomach and duodenal ulcers.
• Chickweed will work to move plaque out of blood vessels and eliminates fatty substances in the system.
• Chickweed strengthens the tissue lining of the stomach and the intestines.
• Chickweed is used in bathing for its "soothing affect" on the body.
• For blood poisoning, use a Chickweed decoction internally and apply a Chickweed poultice to externally affected areas.
• Chickweed has been used to break down cellulite.

Abscesses	BRONCHITIS
ACNE	Bruises
ALLERGIES	BURNS/SCALDS
Appetite depressant	CANCER (FATTY TUMORS)
Appetite stimulant	Carbuncles
Arteriosclerosis	CELLULITE
Asthma	CHOLESTEROL
Bleeding	Circulatory problems
BLOOD POISONING	Colds
BLOOD PURIFIER	Colitis
BOILS	Constipation
BRONCHIAL CONGESTION	CONVULSIONS

COUGHS
Cramps
DEAFNESS
EYES (INFLAMMATION OF)
Gas
GOUT
HAYFEVER
HEMORRHOIDS
Hoarseness
Itching
Impotence
Lungs
Mouth (ulcerated)
Mucus
OBESITY
Peritonitis
Piles

PLAQUE
Pleurisy
PSORIASIS
Rheumatism
Scurvy
SKIN DISEASES
SKIN ERUPTIONS
SKIN RASHES
SKIN (ULCERS)
SORES
Stomach problems
Testes (swollen)
Tissues (inflamed)
TUMORS (fatty)
Water retention
WEIGHT REDUCTION
WOUNDS

CHICORY   (Cichorium intybus)
A.K.A.,: Blue-Sailors, Coffee weed.

BODILY INFLUENCE: Blood Purifier, Diuretic, Laxative, Tonic-mild.
PART USED: The Herb and Root.

Centuries ago, the ancient Romans used Chicory as a blood purifier and for food.

Chicory is so plentiful in North America that you would believe it to be native to this part of the world. It is in fact native to Europe and was imported to this country during the eighteenth century by colonists.

In recent times, herbalists have recommended tonics made from the roots for laxatives and poultices made from leaves to treat inflammations.

It has also been discovered that the juice made from the leaves and the flowering plant can be taken as a tonic which works to stimulate the production of bile, the release of gallstones and the elimination of excessive internal mucus.

• Chicory taken as a tonic helps to eliminate phlegm from the stomach and helps with stomach upsets.

• Chicory helps to reduce uric acid in the body thereby, eliminating the conditions which contribute to gout.

• It helps to treat rheumatics and works to bring relief for joint stiffness.

• The sap of the Chicory stems is used to treat skin irritations that are a result from poison ivy or sunburn.

• Chicory has many of the constituents of Dandelion.

Anemia
Arteriosclerosis
Arthritis
BLOOD PURIFIER
CALCIUM DEPOSITS
Congestion
DIGESTION
Gallstones
Glands
Gout
Infertility

Inflammations
JAUNDICE
Kidney problems
LIVER PROBLMES
PHLEGM (EXPELS)
Poultice
Rheumatism
Spleen problems
Tonic
Uric acid

CINCHONA   (Cinchona calisaya, C. nitida)
A.K.A.,: Jesuit's Bark, Peruvian bark.

BODILY INFLUENCE: Antiperiodic, Antiseptic, Astringent, Bitter, Febrifuge, Oxytocic, Stomachic, Tonic.
PART USED: Bark.

As the Spanish colonies in the Americas developed early in the sixteenth century, one of the Roman Catholic Church missions was to account for new and valuable resources in the New World. Jesuit priests would accompany the Conquistadors, charged to convert Indians to Christianity and make use of their labor wherever resources of value were discovered.

One of the resources cataloged was the bark of the Cinchona tree. The priest's discovered that the Indians would chew the inner bark of the tree and by having done so, were somehow free of malaria.

Later, it was discovered that the bark was the source of quinine. For several hundred years, this constituent of Peruvian bark was a widely prescribed remedy, to combat this disease. Quinidine became a product which resulted from the discovery of quinine. Quinidine is a drug that is prescribed to combat atrial fibrillation, which is a variety of cardiac arrhythmia. It helps to treat irregular pulsation of the heart, headaches caused by muscle stress and to treat muscle cramping.

One of the spin-offs attributed to the discovery of the Cinchona bark is Homeopathy. Samual Hahneman, the father of Homeopathy observed that quinine induced heavy sweating, just as patients did with the disease malaria. He began to experiment with Cinchona and eventually developed his own arsenal of disease combating drugs, based on the principal that triggering the body's immune system is key to curing illness.

• Cinchona is an anti-periodic because of the active ingredient, quinine.

• It treats inflammation making it effective as a treatment for

rheumatic pains.
- Cinchona is effective to treat remittent and intermittent fevers.
- Cinchona works to strengthen the stomach and acts to stabilize the whole nervous system.
- A tonic made of Cinchona has been used effectively to treat chronic intoxication from alcohol.

CINCHONA AND ITS ALKALOIDS SHOULD BE AVOIDED IN PREGNANCIES BECAUSE OF THEIR OXYTOCIC EFFECTS.

Diarrhea
Dropsy
Dysentery
FEVERS (INTERMITTENT)
FLU
Heart palpitations
Hysteria
Inflammation
JAUNDICE

MALARIA
Measles
Menstrual problems
Nervous disorders
PARASITES
Rheumatism
Scrofula
Smallpox
Typhoid fever

CHLORELLA   (Chlorella pyrenoidosa)
A,K.A.,: NONE

BODILY INFLUENCE: Adaptogen, Alterative, Anti-viral, Immuno-stimulant, Nutritive.
PART USED: Whole algae with the cell partially or fully broken down.

Chlorella is an ancient plant that has survived the ages with each cell being self-sufficient and capable of all life-sustaining functions.

Chlorella is a single-celled, fresh-water green algae. Chlorella's name is devised from the fact that it contains pound for pound, the highest concentration of chlorophyll of any known plant.

The hot extract of chlorella stimulates the production of interferon. The substance responsible for this is known as chlorellan, which is a life force stimulant produced by the excitation of macrophage activity. Several studies have been done on the direct and indirect influence of Chlorella on the inhibition and prevention of cancer.
- Chlorella has been shown to be specific treatment for Epstein-Barr and Cytomegalo viruses.
- Chlorophyll in concentrations found in Chlorella have been shown to be helpful in the treatment of pancreatitis.

- Chlorophyll in Chlorella has been shown to tighten the teeth, thus contributing to healthy gums, aids new tissue growth and prevents gums from bleeding.
- Chlorella in a granular form, has been mixed with water and applied to the gums through a water jet device to treat the gums.
- Chlorella has been shown to be an excellent detoxifier of such heavy metals as cadmium, lead, mercury and copper.
- It has been used in the Orient to treat cancerous growths and is anti-viral in nature.
- Chlorella contains all the B vitamins, vitamin C, E, and many minerals.
- Chlorella's biologic coding elements of RNA and DNA, have been found to protect against the effects of ultraviolet radiation.
- Chlorella contains a 'Controlled Growth Factor,' which taken on a regular basis, brings a noticeable increase in sustained energy and immune health.

Allergies	Gastritis
Arthritis	Hangovers
Atherosclerosis	Heart problems
Blood pressure (lowers)	Hypertension
Bowel toxicity	Liver toxicity
Cancer	Skin problems
Cholesterol (reduces high)	Ulcers
Constipation	Weight loss

CINNAMON   (Cinnamomum zeylanicum, C. cassia)
A.K.A.,: NONE

BODILY INFLUENCE: Analgesic, Antibacterial, Anti-fungal, Antiseptic, Astringent, Carminative, Diaphoretic, Emmenagogue, Febrifuge, Fungicide, Sedative, Stimulant, Stomachic, Tonic.
PART USED: The dried bark.

Egyptians included Cinnamon in their embalming mixtures. Thousands of years ago, the Romans were used to paying dearly for it. Cinnamon was first listed in Chinese medicine in the Tang Materia Medica (659 A.D.) It was one of the spices that spurred world exploration.
- Cinnamon works to help calm down the stomach and also reduces milk flow. It also stops uterine hemorrhage and excessive menstrual flow.
- Studies conducted by Japanese researchers has shown that Cinnamon contains a substance that is both anti-fungal and anti-bacterial.

- Cinnamon also helps control other virulent actions by many microorganisms including the one which causes Botulism and Staphylococcus Aureus, a source of staff infections. It devastates the fungi that produces aflatoxin, a potent poison and carcinogen. It has also been shown to suppress E. coli and Candida Albicans.
- Cinnamon is used for discomfort and pain in menopause, chest pain, back and neck pain.

CAUTION: It is not recommended for women who are pregnant.

ABDOMINAL SPASMS	Menstruation (excessive flow)
Arthritis	Nausea
Asthma	Nephritis
Back pain (lower)	Parasites (oil)
Bronchitis	Psoriasis
Cancer	Rheumatism
Cholera	Spasms
Coronary problems	Stomach (calms)
DIARRHEA	Uterine hemorrhage
DIGESTION (IMPROVES)	Vomiting
Fevers	Wart
GAS	

CLOVES (Eugenia caryophyllata)
A.K.A.,: Mother Cloves.

BODILY INFLUENCE: Analgesic, Anodyne, Anti-emetic, Antiseptic, Aromatic, Astringent, Carminative, Disinfectant, Expectorant, Germicide, Rubefacient, Stimulant, Stomachic, Tonic, Vermifuge.
PART USED: Seeds or flower-bud.

Cloves have been well known for a long time. The mild anesthetic property found in the dried under developed flower bud was considered a stand by home-style, toothache anesthetic of some effectiveness. Dentists sometimes used powdered Cloves to disinfect and treat disturbed root canals. Cloves have moderately strong germicidal properties.
- Note that the Cloves found in grocery markets have been found to contain much less strength than those found in herbal stores.
- The oil of Cloves is recommended as a carminative; however, it is suggested that it be used with caution, because of its possible irritant effect. It can be the cause of gastro-enteritis.
- Herbalists world wide have recommended Cloves tea, made by steeping the buds in boiling water, to cure nausea and to rid

the stomach and intestines of gas. In China, the herbalist uses oil of Cloves to treat diarrhea and hernia. Tinctures of Cloves oil have been shown to be effective against such conditions which promote fungi such as those that cause athlete's foot.

- Eugenol is the active ingredient of Cloves and remains one of the major pain relieving agents used by dentists.
- It is also helpful in nausea and vomiting.
- Cloves oil has broad spectrum antibiotic properties therefore, acts as a strong germicide. It is considered by some to be one of the most powerful germicidal agents in the herb kingdom.
- Cloves is considered safe and effective enough to be used for discomfort during pregnancy.
- Cloves is known to increase circulation of the blood, thereby helping to promote digestion and nutrition.

Abdominal pain
Athlete's foot
Backache
BREATH (BAD)
BLOOD CIRCULATION
   (IMPROVES)
Blood pressure (low)
BRONCHIAL CATARRH
Bronchitis
Candida
COLDS
Colitis (mucus)
DIARRHEA
Digestion
DIZZINESS
Dysentery
Dyspepsia

EARACHE
Epilepsy
Flu
GAS
Halitosis
Hiccups
INDIGESTION
Muscle aches
NAUSEA
Pain
Palsy
Parasites (intestinal)
Sexual stimulant
Spasms
Toothache
VOMITING
Warts

COLTSFOOT   (Tussilago farfara)
A.K.A.,: Coughwort, Horsehoof, Calves foot.

BODILY INFLUENCE: Anti-inflammatory, Antitussive, Astringent, Bitter, Demulcent, Diuretic, Emollient, Expectorant, Mucilant, Pectoral, Sudorific, Tonic.
   PART USED: Leaves, Flower, Root.

For more than 2,000 years, Coltsfoot has been regarded as one of the best herbal remedies for coughs. The ancient Greeks called it Bechihon, the Romans called it Tussilago; both words mean "cough plant". It was also called coughwort. Smoking the herb for lung problems was recommended by Dioscorides. Records

throughout history show that people have used Coltsfoot as an asthma remedy. Coltsfoot is very often used as a demulcent against persistent cough such as smoker.s cough.
• The flowers exhibit an ingredient which is expectorant in nature, being very soothing to the mucous membranes, such as the chest and lungs.
• Coltsfoot sedates the cough reflex and resolves wheezing.
• Coltsfoot leaves are sometimes used in a poultice form.
• Coltsfoot used with Horehound and Marshmallow, is one of the best cough remedies.
• Coltsfoot leaves are applied topically to relieve insect bites and stings.
• In recent history, some Herbalists have treated burns and skin problems with the leaves of Coltsfoot.

ASTHMA	MUCUS
BRONCHITIS	Pleurisy
CATARRH	Pneumonia
Chills	Sore throat
Colds	Stings (insect)
COUGHS (DRY)	Swellings
Diarrha	Tracheitis (calms)
Emphysema	Tuberculosis
Hoarseness	Wheezing
Inflammation	WHOOPING COUGHS
LUNG PROBLEMS	

COMFREY (Symphytum officinale)
A.K.A.,: Knitbone, Bruisewort, Woundwort.

BODILY INFLUENCE: Antipyretic, Antitussive, Astringent, Bitter, Cell Proliferant, Demulcent, Expectorant, Mucilant, Nutritive, Styptic, Tonic, Vulnerary.
PART USED: Leaves and Root.

Comfrey has been used as a healing herb since 400 BC. It was known to have the power to encourage body tissue repair. The Greeks used it to stop heavy bleeding and treat bronchial problems. Dioscorides, a Greek physician of the first century, prescribed the plant to heal wounds and mend broken bones.
The Cherokee have used this plant internally for a number of ailments.
• An over abundance of mucilage found in Comfrey, makes it very useful as a demulcent in cases such as colitis.
• Comfrey contains allantoin which is a cell proliferant, stimulates new cell growth which increases cell production and

thus supports more rapid healing. The general rule in Herbology is "If anything is broken, use Comfrey."
- Pouring fluid extract of Comfrey into a wound often closes the wound, thus avoiding stitches.
- Comfrey is indicated when the internal functions are injured or weakened to the degree that bloody discharges are manifested, whether in the sputum, urine or from the bowels.
- Comfrey has been used successfully on any part of the body that might be injured.
- Comfrey is an excellent healer of the respiratory system, especially where there is hemorrhaging of the lungs.
- Comfrey (called the knitter and healer) stops hemorrhaging and bleeding and is particularly useful in treating blood in the urine.
- Comfrey aids in soothing inflammation and when used as a poultice can be applied to sore breasts burns, wounds, swelling, and bites.
- It has been used as a hot poultice in helping ease the pain from bursitis.
- It helps in the calcium-phosphorus balance by promoting healthy skin and strong bones. It feeds the pituitary with its natural hormone and helps to strengthen the skeletal system.
- It helps promote the secretion of pepsin which makes it useful as a general aid to digestion.
- Comfrey has been used with success to arrest all sorts of hemorrhaging or bleeding.
- There have been studies that have said that Comfrey caused cancer in test animals. On close scrutiny of these studies, it was found that the scientists had isolated and extracted out the alkaloids that were in the plant and then massive doses of these alkaloids were given to theses tiny rats that caused tumors and cancer. Scientists that did the original experiments, did tell the news media later that when the product (Comfrey) was given to the rats in its whole and natural state, that this did not happen, though. Should we worry about those alkaloids in Comfrey? If you do, then you better worry about those alkaloids in tomatoes, potatoes or vegetables in the same family, as they have the same alkaloids. Comfrey has earned its title honestly, as being the *knitter, healer* plant. Comfrey is one of the greatest herbs God has ever given to man. The FDA wants to remove Comfrey from the marketplace.

Allergies	BONES (BROKEN)
ANEMIA	Breasts
ASTHMA	Bronchitis
BLADDER PROBLEMS	BRUISES
BLOOD CLEANSER	BURNS
Boils	Bursitis

Cancer	Kidney stones
Colds	Leg cramps
Colitis	Lungs (moistens)
Coughs	Menstruation
Cramps	Mucus (dissolves & expels)
Diarrhea	Pain
Digestive problems	Pancreas
Dysentery	Pleurisy
Eczema	Pneumonia
EMPHYSEMA	Psoriasis
Fatigue	Respiratory problems
Female complaints	Rheumatism
Fevers	Sinusitis
FRACTURES	Skin trouble
Gall bladder	SORES
Gangrenous sores	SPRAINS
Gout	Stomach
Gum disease	SWELLING
Hay fever	Tuberculosis
Infections	Urine (bloody)
Insect bites	

CORNSILK (Zea mays)
A.K.A.,: Mothers Hair.

BODILY INFLUENCE: Alterative, Cholagogue, Diuretic, Demulcent, Lithotriptic, Soothing, Mild Stimulant.
PART USED: The green pistils of the Flower.

Historically, Cornsilk has been mainly used for urogenital infections.

Garilasco de la Vega (1539-1610) made note of its use amongst the Inca's. It is believed that the use of Cornsilk originates from Central America. Maizenic acid is claimed to be the active ingredient, acting mostly as a cardiac solution which stimulates diuretic action in the body. It is known to effect the bladder and kidneys and helps the liver and intestines be treated as well.

• Cornsilk has been used for over a century for kidney problems, for acute and chronically inflamed bladders and the prostate gland.

• Cornsilk has been used when a cardiac weakness was suspected.

• Cornsilk is to be considered for urine retention, catarrh of the bladder, gonorrhea, is useful in controlling inflammation and relieving pain.

• Physicians have used it as a diuretic and conditions of cystitis.

• Cornsilk assists all phosphatic and uric acid build up and is especially useful in treating inflammatory conditions of the urethra, bladder and kidney, which are the cause of most malfunctions of the system due to uric acid retention.

• This is excellent for the aged with urinary troubles and is very helpful for the young troubled with bedwetting due to uncontrollable swollen bladders.

Arteriosclerosis
ALBUMINURIA
Bedwetting
BLADDER PROBLEMS
Blood pressure (high)
Cholesterol
Cystic irritation
Cystitis
Dropsy
Edema
Gonorrhea

HEART TROUBLE
Jaundice
KIDNEY PROBLEMS
Kidney stones
Malaria
Obesity
Prostate problems
Renal cystitis
URINARY TRACT
     (INFLAMMATION OF)
URINATION (PAINFUL)

COUCH GRASS   (Agropyron repens)
A.K.A.,: Witch Grass, Dog grass, Quick grass, Twitch grass.

BODILY INFLUENCE: Antibiotic, Antiphlogistic, Demulcent, Depurative, Discutient, Diuretic, Emollient, Pectoral, Sudorific, Tonic.
PART USED: Root

Couch Grass's primary action is on the urinary system. This gives Couch Grass a urinary demulcent quality. Dr. Thompson claims that Couch Grass will lesson the frequency and pain in cases of escessive bladder irritation from any cause.

The Cherokee and Iroquois used the plant for "gravel" and worms. It has also been found to be used historically for a sore back, painful urination, gravel and discharge of mucus.

• Couch Grass has a history of beneficial use for treatment of the urinary system. It has a soothing, diuretic influence, which acts to increase the flow of the discharge of urine without increasing actual renal secretion. It is used in cystitis and the treatment of catarrhal diseases of the bladder.

• Couch Grass has been known to eliminate kidney stones and pass gravel from the bladder.

• Th extracts of Couch Grass are known to have antibiotic effects and works against a variety of bacteria and molds.

BLADDER INFECTIONS
BLOOD PURIFIER
Bright's disease
Bronchitis

Calculi (dissolving small)
CATARRHAL CONDITIONS
Constipation
CYSITIS

Eyes (strengthens)
Female disorders
Fevers
Gallstones
Gout
Gravel
JAUNDICE
KIDNEY PROBLEMS
Lower back pain
Lungs
Prostate gland (enlarged)
RHEUMATISM
Skin diseases
Stones (Urinary calculi)
Syphilis
Urinary infections

CRAMP BARK   (Viburnum opulus)
A.K.A.,: High Cranberry, Snowball Tree.

BODILY INFLUENCE: Anti-abortive, Antispasmodic, Astringent, Diuretic, Emmenagogue, Nervine, Sedative, Tonic.
PART USED: The Bark, with the inner bark being preferable.

In Russia, it is the berries which are used, fresh or dried for high blood pressure and heart problems. It is also used for coughs, colds, lungs, kidneys, bleeding and stomach ulcers. Externally, for skin conditions and eczema, a decoction of flowers has been used. As its name implies, it is known by the American practitioners to relieve cramps and spasms of involuntary muscles.
• Cramp Bark relieves cramps during painful menstruation. In nature, it is considered one of the best female regulators.
• For the ovaries and uterus, it is considered one of the best relaxants.
• Cramp Bark is good for the heart muscles and it relieves muscle tension and spasms.
• Cramp Bark has been used to prevent threatened miscarriage due to nervous afflictions, rheumatism, colic and headaches.
• Cramp Bark may be used as a tonic for cramps anywhere in the body. It is especially useful for cramps in the abdomen and uterus. Many recommend it for convulsions and spasms.
• Cramp Bark is highly held for its ability to relieve abdominal cramps due to intestinal disturbance.
• Cramp Bark relaxes the uterus and quiets excessive ovarian action.
• Cramp Bark has general application in all spasmodic conditions and is recognized in the National Formulary as a specific antispasmodic for asthma and hysteria.
• Cramp Bark has been recommended to help with nervousness during pregnancy. This condition is usually resultant from after-pains, cramps and the nervous discomforts of pregnancy.

ASTHMA
Colic
Constipation
CONVULSIONS
CRAMPS
CRAMPS (UTERINE)
Debility
Dysentery

Epilepsy
Fainting
Fits
Gall stones
Gas
HEART PALPITATIONS
HYPERTENSION
Hysteria
Jaundice
LEG CRAMPS
Lockjaw

Menstrual cramps
Miscarriage
NERVOUSNESS
Neuralgia
Ovarian irritations
Pregnancy (after-pains)
Pulse (regulates)
Rheumatism
Spasms
Urinary problems

CRESS   (SEE WATERCRESS)

CULVER'S ROOT   (Veronicastrum virgincum)
A.K.A.,: Bowman's Root, Black Root, Physic Root, Culver.s physic.

BODILY INFLUENCE: Alterative, Bitter, Blood Purifier, Cathartic, Cholagogue, Emetic, Hepatic, Laxative, Tonic.
PART USED: Dried Root.

Culver's Root was long an herb in common use among the American Indians. It was first introduced to the white man by Dr. Culver and has since been known favorably as Culver's physic.
• Culver's Root works chiefly on the intestines in chronic constipation due to poor biliary flow. it has a mild action without causing the depression of physical strength common with many other purgative medicines.
• It removes old debris from the bowels.
• Culver's Root has a variety of uses in the body such as in treating pleurisy, removal of morbid matter in the bowels, in fevers and doesn.t weaken bowel tone.
• Culver's Root has a relaxant effect on the body to include a beneficial effect on the liver function.
• Culver's Root is a stomach tonic.
• Culver's Root is helpful for indigestion.
• Culver's Root as a blood purifier helps cleanse obstructions, catarrhal congestion from body passageways without artificial action.
• Culver's Root can be taken with such herbs as Fennel that have gas expelling properties.
• Culver's Root is best used in the dried state. In the fresh state, it has too harsh an action.

CATARRHAL OBSTRUCTIONS
DIARRHEA
Dysentery
Fevers
Food poisoning

LIVER PROBLEMS
STOMACH PROBLEMS
Syphilis
Water retention

CYANI   (Centaurea cyanus)
A.K.A.,: Cornflower, Bachelor's-button, Bluebottle.

BODILY INFLUENCE: Astringent, Diuretic, Tonic.
PART USED: The Whole Herb.

The American Indians used Cyani for snakebites, insect bites and to treat insect stings. It has been used interchangeably with Blessed Thistle. It has been recommended by Herbalist's for its nervine powers. Cyani can be used for such divergent problems as chronic indigestion dermatitis and for ulcers and sores in the mouth. Water distilled from Bachelor.s-button petals has been used to bathe eyes to relieve conjunctivitis and other eye problems. As dried powder, it can be used on bruises. Taken with wine the seeds, leaves or the distilled water of the herb has been used, in years past, to protect against the plague and other infectious diseases.
• Cyani contains important glycosides which have strong antiseptic properties.
• Cyani has been used in an eyewash.
• Cyani's anti-germicidal and anti-bacterial properties have been used as an effective antidote against snake venom and scorpion poisons.

CONJUNCTIVITIS
CORNEAL ULCERS
Dermatitis
EYE DISORDERS
Fevers
Indigestion (chronic)
Infection

Mumps
Nervous disorders
POISONOUS BITES
Sight
STINGS
Toothaches

DAMIANA (Turnera aphrodisiaca)
A.K.A.,: NONE

BODILY INFLUENCE: Aperient, Antiseptic (Urinary), Aphrodisiac, Aromatic, Bitter, Diuretic, Hormonal, Laxative, Nervine, Stimulant, Tonic.
PART USED: Leaves and stems.

Damiana was named mizib-coc by the Maya Indians of Yucatan. Mizib-coc means 'plant for asthma' for which was used by the Indians. It was used by the Maya Indians for pulmonary (lung) disorders, dizziness, vertigo (imbalance) and as a general body cleanser. The herb's reputation for arousing sexual desire is noted by the second part of its botanical name, aphrodisiaca. Damiana is known as a sexual rejuvenator in lose of vitality of the sexual organs, caused by either abuse or senility. Damiana has been recommended for increasing the sperm count in the male.

Damiana is primarily used for treating female problems, in Mexico. It is excellent at restoring an exhausted state of the body and increasing its vital energies. For women, it has been found to strengthen reproductive organs and helps with menopause, by controlling and reducing hot flashes. It has also been used to strengthen the ovum in the female and it also helps to balance the hormones in women. It is one of the herbs of choice for helping with sexual impotency and infertility with both males and females.

• The leaves are a tonic to the nerves and a stimulant in sexual weakness. It is esteemed for its aphrodisiac properties and its excellent effect on the reproductive organs. It overcomes exhaustion and has a tendency to help in the loss of power in the limbs.

• Damiana is a laxative for children.

• Damiana has also been used for cough preparations, helps to relieve cold symptoms, relieves flu symptoms and is a stimulant for the Central Nervous System.

• It stimulates muscular contractions of the intestinal tract.

Anxiety	ENERGY
Asthma	EMPHYSEMA
APHRODISIAC	ESTROGEN (LOW)
Bladder (catarrhal inflammation)	Exhaustion
Brain tonic	Fatigue
Bronchitis	FEMALE PROBLEMS
Constipation	FRIGIDITY
Cough	Headaches
Cystic catarrh	HORMONE BALANCER (MALE
Depression	& FEMALE)
Digestion	HOT FLASHES

IMPOTENCY
INFERTILITY
Kidney inflammation
Lou Gerig's disease
MENOPAUSE
Nervousness
Orchitis (inflammation of a testicle)
PARKINSON'S DISEASE

PMS
PROSTATE (INFLAMMATION OF)
REPRODUCTIVE ORGANS
SEXUAL STIMULANT
Spermatorrhea (Involuntary emissions)

DANDELION (Taraxacum officinale)
A.K.A. - Lion's Tooth, Priest's Cown, Puffball.

BODILY INFLUENCE: Alterative, Anti-rheumatic, Aperient, Bitter, Blood purifier, Calcium solvent, Cholagogue, Deobstruent, Depurative, Diuretic, Galactagogue, Hepatic, Intoxicant, Laxative, Nutritive, Stimulant, Stomachic, Tonic-general.
PART USED: The whole plant, especially the leaves and root.

Dandelion as a potassium rich herb, is a superior natural diuretic which can help support the system's vital potassium levels that are being depleted by the many powerful pharmaceutical preparations being prescribed medically as diuretics which without the use of a Dandelion preparation would create potassium deficiencies. The use of Dandelion helps detoxify the system thus, improving health, increasing mobility and reducing stiffness in the joints.

The common Dandelion is a native of Greece. It thrives under almost any condition and has spread to nearly every part of the world. The first part of the botanical name, Leontodon was derived from two Greek words meaning 'lion' and 'tooth'. It is believed that the name was given to the plant because the jagged leaf looks like the teeth of a lion. Again others say that Dandelion gets its name from the French, 'dent de Leon', meaning teeth of the lion. The Latin name Taraxacum is from the Greek taraxos, meaning disorder and akos meaning remedy.

Dandelion is also known by a number of common names, among them, blow ball, which brings up early memories of a childhood game played in the park. You would give the matured seedhead your best puff of air sending the light seeds off into the air and then counting the seeds remaining to see how many children you were destined to have.

• Dandelion is known for inducing the flow of bile from the liver. It is so effective that the first stages of cirrhosis of the liver has been known to be alleviated by consistent use.

• Dandelion has been used as a poultice for breast cancer. It also has been known to reduce serum cholesterol and uric acid in the system.

- Dandelion is an excellent natural source of potassium. It is an ideally balanced diuretic that can be used safely when such an action is needed. It has been used in conditions where there is water retention due to heart problems. It is a specific diuretic in cases of congestive jaundice. It is also a very valuable general tonic and perhaps the best widely applicable of the herbs as a diuretic and liver tonic.
- The juice of the Dandelion root continues to be used by European herbalists to treat diabetes and liver diseases. They regard Dandelion as one of the best herbs for building up the blood and for helping with anemia.
- The plant is largely cultivated in India as a remedy for liver complaints. In France, the roots are cooked as a vegetable and added to broth and in Germany they are sliced and used in salads.
- Dandelion greens contain 7,000 units of vitamin A per ounce. The Dandelion is so high in vitamin A, that it makes a carrot blush. Whenever or wherever they find cancer, they find a vitamin A deficiency. In Europe, many scientific experiments conducted with the plant have confirmed the traditional belief that its use is beneficial to the health of the liver.
- Dandelion increases the flow of urine. It acts as a gentle laxative and is invigorating and strengthening to the body in general. It's high in organic sodium and with its high potassium content combined, is the balancer of the electrolytes in the blood.
- Dandelion has been used as a high nutrient food. It has been used for calcium deficiencies and is a valuable survival food.
- In situations of severe vomiting, Dandelion restores the gastric balance in patients.
- Dandelion contains all the nutritive salts that are required for the body to purify the blood.
- The juice of the broken stem from the Dandelion can be used to treat warts. When used on a daily basis for about a week, it will dry them up. Dandelion juice from the broken stem is also useful to treat acne, blisters and corns.
- When Dandelion greens are used as a food, it improves the enamel of teeth.
- The Chinese use the seeds as a strong antibiotic in cases of lung infections.
- Inulin, one of the major chemicals in Dandelion, is currently being studied extensively for its immuno-stimulatory functions while also being used to strengthen the kidneys and as a pancreatic acid.
- In testing it against cancer, it has been shown to be active against two tumor systems, stimulating macrophage action. This helps substantiate the Chinese use of Dandelion for breast cancer over thousands of years.

ACNE
Abscesses
AGE SPOTS
ANEMIA
APPETITE STIMULANT
ARTHRITIS
ASTHMA
Bladder
BLISTERS (EXTERNAL)
BLOOD PURIFIER
BLOOD CLEANSER
BLOOD PRESSURE (HIGH)
Boils
Bowel inflammation
Breast cancer
Breast tumors
Bronchitis
Cholesterol (lowers)
Congestion
Constipation
Corns
Cramps
Dermatitis
Diabetes
Digestive disorders
Dropsy
Dyspepsia
ECZEMA
ENDURANCE
Fatigue
Female organs
Fevers
GALL BLADDER

Gallstones
Gas
Gout
Hemorrhage
HEPATITIS
HYPOGLYCEMIA
Indigestion
Infections (bacterial)
Insomnia
Intestines
JAUNDICE
KIDNEY INFECTIONS
Lethargy
LIVER DISORDERS
Metabolism (stimulates)
Pancreas
PMS
Psoriasis
Rheumatism
Scurvy
Senility
Skin eruptions
SKIN PROBLEMS
Sores
Spleen
Stamina
Stomach
Ulcers
Urination
Warts
Water retention
WEIGHT LOSS
Yeast infections

DEVIL'S CLAW   (Harpagophytum procumbens)
A.K.A.,: Grapple plant.

BODILY INFLUENCE: Alterative (blood purifier), Analgesic, Anti-arthritic, Anti-inflammatory, Anodyne, Anti-phlogistic, Anti-rheumatic, Bitter tonic, Cholagogue.
PART USED: Root.

Devil's Claw is found in the Namibian Steppes and the nearby Kalahari Desert of South Africa. The Devil's Claws common name was given because of the thorny, barbed claw arrangement of the seed pod. The root prepared as a tea is highly valued by the Namibian natives who use it for a wide variety of ailments, including arthritis, rheumatism and gout.

Rheumatic patients when taking Devil's Claw tea, found that the tea had to be taken for an extended period of time before its beneficial effects were seen, depending on the severity of the rheumatism.

• Devil's Claw is a valuable plant that has been found effective in the treatment of some cases of arthritis. This action, very likely, is due to a glycoside called harpagoside that reduces inflammation in the joints. This plant also aids in liver and gall bladder problems.

• Devil's Claw is a natural cleansing agent for removing toxic impurities from the system.

• Devil's Claw is will help prevent and overcome the hardening of the veins and arteries and help them to remain elastic. This works to maintain the blood vascular systems circulation, thereby, producing a general over-all-body systems improvement, strengthening and slowing down the aging process.

ARTERIOSCLEROSIS	HEADACHES
ARTHRITIS	INFLAMMATION
ARTHRITIS (RHEUMATOID)	KIDNEY (STRENGTHENS)
BLADDER (STRENGTHENS)	LIVER DISEASES
BLOOD PURIFIER	Malaria
CHOLESTEROL	NEURALGIA
DIABETES	PAIN (LOW BACK)
Gall bladder	POLLUTION (AIR)
Gall stones	RHEUMATISM
Gout	STOMACH DISORDERS

DONG QUAI (Angelica sinensis)
A.K.A.,: Tang-kuei, Woman's herb.

BODILY INFLUENCE: Alterative, Analgesic, Anti-spasmodic, Bitter, Blood tonic, Diuretic, Emmenagogue, Hormonal-female, Laxative, Oxytocic, Sedative, Uterine tonic.
PART USED: The whole plant.

In China and Japan, Dong Quai has a very high reputation. It is second only to Licorice root in sales. Dong Quai has been recorded as being used since 588 B.C. for dysmenorrhea. Its principal use has been used for female problems, especially for ailments affecting the female organs and the smooth muscles of the uterus.

Dong Quai is also used to strengthen and aid in general circulation. Dong Quai has been reported to have antibiotic effects on several bacteria including Escherichia coli,

Streptococcus and Shigella.
- Dong Quai helps to maintain a proper balance of female hormones.
- It has a cosmetic side-affect of enlarging the breasts of some women when taking Dong Quai.
- It helps cleanse and purify the blood, which promotes better blood circulation relieving the pain of traumatic injuries which is caused by the toxic reaction of injured congested intracellular tissue fluid. This improved blood vascular condition helps to relieve tinnitus, blurred vision and palpitations.
- Dong Quai can enhance the use of Vitamin E in cases of vitamin E deficiency, which may be an explanation of its fetus-stabilizing property and prevention of testicular disease.
- Dong Quai calms the nerves.
- Dong Quai is used especially after the delivery of a child, as a post-partum tonic, to regulate menses and as a blood builder.
- Dong Quai used in mixture with Chaparral and Red Clover is effective as a treatment to rebuild the lymphatic system in healing from cancer.
- Dong Quai is a bowel lubricant, thus helping to overcome constipation.

Abdominal pain
ANEMIA
Angina
Arthritis pain
Atherosclerosis
BLEEDING (internal)
Blood pressure (lowers)
BLOOD PURIFIER
Blood vessels
Brain nourisher
Breasts (abscessed)
Bronchitis
Cancer
CHILDBIRTH
Chills
CIRCULATION (poor)
Cramps (menstrual)
Diabetes
FEMALE GLANDS
FEMALE PROBLEMS
Fever
Headaches
Heart
Hormone balancer
HOT FLASHES
Hypertension
Hypoglycemia
Insomnia
Intestines (lubricates)
Laxative (mild)
Liver
Lower back
Lungs
MENOPAUSE
MENSTRUAL DISORDERS
MENSTRUATION
  (REGULATOR)
Migraine headaches
MUSCLE SPASMS
Muscle tension
Nephritis
Nerves (calms)
NERVOUSNESS
Pain reliever
Pituitary gland
Placenta (releases retained)
Plague
Skin problems
Spleen
Stomachache
Tumors (blood)
UTERUS (PROLAPSED)
Vaginal dryness

DULSE   (See Kelp)

ECHINACEA   (Echinacea purpurea)
A.K.A.,: Purple coneflower, Coneflower.

BODILY INFLUENCE: Alterative, Antibiotic, Antiseptic, Antiviral, Carminative, Depurative, Diaphoretic, Immunostimulant, Mucilant, Sialagogue, Stimulant, Vulnerary.
PART USED: Root

Historically, there has been some confusion between at least two varieties of Echinacea and Parthenium integrifolium. All three plants seem to have similar qualities and are easily confused. (See Echinacea integrifolium and Parthenium integrifolium)
Echinacea has been called the King of the Blood Purifiers because it improves lymphatic filtration and drainage. It has been found to help remove toxins from the blood. Some have found it to be good for enlargement and weakness of the prostate gland.

Experiments have shown that the polysaccharides, fatty acids, and glycosides in echinacea strengthen the function of the immune system making it of vital necessity in all health problems.

Echinacea is one of the most useful herbs available to Naturopathics, because it is a natural antibiotics and an alterative. It has been widely used as a retention colonic in ulcerative colitis. Echinacea has benefited toxic headaches with vertigo and a confused mental state when this condition is caused by toxemia (an accumulation of systemic toxins).

Ever since Thomsonians, Echinacea has been known by herbalist as one of the best alteratives for detoxifying the blood. It cleanses the Lymphatic System, supporting the immune system. It is used to increase resistance to bronchitis and other like infections. Other uses are helpful in typhoid fever, cellular abscesses, carbuncles and cancer.

Extensive scientific research has been undertaken on Echinacea in the last twenty years. The results have indicated an antibiotic cortisone-like activity, assistance in synovial membrane healing, support of collagen through hyaluronic acid protection, promotion of wound healing, production of systemic interferon, stimulation of T-cell lymphocytes and tumor suppression.

Echinacea is one of the most potent herbs that support the immune system, and is useful for treating colds and flu. It has anti-biotic like, anti-viral like, and anti-inflammatory like properties.

The active compounds in Echinacea is given to increase the ability of white blood cells to surround and destroy bacterial and viral invaders. Echinacea specifically strengthens the immune system against pathogenic infection by stimulating phagocytosis. T-cell formation; is amongst the most powerful and effective remedies against all kinds of bacterial and viral infections. There are no side effects noted when one takes a high intake of Echinacea.

- Echinacea is an excellent blood cleanser.
- Echinacea works like penicillin in the body with no side effects.
- The use of Echinacea functions especially well in so-called glandular infections and ailments. It is used to treat strep throat and lymph glands.
- Echinacea cleanses the morbid matter from the stomach.
- Echinacea also expels poisons and toxins.
- Echinacea activates the body's defense system against all outside influences and inflammatory conditions.
- Echinacea has antibiotic, anti viral and anti-inflammatory properties.
- Echinacea blocks the receptor site of the virus on the surface of the cell membranes preventing cell infection.

HERB BENEFICIAL DURING PREGNANCY: AN IMMUNE SYSTEM STIMULANT TO HELP PREVENT INFECTIONS

ACNE
Abscesses
ANTIBIOTIC
ANTISEPTIC
BITES/STINGS, internal &
    external
BITES/STINGS, poisonous
Bladder infection
BLOOD BUILDER
BLOOD CLEANSER
BLOOD DISEASES
BLOOD POISONING
BLOOD PURIFIER
BOILS
Bronchitis
Cancer
Catarrhal conditions
Carbuncles
Circulation
COLDS, fight infection
CONGESTION, lymphatic
CONTAGIOUS DISEASES
Digestion
DIPHTHERIA
EAR INFECTION
ECZEMA
Edema
EMPHYSEMA
FEVERS

Flu
GANDRENOUS CONDITIONS
GARGLE
Gingivitis
GLANDS
GUMS, sore
Hemorrhage
IMMUNE DEFICIENCY
IMMUNE STIMULANT
INFECTIONS, external
INFECTIONS, prevents
Laryngitis
LYMPHATIC CONGESTION
LYMPHATIC SYSTEM
Mouth odor
MOUTH SORES
MUCUS
Peritonitis
PROSTATE GLAND
Pyorrhea
SKIN ERUPTIONS
Sore throat
Sores, septic
Syphilis
TONSILLITIS
Tumors
Typhoid fever
WOUNDS

ELDER FLOWER   (Sambucus spp.,)
A.K.A. ; American Elder.

BODILY INFLUENCE: Alterative, Anti-inflammatory, Bitter, Detoxicant, Diaphoretic (mild), Laxative.
PART USED: Aged bark, flowers, berries, leaves.

    The Elder Flower tree provided the wood for Christ's Cross. The Shakers used it as a medicinal herb. It was such a healthy plant that seventeenth-century herbalist John Evelyn called it a remedy "against all infirmities what-so-ever."
    Although Elderberry tea has been employed for generations as a folk remedy for such conditions as colds, coughs, and flus, it has only been in recent years that science discovered that Elderberries contain viburnic acid, a substance which induces perspiration, which is useful in cases of bronchitis and similar ailments.
•   The Elder Flower is used for detoxifying the body tissues at the cell level. It increases blood circulation and promotes sweating.
•   The Elder Flower is known as a fever reducer, blood purifier and cell cleanser.
•   The Elder Flower is an anti-inflammatory agent with an anti-catarrhal action.
•   Elder Flower is used as a sedative for the relief of pain
•   The biggest use of the Elder Flower is in the first stages of colds.
•   The Elder Flower as an herb is used both internally and externally.

ALLERGIES	FEVERS
ASTHMA	Flu
Brain inflammation	Gas
BRONCHITIS	HAY FEVER
Bruises	Hemorrhoids
Cancer	Swollen joints
COLDS	Nerves
Coughs	PNEUMONIA
Deafness (catarrhal)	SINUS CONGESTION
Digestive problems	Skin diseases
Ear infections	Sprains
Eye infections	Ulcers
Eye strain	Wounds

ELECAMPANE   (Inula helenium)
A.K.A. - Scabwort, Elf Dock.

BODILY INFLUENCE: Anti-emetic, Anti-septic, Astringent, Bitter, Blood builder, Carminative, Diaphoretic (mild), Diuretic, Expectorant, Parasiticide, Stimulant, Stomachic, Tonic, Vermifuge, Vermicide.
PART USED: Root , Flower.

Elecampane was widely used by the ancient Romans as a cure for post banquet indigestion. Of this the Roman scholar Pliny wrote many centuries ago; "Let no day pass without eating some of the roots of Elecampane, to help digestion, to expel melancholy, and to cause mirth". American Indians found the plant to be particularly useful in treating bronchial and other lung ailments.

Elecampane is a specific for such conditions as irritating bronchial coughs, where there is copious catarrh formed, such as in bronchitis and emphysema.   Expectoration then is accompanied by a soothing action. This is combined with an anti-bacterial effect.

• Elecampane is widely used by Naturopath's as an expectorant and tonic and is used in chest congestion with excessive catarrhal expectoration.

• Elecampane controls excessive coughing and mucus discharge in bronchitis, respiratory tract inflammation, urinary and menstrual problems.

• Elecampane enhances digestion increasing the appetite, improving assimilation and general well being.

• Elecampane is used internally for intestinal worms.

• Elecampane can be applied externally for skin problems such as scabies and itches.

• Elecampane lessens tooth decay because it has been found to lower excessive sugar levels in the blood. It also provides the necessary nutrients for improving the general health of the mouth and gums.

• Elecampane is used to reduce the retention of water.

• Elecampane is the richest plant source of natural occurring insulin and provides other necessary nutrients to the pancreas to aid in all its vital functions.

• Elecampane is also thought to aid in soothing stomach cramps and other digestive ailments.

• Elecampane is a stimulant, relaxant and tonic to the mucous membranes.

• Elecampane is usually preferred in combination with other herbs.

Appetite	Female problems
Assimilation (poor)	Lungs
Asthma	Menstrual problems
Bladder catarrh	Nausea
BRONCHITIS (CHRONIC)	Poison (counteracts)
Catarrh (intestinal)	Phlegm
Colic	Respiratory inflammations
Consumption	Stomach tonic
Convulsions	Tuberculosis
COUGHS	Urinary tract inflammations
Cramps	Vomiting
Diarrhea (chronic)	Wheezing
Digestion	Whooping cough
Emphysema	Worms

EUCALYPTUS   (Eucalyptus globulus)
A.K.A.,: Blue Gum Tree.

BODILY INFLUENCE: Anti-biotic, Anti-inflammatory, Antiseptic, Anti-spasmodic, Astringent, Deodorant, Expectorant, Rubefacient, Stimulant, Tonic.
PART USED: Bark, Leaves, Seeds.

There are more than 500 species of Eucalyptus,which make up more than three fourths of all the vegetation on the Australian continent. The aborigines and early settlers of Australia, ground and ate the roots of the more diminutive species and later discovered that "lerp" or "manna," a sugary secretion of parasites that infect some of the trees made an excellent base for foods and beverages. The Australian aborigines were probably the first to discover that eucalyptus oil, called eucalyptol, which is very effective in certain medicinal applications.

Eucalyptus may be used externally as a deodorant, in decaying, discharging wounds, in ulcers and in gangrenous or cancerous lesions. In respiratory infections, Eucalyptus may be used as steam inhalation for its antiseptic and stimulatory effects in bronchitis. Eucalyptus is helpful in treating the flu, and pneumonia by facilitating expectoration thereby, relieving congestion.
• Eucalyptus reduced to an oil may be used for pyorrhea, burns and prevention of infections. The oil also clears sinus congestion.
• Eucalyptus may be used to counter some poisonous germs.
• Eucalyptus is a purifier, sweetener and vitalizer.
• To treat a weak stomach or nausea, put a drop of oil on the tongue.
• The oil is an active germicide, possessing antiseptic and astringent qualities.

- The most widely known medicinal use of Eucalyptus oil is for respiratory ailments.
- Herbals recommend inhaling steam laced with the oil to relieve the symptoms of bronchitis, asthma, croup, and chest congestion.
- The oil is a powerful antiseptic. When used as an ointment, it should be rubbed directly on the chest or back to relieve congestion in the lungs.

CAUTION: Eucalyptus oil should not be used in large amounts over a long periods of time since it is difficult to eliminate through the kidneys.

Asthma (vapor)
Boils
Bronchial congestion
BRONCHITIS
Burns (use oil)
Cancer
Carbuncles (external)
Catarrh
Colds
Coughs
Croup
Diptheria
Fever
Flu
Indigestion
LUNGS
MALARIAL DISEASES
Nausea
NEURALGIA
Paralysis
Piles
PYORRHEA (USE OIL)
Pneumonia
Sore throat
STIES
Typhoid
Ulcers (external)
Uterus (prolapsed)
Worms
WOUNDS

EYEBRIGHT (Euphrasia officinalis)
A.K.A.,: Red Eyebright.

BODILY INFLUENCE: Anti-inflammatory, Antiseptic, Astringent, Bitter, Tonic.
PART USED: The whole plant.

Herbalists suspect that the ancients knew of Eyebright's healing powers because the name Euphrasia is of Greek origin, derived from Euphrosyne, meaning 'gladness.' It is believed that the plant acquired this name because of its reputation for curing eye ailments. It brought much gladness by preserving the eyesight of the sufferer. In "Paradise Lost", the poet Milton relates that the Archangel, Michael used Eyebright to cure Adam of the eye infliction suffered by his eating of the forbidden fruit.

For centuries, Eyebright has been depended upon as a herb of choice for various diseases of the eye. Eyebright is used with excellent results for problems relating to mucous membranes. It is most helpful in acute or chronic inflammations of the eye

including, over-sensitivity to light and with stinging and weeping conditions, as well.
• When Eyebright is used as an eyewash, it tends to prevent secretion of fluids and relieves discomfort from eyestrain or minor irritation.
• When the volatile oil is applied in the eye, it becomes activated by sunlight to work on the cornea, ciliary muscle, iris, ligaments, lens, retina and optic nerves. This then, strengthens and soothes these areas, often improving eyesight and has also been used to both retard and reverse cataracts.
• Eyebright works as a vaso-constrictor and astringent to the nasal and conjunctiva mucous. It brings relief in frequent sneezing bouts and rejuvenating to eyes that feel exhausted. Eyebright also helps with eyes that are cloudy and irritated with lacrymation (excessive tears) of watery or stringy mucus.
• Eyebright is known to be a stimulant to the liver and to clean the blood.
• It used for inflammations and has antiseptic properties that fight eye infections.
• It is excellent for weak eyesight.

ALLERGIES
BLOOD CLEANSER
CATARACTS
Catarrh
COLDS
Congestion
CONJUNCTIVITIS
Coughs
DIABETES
Digestive disorders
EARACHE
EYE DISORDERS
EYE INFECTIONS
EYE STRAIN
EYE (STRENGTHENS)
GLAUCOMA
Hay fever
LIVER STIMULANT
Memory
Middle ear problems
PINK EYE
RUNNY NOSE
Sinus congestion
SNEEZING
Sore throat
Sties (dissolves)
Ulcers
VISION AID

FALSE UNICORN   (Chamaelirium luteum)
A.K.A.,: Fairywand, Blazing Star.

BODILY INFLUENCE: Diuretic, Emetic (in large doses), Emmenagogue, Hormonal, Parasiticide, Stimulant, Tonic, Uterine tonic.
PART USED: Root.

The North American Indians used False Unicorn for a variety of uses. Among the uses was to strengthen the body. Pregnant Indian women, chewed the root to prevent miscarriage. It has been used for a variety of female problems. Midwives have successfully used False Unicorn to help pregnant women prevent miscarriages. It is used in cases of infertility and helps to ease the nausea of morning sickness during pregnancy. This herb stimulates ovarian hormones and can be helpful for early menopause, after a hysterectomy or to help the system become normalized after years of contraceptives.

* It can be used by men for impotency and prostate problems.
* It is a good stimulating tonic and strengthener of the reproductive and urinary organs.
* False Unicorn is generally only used for problems existing during pregnancy and is generally not used when pregnancy is normal and healthy.
* False Unicorn has been useful in treating uterine problems in non-pregnant women to help normalize delayed or absent menstruation (amenorrhea). It can be especially helpful where there is a "heavy dragging feeling" in the lower abdomen.
* False Unicorn promotes chemical influences on the kidney which increases urine discharge.
* Herbalist's use it for ridding the intestines of worms and other parasites.
* False Unicorn contains chamaelirin, a strong antiseptic which makes it effective for genito-urinary problems.

Appetite (loss of)
Colic
DIGESTIVE PROBLEMS
Dyspepsia
Edema
Hemorrhage
Impotence
Infertility
KIDNEYS
MENSTRUAL IRREGULARITIES
MISCARRIAGE (PREVENTS)

Morning sickness
Nausea
Nocturnal emissions
Parasites
PROSTATE
Sterility
TAPE WORM
UTERUS (PROLAPSED)
Vaginal discharge
Worms

FENNEL   (Foeniculum vulgare)
A.K.A.,: Sweet Fennel.

BODILY INFLUENCE: Antacid, Anti-inflammatory, Antispasmodic, Aromatic, Carminative, Diuretic, Emmenagogue, Expectorant, Galactagogue, Parasiticide, Stimulant, Stomachic, Tonic.
PART USED: The whole plant.

Historically, the Greek physicians, Hypocrites and Dioscorides, recommended the use of Fennel for promoting milk production in nursing mothers. Culpeper, the British Herbalist, taught that the use of Fennel helped to break up stones in the kidneys.

By helping improve digestion, it quiets hiccups, thus preventing nausea. Its ability to break up uric acid in the tissues helps eliminate gout. This same ability to digest and handle protein digestion and protein waste helps to clear mucus from the liver and lungs. It also works as an antidote to poisonous mushrooms.

Fennel is a rich source of vitamin A, and so is useful in alleviating light sensitivity and improving night vision. Fennel also aids in preventing snow blindness from bright light reflection. Fennel is an aid to digestion and effectively helps in the elimination of intestinal gas, thus reducing the passing of gas and belching. It is considered helpful to clearing phlegm from the lungs.

• Fennel tea is used as a gargle and a breath refresher.
• Fennel can be taken to expel worms.
• Fennel has been applied as an eyewash.
• A Fennel poultice is used to help reduce inflammation and as such, isused to relieve swelling in the breasts of nursing mothers.
• This beneficial herb enriches the quantity and quality of mother's milk which carries over and helps with colic in babies. It is also excellent for children to take. By improving digestion, Fennel reduces the formation and build-up of uric acid tissue, demonstrating it's ability to reduce lumbago, kidney and bladder problems and promoting more normal bowel function.
• Fennel tea helps rid the intestinal tract of mucus.
• Fennel helps in weight reduction by curbing the appetite and alleviating hunger pains.
• Fennel functions as a gall bladder and liver cleanser, due to itsabilities as a tissue cleanser.
• Fennel is very effective for cancer patients after radiation and chemotherapy.

APPETITE (SUPPRESSES)
Asthma
Bedwetting
Bites (insect)
Bronchitis
Cholesterol (lowers)
COLIC
Colon disorders
Conjunctivitis (compress)
Constipation
Convulsions
Coughs
Cramps (abdominal)

DIGESTION (SLUGGISH)
Emphysema
Eyewash
Foodpoisoning
Gallbladder
GAS (EXPELS)
Gout
Hoarseness
INDIGESTION
INTESTINAL PROBLEMS
Jaundice
Kidney stones
LACTATION (INCREASES)

Liver cleanser
Lungs
Migraine headaches
MORNING SICKNESS
Obesity
SEDATIVE (FOR CHILDREN)
Sinus trouble
Snake bites

Spasms (gastrointestinal)
Spleen
Stomach acid
URIC ACID
RETENTION
URINATION (INCREASES)
WEIGHT REDUCTION

FENUGREEK (Trigonella foenum-graecum)
A.K.A.,: Bird's Foot, Greek Hay-seed.

BODILY INFLUENCE: Alterative, Aphrodisiac, Aromatic, Astringent, Carminative, Demulcent, Emollient, Expectorant, Galactagogue, Hormonal, Laxative (bulk), Mucilant, Nutritive, Parasiticide, Stimulant, Stomachic, Tonic.
PART USED: Seeds.

Fenugreek as one of the oldest known medicinal herbs, was used by Hypocrites. It was used extensively in both the Far East and in the West. "The Greatest Medical Discovery since the Dawn of History," so claimed the makers of Lydia E. Pinkham's Vegetable Compound, which was promoted to the American public in 1875 as a treatment for "female complaints." Fenugreek was one of Lydia Pinkham's Vegetable Compound elixirs. major ingredients. The most active compound though, was Black Cohosh.Fenugreek's origin is believed to be in the Mediterranean, but has also been reported as having been used in Asia. Fenugreek is currently being used to treat diabetes in the Middle East. Experimental data indicates that extracts of Fenugreek seeds lower blood sugar levels, thus regulating insulin production.Fenugreek has been shown to soften and dissolve hardened masses of accumulated mucus. Fenugreek as a tea, is a must for those who use, or have used, large quantities of milk, cheese and butter, as they cause large quantities of mucus waste to accumulate in the system that curtail the vital life-promoting processes, to include healthy lung action, free flowing blood circulation and proper lymphatic drainage. It is known to expel certain (accumulated uric acid) toxic waste by way of the lymphatic system. It loosens and expels mucus and phlegm accumulated in the bronchial tubes, soothes mucous membranes in the lungs and gastrointestinal tract and has also been used to treat lung infections.
• Fenugreek has been used to help prevent pregnancies due to it's spermicidal factors.
• Fenugreek seeds are used internally for treating an inflamedgastrointestinal system.

- Due to its containing up to 30% mucilage, Fenugreek poultices are used beneficially on abscesses, boils, inflammations, wounds and other skin problems, because of its drawing power.
- Fenugreek has been used in place of cod liver oil in treating scrofula, rickets, anemia and other disabilities following infectious diseases.
- Fenugreek is a strong stimulator of milk production in mothers and has been said to stimulate development of the breasts.
- Fenugreek can be used as a gargle for sore throats. It also thins mucus.
- Fenugreek contains lecithin which helps to dissolve cholesterol and fatty substances.
- As part of a fiber drink or tonic, Fenugreek seeds expel toxic waste and mucus through the elimination system.
- Some have used Fenugreek with lemon juice and honey to soothe and nourish the body and to reduce fevers.

Abscesses
ALLERGIES
Anemia
Asthma
Blood poisoning
Boils
Bowel lubricant
Breath (bad)
BRONCHIAL CATARRH
Bronchitis
Bruises
Cancer (lymphatic)
CHOLESTEROL (DISSOLVES)
Constipation
COUGHS
DIABETES
DIGESTIVE DISORDERS
EMPHYSEMA
Eyes
Fever
Gallbladder
GAS

Gout
Hay fever
HEADACHE
Healing
Heartburn
Hoarseness
INTESTINES (INFLAMED)
Intestines (lubricates)
Kidney
Lactation (stimulates)
Liver
LUNG INFECTIONS
MIGRAINE HEADACHES
MUCOUS MEMBRANES
MUCUS (DISSOLVES)
Sinus problems
SORE THROAT
STOMACH IRRITATIONS
Ulcers
Vagina
Water retention

FEVERFEW (Chrysanthemum parthenium)
A.K.A.,: Bachelor's-button, Featherfew.

BODILY INFLUENCE: Analgesic, Anti-inflammatory, Anti-microbial, Antipyretic, Aperient, Aromatic, Bitter, Carminative, Emmenagogue, Nervine, Parasiticide, Stimulant, Tonic, Vasodilator.
PART USED: The whole plant.

Since the Middle Ages, Feverfew has been used as an herb to reduce fevers (Febrifuge). Feverfew comes from the Latin febrifugia, which means "driver out of fevers." The ancient Greek physician Dioscorides valued the herb for its effect on the uterus. If contractions were not regular, it was often used in childbirth to help in the delivery of the afterbirth. In the first century A.D., he recommended the herb for "all inflammations and hot swellings," which may have been a reference to arthritis. Recent research is restoring Feverfew's reputation as a pain reliever.

The experiences of migraine sufferers indicate that Feverfew is effective in reducing the number and severity of headaches, as well as alleviating the nausea and vomiting that often accompany them. The word 'migraine' comes to us from the Greeks and means 'half of the skull,' as the excruciating pain usually strikes one side of the head.Researchers have actually shown extracts of Feverfew to have greater activity in inhibiting inflammation and fever than aspirin in experimental studies. Feverfew also decreases the secretion of inflammatory particles from platelets and white blood cells.

• Migraine headaches can also be caused by abuse to the body by consuming heavy white sugar products, coffee, alcohol and tobacco.

• Some of the other possible causes of migraines include mental tension such as grief, rage, anxiety, glandular deficiencies (migraines stop when glandular functions slow down in middle age), wrong eating habits (diet should be low fat, medium carbohydrates), constipation (from autointoxication), certain odors or inhalants can trigger it (paint, smog, perfume, etc.), allergies (from foods or food preservatives, i.e., cheese, milk, chocolate, pork, wine) and liver problems (if the bile thickens from fatty foods, it causes bile ducts to become temporarily congested resulting in nausea and the vomiting of greenish-yellow bile).

• One herbalist stated that "Feverfew needed to be taken dailyas a preventative for migraine headaches, instead of taking it only when they felt a headache coming on.

• Feverfew is used for pain relief, migraine headaches, chills, fevers, colds and inflammation from arthritis.

• Researchers speculate that substances in the Feverfew plant

appear to make smooth muscle cells less responsive to body chemicals that trigger migraine muscle spasms.
- Scientists have determined that extracts of Feverfew have inhibitedthe production of prostaglandins which constrict and dilate cerebral blood vessels which cause migraine headaches.
- Feverfew increases fluidity of lung and bronchial tube mucus.
- Feverfew aids in allowing the body to heal itself and is a natural way to strengthen the body.
- Feverfew has been used to restore normal liver function.
- Alcohol destroys Feverfew's benefits.

Aches	HAYFEVER
Ague (Malaria)	HEADACHES
Allergies	Hot flashes
Appetite stimulant	Hysteria (nervous)
ARTHRITIS PAIN	Indigestion
Arthritis (rheumatoid)	Insect bites (external)
Asthma	Lungs
Bronchitis	Menopause symptoms
CHILLS	Menstrual cramps
Circulation	Menstruation (promotes)
COLDS	MIGRAINE HEADACHES
Digestive problems	Muscle tension
Dizziness	Pain
Fevers	SINUS HEADACHE
Female problems	Tinnitus
Flu	Vertigo

FIGWORT   (Scrophularia nodosa)
A.K.A.,: Scrofula plant, Carpenter's Square.

BODILY INFLUENCE: Alterative, Anodyne, Anti-inflammatory, Bitter, Demulcent, Diuretic, Laxative, Parasiticide, Circulatory Stimulant, Tonic.
PART USED: The whole plant.

Herbalist's have also called the plant Scrofularia, after its use as a remedy for "scrofulous ailments," such as tuberculosis of the lymph glands and other diseases characterized by swellings and eruptions.
- Figwort finds most use in the treatment of skin problems.
- Figwort will work to aid the digestive organs and being a diuretic,helps to maintain clean kidneys.
- Figwort provides hormone-like materials into the system to help soothe the digestive organs.
- In Britain, Figwort is used to treat circulatory disorders and is helpful in treating varicose veins.

- Figwort is believed to be helpful at reducing high blood pressure, and is a diuretic as well as an efficient pain killer when nothing stronger is at hand.
- Figwort may be used as a cosmetic skin medication to treat eczema, scabies, some tumors and rashes. It can also be made into anointment or fomentation for use on scratches, bruises and wounds on the surface of the skin.

ABRASIONS
ATHLETE'S FOOT
Bruises
Constipation
CRADLE CAP
Cuts
Digestive organs
Dropsy
Eczema
Fevers
Gout
Hemorrhoids
IMPETIGO
Insomnia
Kidneys

Liver conditions
Menstruation (promotes)
Psoriasis
Rashes
RESTLESSNESS
Ringworm
Scabies
SKIN DISEASES
Sores
Toothaches
TUMORS (SKIN)
Ulcers
Worms
Wounds

FOXGLOVE (Digitalis purpurea)
A.K.A.,: Witch's Bells.

BODILY INFLUENCE: Cardiant, in overdose, it is a nauseate and emetic.
PART USED: Leaves.

An English doctor, by the name of Withering, found digitalis in the tea mixture of an old woman herbalist who used it to cure dropsy and what we term today as congestive heart condition. He had heard of the old woman and that she practiced folk medicine with herbs gathered in the countryside. At the time that he visited her she was treating a patient afflicted with excessive fluid retention. Withering, upon seeing this patient expected him to die. The patient in fact was cured with what Withering concluded was a bag of useless weeds. Later Withering identified Foxglove as an element in this bag of weeds, Withering later identified Foxglove as an ingredient useful for treating inflammation, or edema, which is associated with congestive heart condition.

He also learned that Foxglove is a deadly poison, when taken in large excessive doses, and as likely to stop the heart as to keep it going. This discovery took place in the 1775. Digitalis has been used ever since 1875 the year that Dr. Withering reported his experience with the old Indian Herbalist and his later discoveries.

The name Foxglove is derived from the shape of the blossoms, which bear a resemblance to glove fingers. As long ago as the Middle Ages, Lily of the valley was held in high esteem as a heart medicine. Later, however, when the more potent digitalis, or Foxglove, was discovered, Lily of the valley fell into disuse. As a toxic substance Lily of the Valley, does not pose the same danger as does Fox Glove, since within four hours the glycosides, the active substance, is broken down by the body, rendering it non-toxic. However the medicinal effects continue much longer.

CAUTION; Fox Glove Can be Poisonous. Do not use without direction.

FUMITORY   (Fumaria officinalis)
A.K.A.,: Earth Smoke.

BODILY INFLUENCE: Alterative, Cholagogue, Diuretic, Laxative, Stomachic, Bitter Tonic.
PART USED: The flowering herb.

Fumitory has been used historically in the treatment of skin problems due to it being a general cleansing agent. Fumitory is also used as an eyewash to ease conjunctivitis. Today, Fumitory is used as an internal tonic principally for liver and gallbladder problems. Large doses can work as a laxative and diuretic, but excessive doses can cause stomach ache. It can also be used for scabies and other skin problems. Because of its diuretic principles, it helps with high blood pressure.

Acne
Arteriosclerosis
BLOOD PRESSURE, HIGH
Bronchitis
Conjunctivitis
Constipation
Dermatitis
Eczema
Hemorrhoids
Hysteria
KIDNEYS
LIVER CONGESTION
Rheumatism
Scurvy
Skin diseases
Stomach disorders

GARCINIA (Garcinia cambogia)
A.K.A.,: Mangosteen, Brindall Berries.

BODILY INFLUENCE: Astringent, Anti-catarrhal, Demulcent, Thermogenesis.
PART USED: Fruit.

Scientific studies suggest that Garcinia, a fruit indigenous to India and Thailand, can be helpful in controlling appetite. The effect is to stifle the body's ability to turn over-supply of carbohydrates into fat and augment calorie-burning.

It is known to subdue appetite, slowing down the conversion of excess carbohydrates into fat. In this process, it will build additional stores of body energy (glucose).

Research indicates that Garcinia triggers fatty acid oxidation in the liver, preventing excess carbohydrates from turning into fat. Garcinia has been shown to inhibit fat storage and is active as an appetite suppressant, burning fat via thermogenesis. Subsequently, the liver can efficiently compound glucose and build up glycogen stores. The result is less hunger, a reduction in fat and the experience of more energy.

Garcinia is composed of more than 50% hydroxycitric acid, making this ingredient, Garcinia's key active constituent. Fatty tissue growth and function is altered by the ingestion of hydroxycitric acid. It is said to block the formation of certain functions so as to prevent the formation of fatty tissue formation. Tests have been run to show that it has great results in weight reduction.

As a result of the studies on Garcinia, one researcher determined that the herb may affect the way the body stores fat and if combined with a knowledgeable program of eating and exercise, could have great potential as weight control management.

- It helps reduce the body's ability to store fat.
- It lowers body weight through appetite control.
- It lowers serum triglycerides.
- It creates a process in the body called thermogenesis.
- It helps with catarrhal conditions of the throat, urinary system and uterus.
- It has been found to have no adverse or toxic side effects.

GARLIC   (Allium sativum)
A.K.A.,: Clove Garlic, Poor-man's-treacle.

BODILY INFLUENCE: Alterative, Anti-bacterial, Anti-biotic, Anti-catarrhal, Anti-fungal, Anti-pyretic, Antiseptic, Antispasmodic, Anti-viral, Aromatic, Carminative, Cholagogue, Depurant, Diaphoretic, Digestant, Diuretic, Emmenagogue, Expectorant, Fungicide, Hypertensive, Hypotensive, Immunostimulant, Nervine, Parasiticide, Prophylactic, Rubefacient, Stimulant, Stomachic, Tonic, Vulnerary.
PART USED: The whole plant.

Garlic is first noted by Chinese literature in the Collection of Commentaries on the Classic of the Materia Medica (500 A.D.). According to a 3,500 year old Egyptian scroll, healers even then believed garlic could help a person fight cancer. Dioscorides who lived in the first century A.D. was a surgeon and physician in the Roman armies. He described Garlic with regard to the Doctrine of Signatures. This is the notion that the medicinal properties of the plant are revealed symbolically by its outward form. Thus, a plant such as garlic, with a long hollow stalk, would be good for all diseases of the windpipe.

When the plagues ravaged Europe, the populace ate garlic daily as a protection against the disease. Garlic is known as a natural anti-biotic, without the deleterious effects of the drugs that kill all life within the body. It was reported that garlic may have worked as a preventive simply by keeping others at a safe distance, but it did work, and it saved many lives. When it was discovered that garlic would prevent the plague, there were those who protected themselves by using it. Some of them later took advantage of this protected state and robbed those that were dead or dying. When caught, they were executed for their crimes, which was an ironic turn of events for having missed the angel of death.

As a medicinal plant, Garlic can be used extensively for disease prevention. Internally, it can be used against infection of all kinds. Externally, is has been used for eye, ear, nose and throat infections and because of the thiamin content, it is used to prevent mosquito bites. Garlic has measurable amount of germanium (a mineral which strengthens the immune system), an antioxidant for aiding in physical endurance and is of excellent benefit in wound healing.

Nutritionally, Garlic has been found useful for some control in glucose tolerance for both hypoglycemia and hyperglycemia, possibly by helping to reduce insulin requirements. It is useful in orchestrating and blocking atherosclerosis and in reducing blood cholesterol. Garlic has also been shown to lower serum cholesterol and triglycerides, while also raising HDL levels in both healthy individuals and patients of coronary heart disease. It helps protect against narrowing of the arteries. Garlic is known to dissolve LDL (harmful) cholesterol and to lower triglycerides, while increasing HDL (beneficial) cholesterol levels.

Garlic owes most of its strong aroma to allicin, which is produced by the enzymatic action of allinase on alliin (a sulphur-containing amino acid). This action does not take place until garlic is bruised, thus the aroma of fresh garlic is not offensive until it is crushed or cut. There are some that have discovered a way to prepare a garlic product devoid of the sulfur smell by removing the allicin, however it is the consensus of opinion that allicin is the ingredient that destroys fungus and possesses other medicinal benefits.

Most of the beneficial effects of garlic are thought to be the result of its sulfur compounds. The plant is easy to grow and its strong odor serves a useful purpose in the garden. It helps to discourage insects that might prey on other plants.

Researchers at Loma Linda University have found compounds in Garlic that activate enzymes in the liver that destroy alfa-toxin, a potent carcinogen produced by mold that can grow on peanuts and grains. Alfa-toxins are claimed to be a leading cause of liver cancer.

- It is known for being able to stimulate the lymphatic system to throw off waste materials.
- It works to relieve pain resultant from insect bites.
- Garlic rids the respiratory tract of phlegm and works to rid the bowels of parasites.
- Because it is a natural anti-biotic, it helps to control fevers and works to combat viruses.
- Garlic helps to control disorders of the blood. It is even good for expelling thread worms from the body.
- Garlic has been used in enemas and colonics, having the ability to rid the colon of intestinal parasites.
- Garlic also has the ability to destroy harmful bacteria and at the same time leave behind beneficial bacteria for the body to utilize.
- Garlic strengthens blood vessels and is a powerful detoxifier providing protection against pollutants and heavy metal toxicity.
- Evidence continues to mount that of the 50 compounds in garlic, 10 are active in reversing cancer development.
- Garlic has been used in cough remedies for centuries.
- Externally, Garlic has often been used as a drawing poultice. IT HAS BEEN RECOMMENDED TO APPLY A LAYER OF OLIVE OIL BEFORE APPLYING GARLIC DIRECTLY ON THE SKIN.
- In India, Garlic is used to wash wounds and ulcers.
- Garlic strengthens the heart, it also nourishes and has a positive effect on the stomach, spleen and lungs.

- Garlic protects against cancer-causing agents as found in cigarette smoke, char-broiled meat and polluted air. It is a specific anti-tumor agent used as a preventive for many types of cancer and other degenerative diseases.
- Garlic improves circulation, while it stimulates the immune system. It contains an anti-coagulant which normalizes blood platelet adhesion by reducing the "stickiness of the blood" thereby improving circulation.
- Garlic is effective in treating arthritis and may help prevent breast cancer, heart disease, strokes and some viral infections.
- The Russians call Garlic, a natural antibiotic and have referred to it as Russian penicillin.
- Paavo Airola, a leading authority on biological medicine, described Garlic as the "King of the Vegetable Kingdom".
- Aged garlic is good for use as an anti-oxidant, anti-tumor agent, immune enhancer, liver protective agent and anti-stress agent.
- Garlic is good as mosquito repellent, when applied to the body with olive oil.
- It is also good for avoiding mosquitoes when taken internally with liquid capsules of B-1 and B-12, one hour before going outside.
- Garlic powder is good on open wounds and works to promote the healing process.
- Research in the 1970's, has shown that oils extracted from Garlic inhibited blood clotting.
- Garlic is one of many Super foods that some consider to be one the most potent healing herbs in the world.
- Allicin is active against fungi which includes Candida Albicans. It is even more effective than Nystatin. There are also microbes that are inhibited by Allicin-rich garlic, including the influenza viruses.
- The activities of the parasitic fungus, that is associated with AIDS, is inhibited by the presence of Garlic.
- Garlic is effective in treating respiratory conditions such as asthma, bronchial and lung problems. It is a superior expectorant, helping to expel phlegm from the lungs.
- Garlic with Capsicum and Vitamin C taken internally at the first notice of a cold can help.
- Inserting one capsule of Garlic in the rectum can relieve the pain of hemorrhoids by helping to shrink hemorrhoidal tissue.

Acne
Allergies
Anemia
ANTIBIOTIC (NATURAL
   PENICILLIN)
ANTI-FUNGUS

ANTI-VIRAL
ARTERIOSCLEROSIS
ARTHRITIS
ASTHMA
Athlete's foot
BLOOD POISONING

BLOOD PRESSURE (HIGH)
Blood cleanser
BLOOD PURIFIER
BRONCHITIS (CHRONIC)
CANCER IMMUNITY
CANDIDA ALBICANS
Childhood diseases
CHOLERA
CIRCULATION (POOR)
COLDS (FIGHTS INFECTION)
COLITIS
CONTAGIOUS DISEASES
COUGHS
Cramps
Diabetes
Diarrhea
DIGESTIVE DISORDERS
Diverticulitis
Dropsy
EAR INFECTIONS
Emphysema
FEVER
FLU
FUNGUS PROBLEMS
Gallbladder
GAS

HEART
Hypoglycemia
INFECTIONS
INFECTIOUS DISEASES
Insomnia
INTESTINAL INFECTIONS
Intestinal worms
Kidney function (promotes)
LIVER (DETOXIFIES)
Lumbago
LUNGS
Mucus
PARASITES
PINWORMS
Pneumonia
PROSTATE GLAND PROBLEMS
Rabies
RESPIRATORY CONGESTION
Rheumatism
Sinus problems
Staph & Strep
Ulcers
Warts
Worms (expels)
YEAST INFECTIONS

GENTIAN   (Gentiana lutea)
A.K.A.,: Bitterwort, Sampson's Snakeroot.

BODILY INFLUENCE: Alterative, Anti-bilious, Anti-inflammatory, Anti-pyretic, Antiseptic, Bitter, Cholagogue, Digestant, Laxative-mild, Parasiticide, Sialagogue, Gastric Stimulant, Stomachic, Tonic.
PART USED: Root.

Gentian was named after Gentius, King of Illyria. Gentius was also a botany student. It is generally believed that King Gentius was the first to discover the remedial value of the plant which bears his name.

Gentian is popular in Appalachia, where some people carry a piece of the root to energize and to increase physical strength. Gentian is useful as a blood-builder and has been popular to use during convalescence.

The custom of employing Gentian, as a bitters for stomach tonic, goes back in history to the begining of the use of Gentian itself. The ancient Romans, notorious for their food orgies, were convinced that bitters were important for digestion.

Father Kneipp, a nineteenth century German who was a natural healer and well known in Europe, strongly advocated the use of Gentian bitters. He is quoted from his journals as saying, "If the food is felt to be heavy in the stomach, and is troublesome, a little cordial made with a teaspoonful of Gentian extract in a half a glass of water, will soon stop the disorder."

Gentian strengthens the entire human system. Gentian can do all this even when given in moderate doses. Because it stimulates the appetite, this herb is useful in treating anorexia and exhaustion.

Gentian is beneficial to the digestive process due to its ability to improve the blood vascular system, insuring that the abdominal organs receive a rich supply of blood.

Another attribute of Gentian is that it appears to have a mild cleansing effect on the bowel and is effective for slowly cleansing hardened morbid matter from the colon.

Gentian stimulates the pancreas and this makes it a valuable herb for the diabetic or pre-diabetic. It also has a normalizing effect on the thyroid gland.

• Gentian strengthens the digestive organs, increases circulation and is good for the female organs.

• Gentian is a fortifying tonic particularly useful for jaundice, bile production and for liver malfunction.

• Gentian is a stimulator of the general circulation which in turn is a strengthener of the total system.

• Gentian is high in simple energy producing sugars and is beneficial to the digesting organs, the stomach and pancreas, as well as being an aid to the well-being of both the kidney and spleen.

• It has also been found that Gentian root increases the activities of many glands and organs giving much of the stimulating effect of adrenalin, the hormone that is secreted when the body needs quick energy in an emergency situation.

Anal itch	Gas
APPETITE STIMULANT	Gastritis
Blood purifier	Gout
Circulation	Heartburn
Colds	Hepatitis
Constipation	HYSTERIA
Convulsions	JAUNDICE
Diarrhea	LIVER DISORDERS
DIGESTION (STRENGTHENS)	Nausea
Dysentery	Spleen
Dyspepsia	Urinary tract infections
Female weakness	Vaginal rashes & discharges
Fever	Worms (expels)

GINGER   (Zingiber officinale)

A.K.A.,: African Ginger.

BODILY INFLUENCE: Analgesic, Antacid, Anti-emetic, Anti-inflammatory, Antispasmodic, Aperitive, Aromatic, Carminative, Diaphoretic (if taken hot), Diuretic, Emmenagogue, Nervine, Rubefacient, Sialagogue, Stimulant, Stomachic, Tonic.
PART USED: Root.

It was the Spaniards who introduced the Americas to the Ginger plant in the early part of the 16th century. Ginger became so popular among Europeans that in 1884, Great Britain imported over 5 million pounds of the root.

Research conducted at Cornell University Medical College has found that Ginger may help prevent strokes and hardening of the arteries. This active ingredient of Ginger, Gingerol, is proven effective in preventing recurrences of so-called "little strokes." It is believed that this substance, Gingerol, inhibits an enzyme that causes cells to clot.

Aspirin has currently been lauded medically for its blood thining properties which help prevent heart problems. What has not been addressed however, is the fact that the Aspirin has serious side effects such as causing stomach and intestinal ulcers, which often hemorrhage causing death.   Also it is said that Aspirin blocks Ginger's action to prevent blood platlets from clumping.   So although Aspirin can prevent the clotting that prevents strokes, it also prevents Ginger from naturally doing a better job of preventing harmful problems.

Ginger thins the blood and lowers blood cholesterol. It is known to work to reduce fevers. It can be used to relieve vomiting and to soothe the stomach and spleen in the process.

Ginger is a warm blood vascular stimulant and body cleansing herb and is used in respiratory and lung/chest clearing combinations.   It is system alkalizer and a stimulant of the digestive system.   It is a catalyst in nervine and sedative formulas. It has a variety of uses such as in a gargle preparation and as part of sore throat syrups.   It is used as a diaphoretic encouraging profuse sweating helping in the removal of toxic waste.   It is a kidney stimulant to increase kidney filtration.

Ginger has a reducing effect on migraine headaches without the side effects found with drugs. Ginger has been found effective in combating nausea caused by motion sickness.

• Ginger is most often used as a carminative, usually mixed with a variety of other herbs, because of its great ability to stop griping and cramping especially in the abdominal and intestinal area.

• Ginger has long been recommended by herbalists as a regulator of blood cholesterol to improve blood circulation,

especially to the extremities (hands and feet).
- In China, Ginger is used in the first stages of the common cold.
- With the stress and strain found in modern women, Ginger is remarkable in alleviating menstrual cramps. It has been found to be effective in arresting excessive menstrual flow and to increase the flow of urine, when taken as a hot infusion.

GINGER IS BENEFICIAL DURING PREGNANCY:
IT IS EXCELLENT FOR MORNING SICKNESS
AND HAS LOTS OF MINERALS.

Bowels
BRONCHITIS (CHRONIC)
Chicken pox
CHILDHOOD DISEASES
CIRCULATION (POOR)
COLDS
COLIC
COLITIS
Colon spasms
Constipation
COUGHS
CRAMPS
DIARRHEA
DIGESTIVE DISORDERS
DIZZINESS
FATIGUE
FEVERS
FLU
GAS
Gout
HEADACHE
Hemorrhage
INDIGESTION

Influenza
Kidneys
LEARNING PROBLEMS
Menstrual cramps
MORNING SICKNESS
MOTION SICKNESS (TO
    PREVENT)
Mumps
NAUSEA
PARALYSIS
Pelvic circulation
Pneumonia
Shock
Sinus congestion
Sinusitis
SORE THROAT
STOMACH (SETTLES
    STOMACH)
Tongue paralysis
TOOTHACHE
Vagina
VOMITING
WHOOPING COUGH

GINKGO   (Ginkgo biloba)
A.K.A.,: Maidenhair Tree.

BODILY INFLUENCE: Adaptogen, Anti-fungal, Anti-oxidant, Anti-tussive, Astringent, Bitter, Expectorant, Nervine, Parasiticide, Sedative, Circulatory Stimulant, Vaso-dilator.
PART USED: Leaves, seeds.

The Ginkgo biloba tree is known as the oldest species of tree in the world today. It is a hardy tree being the only tree to survive the Hiroshima atomic blast and it is still alive today. They have been known to live well over an average of 1,000 plus years. The strain goes back as far as written history in the Orient. The claim is that the Chinese protected the tree and nurtured it through the Ice age. It is a tree planted today in the monasteries in the Orient by the monks and looked after dutifully.

It is today being planted in groves to be used as a medicinal plant for the Ginkgo extract to be harvested from. The Ginkgo biloba tree is extremely resistant to all kinds of pollution, viruses and fungi and therefore, was extensively planted throughout Asia and later in Europe. Today, Ginkgo biloba is used in landscaping and planted wherever it's gentle fern-like leaf is appreciated for the beauty inherent to this particular plant. The plants' main use can be said to be extending the functional life of many people. Ginkgo is an herb of longevity. Its recorded history dates way back in plant antiquity. Considered to be possibly the oldest living tree species, having survived for thousands of years, Ginkgo-biloba has been termed as a living fossil.

In China, the curative powers of Ginkgo have been known for thousands of years. It has been used as an aid in the treatment of many of the problems typically associated with aging, such as poor blood circulation, mental confusion, memory loss, and many of the disruptions expected with the onset of senility. Ginkgo has been shown to increase mental alertness and memory significantly.

Ginkgo was found to inhibit free radical scavengers from destroying cells. The elixir in Ginkgo has been found to be effective in reducing blood cell clumping. It is in the clumping of blood that modern medical science has discovered can bring on congestive heart disease. Ginkgo is responsible for an increase in acetyl-choline levels, therefore, the extract taken from Ginkgo enhances the ability of the body to better transmit body electrical impulses.

• Ginkgo, by improving blood circulation to the central nervous system, aids in the treatment of dementia and Alzheimer's disease.

• By strengthening the blood vascular system and decreasing the possibilities of clots, there is a strong possibility of strokes being prevented.

• Hearing is improved with this improved circulation. It increases tissue oxidation and improves vital nutrients being delivered to the body tissues. Use of the herb, improves ear problems as it improves blood flow to the nerves of the inner ear. It has also been found to help Tinnitus (ringing in the ear).

• Ginkgo also improves blood circulation in the eye and related eye structures such as the retina which helps prevent macular degeneration.

• By improving blood flow, Ginkgo reduces the frequency of asthma attacks and even helps in preventing organ transplant rejection.

- In some disciplines involving healing, Ginkgo is used primarily as a brain and mental energy stimulant. The plant is known to increase both peripheral and cerebral circulation through vaso-dilation.
- Ginkgo has been used to increase the quality of blood flow to the brain to improve memory. This is especially true when memory loss is due to strokes, thus, it is helpful in the treatment of strokes by preventing blood clot formation. The herb also helps arteries in the legs and relieves pain due to circulatory problems.
- Ginkgo biloba stimulates cerebral circulation and oxygenation of cells; hence, mental clarity and alertness is experienced.
- Part of the reasoning in explaining improved circulation by using Ginkgo, is that it dilates the blood vessels, facilitating improved blood flow to the tissues.
- Because of its high flavonoid content, the first area of scientific study was the vascular system. In several studies, Ginkgo biloba has been shown to protect the body from arterial blockage, while increasing levels of glucose and ATP at the cellular level. The effect is to maintain energy within individual cells that might be affected. In persons recovering from blood clots in the arteries of the heart, Ginkgo biloba was found to lower blood pressure and dilate peripheral blood vessels, including the capillaries.

Alertness
Allergies
ALZHEIMER'S
Arthritis
Anxiety attacks
Asthma
ATTENTION SPAN
Cancer
CIRCULATORY DISORDERS
Coughs
Depression
DIZZINESS
Equilibrium
Eye problems
Headaches
Hearing

HEART PROBLEMS
Impotence
LONGEVITY
Lung problems
MEMORY LOSS
Mental clarity
Mood swings
Muscular degeneration
Shock (toxic)
Senility
STROKES
Tinnitus
Varicose veins
Vascular disorders
Vertigo
Visual acuity

GINSENG (Panax schinseng)

A.K.A. PANAX quinquefolium (American Ginseng), PANAX schin-seng (Korean or Asiatic Ginseng), PANAX pseudoginseng (Tienchi Ginseng).

BODILY INFLUENCE: Adaptogen, Alterative, Aphrodisiac, Cell Proliferant, Demulcent, Digestant, Diuretic, Expectorant, Nervine, Nutritive, Rejuvenative, Immuno-Stimulant, Cardiotonic, Tonic.
PART USED: Root.

The herbs botanical name, Panax is derived from the Greek word "panacea" meaning all healing. Panax, having been taken from the Greek word Pan, which means Power and when combined with the Greek word akos or ills, it takes on a meaning of a plant that cures all ills. The species name, Ginseng, is Chinese for "man plant", which is attributed to the shape of the root that resembles a man.

Ginseng is stimulating for physical activities and can be used as a aphrodisiac, believed as such because of its healing qualities on the prostate. In women, Ginseng is known to produce testosterone; therefore its use for them is not recommended over long periods.

Ginseng is good for the digestive system, aiding in the recovery of certain illnesses and is combined with other tonics for building strength. Ginseng supports adrenal function, reduces stress and regulates blood sugar.

Ginseng is considered by some as the most effective adaptogen of all tonic herbs. Ginseng has measurable amounts of germanium, providing energy to all the body systems. It promotes regeneration of the body suffering from stress and fatigue. It is known to aid in the rebuilding of body strength. It has long been found to be particularly nourishing to the male reproductive and circulatory systems. Ginseng has found new usefulness for women as a stimulant for brain and memory centers. As stated earlier, women should not prolong the use of Ginseng. Ginseng benefits are found to be cumulative in the body. Taking this herb for several months to a year is far more effective than short term doses.

All varieties of Panax Ginseng do endow an individual with more energy and help to improve brain function and build up cells throughout the body. It has been known to raise blood pressure when found to be low and conversely, it has been found to lower the blood pressure when it is higher than desired.

It is held by many, that the Manchurian Ginseng from the mountains of China is the best Ginseng and some old roots have been known to sell for as much as $20,000.00. In 1976, a four hundred year old root from this particular variety was found on an island off the shores of Korea. It was reported to have been sold for an incredible $10,000.00 per ounce. Its total weight was fourteen and a half lbs., which meant that its total value was no less than $1,320,000.00! This would make the sale of Ginseng in Korea as being the most expensive transaction of this root in modern history and probably in all times.

American Ginseng is preferred by the majority of the common people in both China and Japan, while the Korean and Chinese variety is preferred in North America.

The age of the Ginseng root is of utmost importance; hence, its greater value as a medicine of old roots. It is rumored that extremely old roots glow in the dark, giving off a peculiar type of illumination. The shape of the root is another important factor according to ancient Chinese lore. Legend holds that a superior root has the shape of a man walking at a comfortable gait.

The Panax variety of Ginseng increases male hormone production. This is the reason its long term use is not suggested for the female. Over a two month period, it may bring about the emergence of secondary male sexual characteristics. Many herbalist's suggest that females should use the Panax variety for no more than 6 weeks at a time, with a 6 month break in-between.

Panax Ginseng should never be allowed to come in contact with metal as this has been observed to decrease its strength.

Chinese Ginseng has a tonic effect on the pituitary gland and a stimulating effect on the adrenals, giving it its adaptogen effect. By speeding up the nervous reflexes, this herb increases analytical and overall mental performance, while diminishing fatigue.

A Chinese text dating from the first century A.D. describes Ginseng as "enlightening to the mind and increasing the wisdom. Continuous use, it is said, leads to longevity."

• Ginseng helps to fight against fatigue and depression in men by eliminating stress and thus enhance physical well-being. It also works to reduce nervous reaction due to stressed-out conditions.

• Ginseng has a history of improving normal adrenal flow from the adrenal glands, therefore, making it effective at combating male impotence.

• Ginseng is safe and may be used by men as a preventive medicine.

• Ginseng acts on free radicals in the body which slows down the effects of aging.

• Ginseng also effects the pituitary gland, helping to regulate body tissue and vascular tone.

AGE SPOTS
Aging
ANEMIA
Antidote (for some drugs)

APPETITE (STIMULATES)
ASTHMA
Bleeding (internal)
Blood diseases

BLOOD PRESSURE
Bronchitis
Cancer
Collapse
Concentration (lack of)
DEBILITY
DEPRESSION
DIABETES
Digestive problems
DYSPEPSIA
ENDURANCE (INCREASES)
FATIGUE (CHRONIC)
FEVERS (CHRONIC)
HEMORRHAGE
HORMONE IMBALANCE
Hyperglycemia
Hypoglycemia
Hypotension
Impotence
Insomnia
Liver diseases
LONGEVITY
Lung (strengthens)
Malnutrition
Nausea
NEUROSIS
Palpitation
Radiation protection
SEXUAL STIMUALNT
Shock
STRESS
THIRST
Ulcers
Vitality (mental)
VITALITY (PHYSICAL)
WEAKNESS

GINSENG, WILD AMERICAN   (Panax quinquefolium)

BODILY INFLUENCE: Adaptogen, Alterative, Aphrodisiac, Cell Proliferant, Demulcent, Digestant, Expectorant, Nervine, Nutritive, Rejuvenative, Immuno-Stimulant, Cardiotonic, Tonic.
PART USED: The Root.

In America, Ginseng was valued by the American Indians long before the coming of the Europeans. It began to acquire universal acclaim in the 1700's, when the Jesuits found it being used and began to export it to China. George Washington is credited with documenting this information having met with many pack horses carrying Ginseng. Daniel Boone and Davy Crockett are said to have made large sums of money in Ginseng trafficking.

The American Ginseng has many of the properties as those from China and Asia and are listed under their label above, except that the American variety acts to tranquilize the brain, while moderately stimulating the vital organs. It also helps to relieve fatigue. It is particularly good for increasing body fluids.

GINSENG, SIBERIAN   (Eleutherococcus senticosus)
A.K.A.: Taiga root, Touch-Me-Not, Devil.s Bush.

BODILY INFLUENCE: Adaptogen, Alterative, Anti-rheumatic, Antispasmodic, Aperitive, Aphrodisiac, Calmative, Cardio-tonic, Hypertensive, Immuno-Stimulant, Prophylactic, Tonic, Vasodilator.
PART USED: Root.

While this plant is called Ginseng, it is substantially different than the Panax variety. One of the major differences is that it may be taken by both males and females over a long period of time. From research done in Russia, it has been determined that Siberian Ginseng is an excellent adaptogen, working very good when the body is under chemical or physical stress. This would assist the body when breaking some drug dependencies or aid in the case of emotional suffering.

Siberian Ginseng helps in many nervous disorders and helps when under mental or physical exhaustion. It will curb irritability. It improves appetite, sleep and reflex action, in those suffering from chronic anxiety. It also hastens recovery from surgery. It protects against the danger of radiation, including atomic fallout, microwaves, and x-rays.

• Siberian Ginseng has been found to improve cerebral circulation, thereby, increasing mental alertness.

• Siberian Ginseng is effective at improving health. As such, it helps to improve physical and mental alertness.

• Siberian Ginseng works to detoxify the blood thereby, improving circulation. It has proven value in treating early stages of atherosclerosis.

• Russian athletic coaches prescribed Siberian Ginseng for their Olympic contenders. It was also prescribed for military officers that were in senior levels of command, to offset the effects of aging.

• There was a study done in East Germany and Russia in the 50's. Eleven thousand were people in the study, with 14 PhD.'s writing their papers on the subject. Their conclusions by consensus showed that when 500 mg. of Siberian Ginseng was consumed every day without let up, those studied had 100% protection from every viral infection known to man.

Acne	BLOOD PRESSURE
Adrenals	Cancer
Aging	Chest problems
Anemia	Childbirth (bleeding)
Anxiety	Colds
Appetite stimulant	Constipation
Asthma	Coughs
Bleeding	DEPRESSION

Diabetes
Diarrhea
Digestive disorders
ENDURANCE (INCREASES)
Energy
Fatigue
Fevers
HEMORRHAGING
Hormones (balances)
Hyperglycemia
Impotence
Irritability (curb)

Lung problems
LONGEVITY
Lung problems
Memory
Pancreas
PITUITARY GLAND
PROSTATE GLAND
Radiation protection
Stomach problems
Stress
Viruses

GINSENG, TIENCHI (Panax pseudoginseng)

BODILY INFLUENCE: Alterative, Anodyne, Cell Proliferant, Digestant, Emmenagogue, Hemostatic, Immuno-Stimulant, Nutritive, Tonic.
PART USED: The Root.

Ginseng is usually classified as a homeostatic and a trauma herb which is frequently used as a tonic. It is often preferred over the other Ginseng's for those under the age of 40 or one active in sports. This is due to its ability to increase stamina. However, there is not the danger of overtonification as can occur with regular Ginseng.

Tienchi Ginseng is most used for traumas and injuries due to its strong tonic properties and its strong hemostatic action for acute conditions. This Ginseng is also used externally in a trauma liniment to reduce swelling and pain caused by traumatic injuries to muscles, tendons, connective tissue and other soft tissues. It is also taken internally, alone or in combinations with other herbs, for all types of traumatic injuries, even gunshot wounds. It is effective in dissolving blood clots when taken internally. As with Panax Ginseng, it may be taken as a blood and energy tonic and is as effective. It is preferable for younger people, as it moves the chi better than the common American or Oriental Ginsengs. It is a heart strengthener and improves athletic abilities. It is the tonic of preference in sports medicine.

Athletic performance
Bloot clots
Boils
BRUISES
CUTS
Dysmenorrhea
GUNSHOT WOUNDS
INJURIES (ACUTE)

INJURIES (SPORTS)
NOSEBLEED
POST-PARTUM
SPRAINS
SWELLING
TRAUMAS
WOUNDS

GLUCOMANNAN   (Amorphophallus konjak)
A.K.A.,: None

BODILY INFLUENCE: Bulking agent, Digestant.
PART USED: Root.

Glucomannan is taken from the extracted mucilage of the Konjak root. Its principal use is found in its application as a bulking agent to promote the feeling of being full, reducing the eating of less food.
•   Glucomannan serves to pick up fat from the colon wall and transports it through the colon and discharges it from the system. This effectively eliminates contamination of the bloodstream. This would help reduce obesity. Because it dramatically expands when ingested, it must be followed by substantial amounts of water.
•   Glucomannan is effective at absorbing toxicity resultant from improper food combining or other problems which would produce toxic waste from an ingestion of poor food or poor food combining.

Blood pressure (high)
CONSTIPATION
Diabetes
DIGESTIVE PROBLEMS
DIVERTICULAR PROBLEMS

HEMORRHOIDS
Hypoglycemia
OBESITY
Pancreas

GOLDEN ROD   (Solidago canadensis)
A.K.A.,: Blue Mountain Tea.

BODILY INFLUENCE: Anti-catarrhal, Anti-inflammatory, Astringent, Carminative, Diaphoretic, Diuretic.
PART USED: Flowering tops, leaves.

When experiencing upper respiratory catarrh, Golden rod is perhaps the first plant to consider, whether the problem is acute or chronic. For ailments of congestion in the upper respiratory area, its most effective use is in combination with other herbs for treatment of congestion such as experienced from a flu condition. It is also used to promote healing of certain types of wounds.
Another application of Golden Rod is found in using it for kidney problems, such as, when experiencing dark, cloudy urine. It is also effective in clearing up kidney and bladder stones. Its astringent action makes it useful against diarrhea and intestinal hemorrhage.

Arthritis
Bladder stones
CATARRH (UPPER
    RESPIRATORY)
DIARRHEA
Eczema
Flu
GAS

Indigestion
Intestinal hemorrhage
Kidney stones
Kidney problems
Laryngitis
Nephritis (chronic)
Urinary problems

GOLDEN SEAL   (Hydrastis canadensis)
A.K.A.,: Seal-all, Golden Thread, Yellow Root, Indian Dye.

BODILY INFLUENCE: Alterative, Antacid, Anti-bilious, Anti-bacterial, Antibiotic, Anti-catarrhal, Anti-periodic, Antiseptic, Antispasmodic, Anti-syphyilitic, Aperitive, Astringent, Bitter, Cholagogue, Depurant, Diuretic, Emmenagogue, Hemostatic, Hepatic, Laxative, Nervine, Ophthalmic, Pectoral, Prophylactic, Immuno-Stimulant, Stomachic, Tonic.
PART USED: Root.

Golden Seal is used as an herb specifically for the mucous membranes, (sometimes referred to as "the King of the Mucous Membranes"). It thus finds its use in the treatment of congestion and chronic inflammation of the respiratory and urogenital tracts, catarrhal affliction of the nose and chronic gastritis and enteritis. It has been used for catarrh of the bladder, hepatic congestion and has also been applied in conditions effecting eye inflammation. Golden Seal sometimes finds use in the treatment of female problems relating to inflammation of the vagina, uterus and urethra.

Golden Seal was discovered and is found primarily in eastern North America (Canada and United States). It is found most plentifully in the woods of Ohio, where the Cherokee Indians introduced Golden Seal as a medicine for the treatment of ulcers and arrow wounds. It has been considered useful for arresting bleeding from the uterus and for profuse menstruation. Golden Seal is an effective treatment, specific in female applications for uterine contractions and menstrual disorders.

• The most active ingredient of Golden Seal, and the one that accounts for its chemical effectiveness, is hydrazine.

• The British Pharmaceutical Codex 1934 states that Golden Seal is useful in controlling uterine hemorrhage. Golden Seal is valuable for disorders of the uterus as it causes "uterine contractions."

• Another constituent of Golden Seal is Berberine which has been shown useful against a variety of microbes. It has demonstrated effectiveness as an immuno-stimulator, as a result of increasing blood supply to the spleen. Also it has shown to activate macrophages and has tumor inhibitory action.

- Applied externally, Golden Seal has been shown to be valuable for chronic inflammation of the mucous membranes. It is an effective treatment for cracks in the skin and fissures such as those occurring in the nipples. Some have found Golden Seal good in the treatment of indolent ulcers.
- Golden Seal used as an eyewash mildly antibiotic and astringent helping to reduce inflammation of the eye. Golden Seal is very gritty so always strain it through cheese cloth before using it in solution for the eye.
- Golden Seal stimulates the bowels and acts to increase the flow of urine.
- Golden Seal acts as an antiseptic and can be used to cleanse boils, wounds and ulcers.
- Golden Seal helps reduce sugar in the blood when used in combination with Licorice. Myrrh may be used as an alternate, if low blood sugar is a problem.
- Golden Seal also reduces swelling, when such is caused by high sugar levels.
- Golden Seal strengthens the immune system through its antibiotic and anti-bacterial properties.
- Golden Seal helps promote good heart and respiratory function.
- Golden Seal has also been found effective in its use for the treatment of worms and infections.
- Early on, the pioneers followed the Indians' example in using Golden Seal to treat watering eyes, wounds and rashes. They also chewed it to relieve mouth sores.
- More recently, it has been used to prevent morning sickness, for liver and stomach complaints, to check internal hemorrhage, to increase appetite and the secretion of bile, as a mouthwash, and for urinary and uterine problems.
- Golden Seal can be helpful in preventing pitting of the skin in smallpox and to cure ringworm.
- Golden Seal is useful in treating stress and anxiety resultant from high blood sugar.
- Golden Seal is reported to strengthen the immune system through its antibiotic and antibacterial properties.
- Golden Seal contains the natural antibiotic, Berberine, which find its use in mouth and gum problems.
- Golden Seal is also said to help promote heart and respiratory function, increasing its capacity, because of its ability to clean mucous membranes and counter infection.

Allergies
Asthma
ANTIBIOTIC
ANTISEPTIC
BLADDER INFECTIONS
BLADDER PROBLEMS
BLEEDING (INTERNAL)
Bowel problems
Breath freshener
Bright's disease
BRONCHITIS
Burns
Chicken pox
CHOLERA
CIRCULATION
COLDS (FIGHTS INFECTION)
COLITIS
COLON INFLAMMATION
Conjunctivitis
Constipation
CONTAGIOUS DISEASES
COUGHS
DIARRHEA
Digestive disorders
Diphtheria
Dyspepsia
Earaches
Eczema
EYE INFECTIONS
EYE WASH
Fever
Flu (stomach)
Gallbladder
Gastritis
General cleanser
Glands (swollen)
GONORRHEA
GUM DISEASES
Hay fever
Heart trouble
HEMORRHAGE (INTERNAL)
HEMORRHOIDS

Hepatitis
Herpes (genital)
Hoarseness
INFECTIONS
INFLAMMATION
INSULIN
INTESTINES
Itching
KIDNEYS
LIVER PROBLEMS
MEASLES
MENSTRUATION (EXCESSIVE)
Morning sickness
MOUTH SORES
MUCOUS MEMBRANES
NASAL PASSAGES
Nausea
Nervous disorders
NOSEBLEEDS
Obesity
PANCREAS
Poison ivy/oak
PROSTATE GLANDS
Psoriasis
Ringworm
Scarlet fever
SINUS CONGESTION
SKIN DISORDERS
Small pox
SORE THROAT
Spleen
Stomach problems
Syphilis
Thyroid
Tonsillitis
TYPHOID FEVER
Ulceration (skin)
Urethritis
VAGINITIS
Venereal disease
WOUNDS

GOTU KOLA   (Hydrocotyle asiatica)
A.K.A.,: Indian Pennywort.

BODILY INFLUENCE: Adaptogenic, Alterative, Anti-pyretic, Anti-spasmodic, Aphrodisiac, Astringent, Blood Purifier, Diuretic, Nervine, Sedative, Stimulant, Brain Tonic.
PART USED: The whole plant.

Historically, Gotu Kola is considered to be one of the best herbal nerve tonics. Many people use Gotu Kola to improve their learning ability by facilitating better recall. Because Gotu kola acts as a cleanser of the blood, it follows that it strengthens the heart, balances the hormones and the nervous system and has been used to help menopausal problems in women.

As a result of improving blood circulation, it is good when used pro-actively to avoid and treat a nervous breakdown. This is due to its effect as an energy enhancer on the cells of the brain.

In India, the herb is known for its calming effect. In Sri Lanka, it was discovered to be a favored food for elephants, therefore, it was believed to be a life enhancer which contributed to long life. The herb gained a reputation as a longevity promoter and a Sinhalese proverb advised, "Two leaves a day keep old age away."

• Gotu Kola is valued as a nervous system restorative. It also has been found to exhibit wound-healing capabilities.

• Gotu Kola was found to increase mental activity, while act as a mild tranquilizer.

• Gotu Kola is used to combat fatigue and to improve memory. It has also been used as a blood cleanser for skin disease.

• In the Far East, Gotu Kola has been employed for leprosy and tuberculosis. In both China and India, Gotu Kola can be found as being used to increase energy.

• Gotu Kola is a "brain food" which promotes memory and as an energy enhancer, it acts to prevent aging.

• Gotu Kola is effective in the treatment of mental problems dealing with anxiety and loss of memory. It is sometimes known as the memory herb because it is known to stimulate circulation to the brain.

• Gotu Kola is beneficial in the treatment of high blood pressure.

Age spots	DEPRESSION
AGING	Dysentery
ARTERIOSCLEROSIS	ENERGY (INCREASE)
BLISTERS	Exhaustion
BLOOD PRESSURE (HIGH)	FATIGUE (MENTAL &
CIRCULATION TO BRAIN	PHYSICAL)
Clear voice	Fever

Headaches
HEART (STRENGTHENS)
HYPOGLYCEMIA
INABILITY TO CONCENTRATE
Insomnia
LEARNING PROBLEMS
LEG CIRCULATION
LEPROSY
Liver
Longevity (promotes)
Measles
MEMORY PROBLEMS
MENOPAUSE
MENTAL TROUBLES
NERVOUS BREAKDOWN
PITUITARY GLAND
PSORIASIS

Rheumatism
Schizophrenia
Scrofula
SENILITY
Skin conditions (inflammatory)
Sore throat
SPINAL MENINGITIS
Stamina
Stomach problems
Stuttering
TONIC
Tonsillitis
ULCERATIONS
Ulcers
Varicose veins
WOUND HEALING

GRAPEFRUIT SEED (SEE SECTION ON EXTRACTS)

GUMWEED (Grindelia spp.,)
A.K.A.,: Tar Weed.

BODILY INFLUENCE: Anti-spasmodic, Bitter, Demulcent, Diuretic (moderately), Expectorant, Respiratory Stimulant, Sedative.
PART USED: Flowering Top and Leaves.

Gumweed has a wide variety of uses, such as treating respiratory problems associated with colds and bronchial wheezing due to asthmatic conditions.

Another use for Gumweed is as a treatment for inflammation, irritation and wounds to the skin, such as would be found with burns, rashes and other skin problems that can be treated with a poultice.

• Gumweed is an effective antidote for a variety of skin problems due to allergic reaction or wounds.

• Some uses of Gumweed are to control spasms resulting from asthma and whooping cough, for bronchial problems and nasal congestion.

• Gumweed should not be used internally with patients that have a history of heart problems.

ASTHMA
BLADDER INFECTIONS
Blisters

Bronchial irritation
BRONCHITIS
Burns

Coughs	Nasal congestion
Coughs (spasmodic)	POISON IVY/OAK
Dermatitis	PSORIASIS
Eczema	SKIN DISORDERS
Flu	UTERUS INFECTIONS
Impetigo	WHOOPING COUGH

GUARANA   (Paullinia cupana)
A.K.A.,: Brazilian Cocoa.

BODILY INFLUENCE: Aphrodisiac, Febrifuge, Narcotic (slightly), Nervine, Nutritive, Stimulant.
PART USED: Crushed seeds.

At this time, Guarana is considered to be the richest source of caffeine world- wide. Like all plants containing caffeine, Guarana is addictive and can cause all the unpleasant symptoms such as found with heavy coffee drinking. Like coffee, this plant is also native to South America. Sometimes referred to as Brazilian cocoa because the beverage made from the plant tastes remarkably similar to that of ordinary cocoa.

The Maues and Murdurow Indians are able to travel through jungles and across mountains for miles at a steady pace, with a stick of Guarana as their only food. The sticks look like licorice and are consumed in small quantities by the Indians who scrape off small fragments which they chew and swallow.

According to South American legend, its nutritious and stimulating qualities were first discovered by the Incas centuries before the European first set foot on the American Continent.

Guarana has even recently been a substance brought to market by traders from the Amazon jungles. Guarana is made from seeds taken off the Paullinia vine. Indians pound the seeds into a meal and make a paste which is formed into rolls. When dried Guarana becomes hard and of a dark color, resembling large sausages.

Guarana's virtues consist in its stimulating principle similar to the caffeine in tea or coffee. Guarana has been reported to have been used by the Japanese soldiers in World War II. They were supplied with Guarana, using it by chewing. Reports claim it was effective in maintaining stamina and was found to aid in alertness and keeping courage.

Guarana, of course, should be avoided where the consumption of caffeine is to be stopped. Guarana has been found to contain between 2.6 to 7% caffeine and its action is very similar to both coffee and cocaine combined. This is due to the caffeine which is found in abundance and chemicals similar to cocaine. It certainly has a stimulant nervine effect and is therefore often found to be used by truck drivers and students who seek to stay awake.

While Guarana is touted as a natural stimulant by many people, it is a stimulant, like coffee, kola nuts and Chinese tea. It must be remembered that natural does not necessarily mean non-addictive or safe. Guarara is one of the richest plant sources of caffeine in the plant kingdom. It has 2.5 times the caffeine content of coffee. Extracts or concentrates of the plant can enrich the caffeine content 13-21 fold.

Caffeine is, of course, quite harmful and addictive when taken in concentrated doses or large quantities. It has been used by some for headache or depressions that accompany menstrual problems. It is also useful for decreasing restlessness, improving alertness and as a general tonic for headache and sore muscles. Some have used it to overcome menstrual problems due to stress and tenseness.

It should always be remembered that Guarana also exerts stimulation to the heart and increases blood flow.

When used in combinations of ingredients, as in the presence of ephedrine, there should be caution. There is research which shows that caffeine has a thermogenic (heat producing or calorie burning effect) in the presence of ephedrine (a chief alkaloid in Ma Huang or Chinese Ephedra). However, any potential benefits in weight loss with such a combination should be measured against the potential for addiction and possible harmful side effects of these two herbs when used in combination with each other. Any use of this herb should be considered the same as using medically prescribed drugs.

Guarana is a rich, natural source of rain forest Guaranine, and can be used for long, slow endurance energy that may be obtained without coffee's heated hydrocarbons, which have been known to be a source of health problems. This does not preclude the harmful effects of the high caffeine content.

GUAR GUM   (Cyamopsis tetragonoloba)

BODILY INFLUENCE: Laxative (mildly), Mucilant.
PART USED: Bean.

Commercially, Guar gum is a plant cultivated in India for livestock feed. There exists growing interest in the use of Guar gum for the treatment of diabetes and to assist in curbing appetite. It is not recommended for use by those who have difficulty swallowing or who have had gastrointestinal surgery. Some persons with colon disorders may have trouble using Guar gum. This root also has the ability to reduce cholesterol, triglycerides, and low-density lipoprotein levels. It also binds to toxic substances, which makes possible their elimination from the body.

Guar-gum is a water soluble dietary fiber, like Oat gum (Oatbran) and pectin. Guar gum has been clinically demonstrated to reduce low-density-lipoprotein (LDL) cholesterol levels by as much as thirty five percent and serum cholesterol by up to twenty percent. This is according to an article in Longevity magazine (February 1988).

An additional advantage found with Guar gum is its ability to reduce blood glucose and serum insulin levels; thus, making it effective in the treatment of diabetes.

GRAVEL ROOT   (SEE QUEEN OF THE MEADOW)

GUGGUL   (Commiphora mukul)
A.K.A.,: Gum Gugul.

BODILY INFLUENCE: Anti-inflammatory, Anti-rheumatic, Cardiotonic, Diuretic.
PART USED: Gum resin.

Guggul is a gummy yellowish resin extract from India used primarily for reduction of cholesterol. It also reduces platelet stickiness and helps to eliminate blood clots, which may make it effective in preventing strokes as well as preventing other cardio-vascular problems. Gum Guggul is an Indian herb which has been used in Ayurvedic medicine for thousands of years. It is a natural alternative to drugs for reducing cholesterol. It has been used to increase HDL cholesterol which is known as the good cholesterol which is needed by the body. HDL-cholesterol has been shown to offer protection against heart disease due to atherosclerosis.

Gugulipid has its cholesterol-lowering action due to its ability to increase the liver's metabolism of LDL-cholesterol. As for example, guggulsterone has the ability to increase the uptake of LDL-cholesterol from the blood by the liver. Another very important ability of guggulsterone is that it stimulates thyroid function. It is possible that this thyroid-stimulating effect is responsible for the extract's lipid-lowering activity.

Guggul has been used for weight loss with great success. It also is very beneficial as a heart tonic and for increasing energy. It has been used for blood disorders that show up with skin problems such as psoriasis, eczema and boils. It seems to have the ability to strengthen the skeletal part of the body by giving strength to the bones, nerves, it cleanses bone tissue and improves flexibility helping to keep that youthful mobility. It has anti-inflammatory properties and helps to boost the immune system.

- Guggul increases HDL cholesterol and reduces LDL cholesterol.
- It lowers triglyceride levels.
- It is a relaxant of the muscles which helps relieve menstrual pain.
- It is a blood detoxifier which breaks up stagnation in the body.
- It is a heart tonic which strengthens the heart.

Arthritis pain	Energy
Blood cholesterol (lowers)	Menstrual pain (relieves)
Boils	Psoriasis
Carbuncles	Skin rashes
Circulation (stagnation)	Traumatic injuries
Dermatitis (contact)	Weight management
Eczema	

GYMNEMA SYLVESTRE
A.K.A.,: None

BODILY INFLUENCE: Digestant, Tonic.
PART USED: The whole plant.

Used primarily in combination with other herbs, it has been shown to be effective in toning the blood and strengthening the body in general. The Hindu name for this herb is 'Gurmar,' meaning 'sugar destroyer.' Gymnema is effective at blocking the taste of sugar from the system. Taken before sugar, the Gymnema molecule blocks the passages through which sugar is normally absorbed, so that fewer sugar calories are assimilated. Both sugar and Gymnema are digested in the small intestine, but the larger molecule of Gymnema cannot be fully absorbed. The remaining sugar is eliminated as waste.

The active ingredient in Gymnema Sylvestre is 'gymnemic, an organic acid.' Gymnemic acid is composed of molecules with a similar atomic arrangement to glucose molecules. These molecules fill the receptor locations on the taste buds temporarily from one to two hours, preventing the taste buds from being able to taste any sugar molecule in the food. This action is repeated in the intestines when the gymnemic acid fills the receptors located on the absorptive external layers of the intestines, blocking temporally, the absorption of the sugar molecules.

A taste test can show how Gymnema works. First, taste something sweet, then swish a sip of Gymnema Sylvestre tea around in your mouth. Finally, taste something sweet again. You will not be able to taste the sugar, because Gymnema has blocked the taste of the sugar in your mouth in the same way it blocks sugar in digestion. Gymnema won't affect food from tasting good, but will suppress the desire for sweets. This sugar blocking action of Gymnema works well in cases of diabetes.

• When used for hyper-insulin, Gymnema is recommended to be taken with GTF Chromium in order to stabilize blood sugar.

• Gymnema is an herb that reduces blood sugar levels after sugar consumption.

• Gymnema has a molecular structure similar to that of sugar that can block absorption of up to fifty percent (50%) of dietary sugar calories.

Allergies	Hyperactivity
Anemia	Hypoglycemia
Cholesterol	Urinary tract infections
Diabetes	Weight management
Digestion	

HAWTHORN (Crataegus oxycantha)
A.K.A.,: English Hawthorn, Mayflower, May Bush, Mayblossom.

BODILY INFLUENCE: Anti-spasmodic, Astringent, Cardiac, Digestant, Diuretic, Emmenagogue, Hypertensive, Hypotensive, Sedative, Cardi-tonic, Tonic.
PART USED: Berries and Bark.

The Hawthorn tree has been regarded as sacred according to Christian tradition, that the crown of thorns placed on the head of Christ was of its origin. In fact, a grove of Hawthorn trees still stands outside of Jerusalem on the Mount of Olives.

Hawthorn has a variety of ways in which it has been shown to be beneficial.

It has the ability to increase oxygen utilization by the heart, it increases enzyme metabolism in the heart muscle, it acts as a very mild dilator of coronary vessels and serves as a peripheral vasodilator (dilating the blood vessels away from the haert, thereby lowering the blood pressure and reduces the burden placed on the heart).

Hawthorn is used primarily as a cardiac tonic and considered valuable for improvement of cardiac weakness, angina pectoris, valve murmurs from heart valve defects, an enlarged heart, sighing respiration, nerve depression or unexplained chronic fatigue. There is evidence that it is effective as facilitating mitral regurgitation, easing cardiac pain, regulating rapid or feeble heart beat, helping with difficulty in breathing owing to ineffective heart action, lack of oxygen in the blood, helping heart strain due to overexertion and useful in cholesterol reduction.

• Scientists have discovered that Hawthorn increases coronary blood flow and improves myocardial metabolism allowing the heart to function with less oxygen. Hawthorn dilates blood vessels, allowing blood to flow more freely and thus, is effective at lowering blood pressure. In addition, it acts directly on the heart muscle to help a damaged heart work more efficiently. Recent knowledge concerning the action of Hawthorn on the circulatory system seems to indicate its active principle is provided by its flavonoids which act on cardiac and circulatory problems by its dilation effect on the blood vessels which causes some reduction in blood pressure.

- It is very effective in relieving restlessness and insomnia.
- Studies have shown that Hawthorn is excellent for both the prevention and and treatment of coronary heart disease when used on a regular basis.

ADEMIA
Adrenal weakness
ANGINA PECTORIS
ARRHYTHMIAS
ARTERIOSCLEROSIS
Arthritis
Blood clots
BLOOD PRESSURE (HIGH OR LOW)
CARDIAC SYMPTOMS
Dropsy
EDEMA
ENLARGED HEART
HARDENING OF THE ARTERIES
HEARTBEAT (IRREGULAR)
HEART DISEASE
Heart fibrillation
HEART PALPATATIONS
HEART VALVES
HEART WEAKNESS
Hypertrophy
Hypertension
Hypoglycemia
Liver
Menopause
Nephritis
Rheumatism
Sleeplessness
Sore throat
Stomach
Stress
Vibrancy

HOPS (Humulus lupulus)
A.K.A.,: NONE

BODILY INFLUENCE: Anodyne, Anti-spasmodic, Aromatic, Bitter, Calmative, Carminative, Cholagogue, Diuretic, Febrifuge, Nervine, Parasiticide, Sedative, Soporific, Stomachic, Tonic.
PART USED: Flowers, leaves.

Hops, a natural preservative, has been used in the brewing of beer and contributes to its distinctive flavor and aroma. Another use of Hops has been to fill a muslin pillow with it to help provide non drug-induced sleep and has been known to calm the nerves and prevent nightmares.

It is known to be a nerve tonic, especially for relaxing excited cerebral conditions. Hops has been found to be an excellent nervine that is fast acting and will produce sleep when insomnia is a problem. Hops has been given for jaundice, being known to increase bile secretion, and will help to tone up the liver and gall-bladder. As an enema, Hops can be beneficial because of its relaxing, calming nature.

- Hops has a sedative effect and serves to calm and soothe the nerves thus, relieving muscle spasms. It also relieves pain and reduces fevers.
- Hops is an excellent herbal source of niacin.
- Hops has been used successfully to decrease the desire for alcohol.
- Hops increases the flow of urine, assists a sluggish gallbladder and tones the liver.
- A poultice of Hops soothes inflammations, including boils, relieves the pain of facial neuralgias, sciatica and other rheumatic pains and helps reduce the pain of a toothache. The Lupulon and Humulon properties found in Hops help to prevent infections.
- Hops specifically works to tone the muscles of the stomach controlling the hyper-excitability of the gastric nerves.
- Hops will work to clean the liver, increasing the flow of bile.

Alcoholism (curbs)
Anxiety
APPETITE STIMULANT
Bedwetting
BRONCHITIS
Coughs
Cramps (intestinal)
DELIRIUM TREMENS
DIGESTION
Dizziness
Earaches
FEVERS
Gas
Gonorrhea
HEADACHES
Heart conditions (nervous)
Hoarseness
HYPERACTIVITY
Hysteria
Indigestion
INSOMNIA

Jaundice
Leg cramps
Liver congestion
Menstruation
Morning sickness
Colitis (mucous)
NERVOUSNESS
Neuralgia
PAIN
Restlessness
Rheumatism
Ringworm
SEXUAL DESIRES (EXCESSIVE)
Shock
Sleeplessness
Stomach tonic
Toothache
Ulcers
Urinary tract infections
Water retention
Worms (expels)

HOREHOUND (Marrubium vulgare)
A.K.A.,: NONE

BODILY INFLUENCE: Anti-inflammatory, Anti-tussive, Aromatic, Bitter, Diaphoretic, Diuretic-mild, Expectorant, Laxative, Parasiticide (large doses), Stimulant, Stomachic, Tonic.
PART USED: The Herb.

Horehound has long been known as a soothing syrup and tonic candy. Horehound candy used to be on sale in most grocers shops in Victorian times and a favorite with the children. This was a well-known throat and lung remedy.

• As an expectorant, Horehound works to treat coughs and croup, common to children with colds. It will help to expel phlegm from the respiratory bronchial system. It affects the respiration directly by dilating vessels.

• Singers will find Horehound sustains vocal cords and helps with hoarseness, laryngitis and congestion.

• As a poultice, the herb can be effective in treating some wounds. Internally, it helps to promote healthy bile secretion.

• Horehound can be used as a tonic for treatment of many conditions peculiar to ailments of the stomach.

• People have also believed it capable of removing obstructions from the liver and the spleen.

• It can be used as a wash for skin dermatitis conditions to promote healing.

ASTHMA
Bronchitis
Catarrh
COLDS
COUGHS
CROUP
Dermatitis
Dyspepsia
Earaches
Eczema
Fevers
Hepatitis (chronic)
Herpes
HOARSENESS
HYSTERIA
Infectious diseases
Jaundice
LUNGS
Menstruation (promotes)
PHLEGM
Shingles
Sore throats
STOMACH TONIC
Sweating promoter
RESPIRATORY ORGANS
Tonic
Tuberculosis
Typhoid fever
Worms
Wounds

HORSERADISH   (Cochlearia armoracia)
A.K.A.,: NONE.

BODILY INFLUENCE: Antibiotic, Antiseptic, Carminative, Diaphoretic, Digestive, Diuretic, Expectorant, Laxative (mild), Parasiticide, Rubefacient, Sialagogue, Stimulant, Stomachic.
PART USED: Root.

The volatile oil works as a nasal and bronchial dilator and local irritant. This process has been used for cleansing the sinuses. The vapor has been shown to inhibit microorganisms. Internally, it works as a stimulant for digestion.

Horseradish has a wide variety of applications for which it will facilitate healing. Internally, it has been used for sinus problems, digestion, a strong diuretic, dropsy, for fevers and chronic rheumatism. Externally, it has been used as a rubefacient, applying it to the skin over the liver or spleen to help in detoxification of those organs.

Horseradish is effective for promoting stomach secretions and has been found effective as an aid to digestion.

• Horseradish has been found to help all bronchial and lung disorders.

• Externally, chopped or grated fresh Horseradish has been mixed with a little water and applied as a heat-producing and pain-relieving compress for neuralgia, stiffness, and pain in the back of the neck.

• The classic internal use of Horseradish is to treat kidney conditions in which excessive amounts of water are retained.

• Horseradish is a natural anti-biotic and may be used to help many internal conditions of illness, most specifically, upper respiratory problems and infections of the urinary tract.

• It has been used as a parasiticide for parasitic involvement within the human body.

APPETITE STIMULANT	EXPELS WORMS
Arthritis	Fevers
ASTHMA	Flu
Bladder trouble	Gout
Bronchitis	Hoarseness
CATARRH	Hypoglycemia
CIRCULATION	Liver
Colds	Lungs
Congestion	Mucous membranes
COUGHS	Nasal passages
DIGESTIVE DISORDERS	Neuralgia (external)
DROPSY	Respiratory congestion

Rheumatism
Sciatic nerve
SINUS PROBLEMS
Spleen
Sweating (promotes)

TUMORS (SKIN & INTERNAL)
Water retention
WORMS (EXPELS)
Wounds

HORSETAIL   (Equisetum arvense)
A.K.A.,: Shavegrass, Bottlebrush, Dutch Rushes.

BODILY INFLUENCE: Astringent, Carminative, Diuretic, Emmenagogue-mild, Galactagogue, Hemostatic, Lithotriptic, Nutritive, Parasiticide, Vulnerary.
PART USED: The whole plant.

Its botanical name is derived from two Latin terms, equus, meaning horse, and seta for bristle. The name resulted from its peculiar bristled appearance at the stem joints. Horsetail is strongly astringent and is therefore used for both internal and external wounds. It has been used for centuries, as a diuretic aiding in kidney infection, dropsy, and gravel. It is also beneficial as a wash for swelling eyelids. In Guatemala, American Indians have used it for cancer. Decoctions, poultices and infusions were used for polyps, abdominal and oral cancer.

Horsetail has large amounts of silica. Children have large amounts of silica in their body which makes children so supple and limber. As we age, we allow our bodies to become heavy with calcium and thus, lose our ability to bend, becoming stiff and immobile.

• Horsetail helps facilitate the use of calcium in the body.
• It has a high silica content, helps to strengthen fingernails, increases the flow of urine and helps to hold calcium in the body.
• Horsetail is also good for preventing split-ends (hair).
• It kills eggs of parasites and dissolves tumors.
• Horsetail increases the production of urine and shrinks inflamed mucosal tissue, particularly the prostate.
• Studies have shown that fractured bones will heal much faster when Horsetail is taken.
• It has been found to be good for eyes, ear, nose, throat and glandular disorders.
• Silica found in Horsetail, is helpful in aiding circulation.
• Using Horsetail in solution for bathing will produce an accelerating and invigorating effect for the body. It increases the metabolic rate of the body by feeding the system through the skin, improving circulation, swelling due to injury or dropsy and is useful in treating mending bones and chilblains.

- It is used as a poultice to reduce menstrual bleeding, Horsetail is effective because it promotes coagulation; hence, decreases bleeding.
- Horsetail has been used historically for diabetes.
- It is used as a diuretic and tonic for body 'spring cleaning' and detoxification.

ARTHRITIS
Bedwetting
Bell's Palsy
BLADDER
BLEEDING (INTERNAL)
Chilblains
CIRCULATION PROBLEMS
Conjunctivitis
Convulsions
DIABETES
Dropsy
Eyes
Fingernail biting
Gas
GLANDULAR DISORDERS
HAIR LOSS
Hair (split ends)
Heart
Hemorrhage

Incontinence
KIDNEY STONES
Liver (overactive)
Menstruation (excess)
Mucus
Muscle cramps
NAILS (WEAK OR BRITTLE)
NERVOUS TENSION
NOSEBLEEDS
Osteoporosis
PARASITES
Prostatitis
Skin problems
Sty
Tumors
URINARY ULCERS
URINATION (SUPPRESSED)
Worms

HO-SHOU-WU (Polygonum multiflorum)
A.K.A.,: Fo-Ti.

BODILY INFLUENCE: Adaptogen, Alterative, Aromatic, Astringent, Bitter, Blood Purifier, Diuretic, Hormonal, Nervine, Sedative, Stimulant, Tonic.
PART USED: Root.

Ho-Shou-Wu has been claimed by the Chinese to be an herb for longevity and restoration. It is a flavonoid-rich herb with particular success in longevity formulas. Also used as a cardio-vascular strengthener, it increases blood flow to the heart. It should be used with large amounts of water to be effective and needs to be used for a long period of time to get the desired results.
- Ho-Shou-Wu is a rejuvenator having an influence on the endocrine glands, which in turn, strengthens the body.
- Ho-Shou-Wu used as a tonic will help tone the liver and kidneys simply by promoting healthy blood.

- It may be used to treat unexplained chronic fatigue and traumatic bruises.
- It is also helpful to many of the effects of aging, such as loss of muscle tone and loss of hair color.

Aging
Anemia
Arteriosclerosis
Arthritis
Backache
Blood vessels (dilates)
Cancer
Circulation (poor)
Colds
Colic
Diarrhea
Diabetes
Dizziness
Enteritis
Gout
HAIR (PREMATURE GRAYING)

Heart problems
Hemorrhoids
Hypoglycemia
IMPOTENCY
INFERTILITY
Inflammation
Knee (pains & ligaments)
Liver weakness
LONGEVITY
Menstrual problems
MUSCLE TONE
NERVOUS DISORDERS
Post-partum
Spleen weakness
Tumors
Ulcerations

HYDRANGEA (Hydrangea arborescens)
A.K.A.,: Seven Barks.

BODILY INFLUENCE: Anti-lithic, Bitter, Calcium Solvent, Cathartic, Diuretic, Lithotriptic, Tonic.
PART USED: Leaves and Root.

- Hydrangea increases the flow of urine and will remove bladder stones and the pain caused by them.
- Hydrangea will also relieve backache caused by kidney trouble.
- The curative principles attributed historically to Hydrangea are remarkable in content. Its effectiveness is due to its alkaloids that behave like cortisone without the deleterious side effects. As a blood cleanser, it may be as effective as Chaparral.
- Hydrangea's ability to maintain blood, makes it useful to treat lymphatic conditions caused by poor blood. It is helpful in preventing the formation of gravel and will help deposits to pass through the ureters from the kidneys to the bladder.
- Hydrangea works wonderfully for those with severe rheumatism.
- It also helps correct bedwetting in children.
- As a diuretic herb, it is particularly helpful for prostate

infection and inflammation and for kidney fluid retention. It is also effective for arthritis swelling and bladder infections.

ARTHRITIS (CALCIUM DEPOSITS)
Backache
BLADDER STONES
BLADDER INFECTIONS
Calcium deposits
Dropsy
GALLSTONES
GONORRHEA
GOUT
Inflammation (shrinks tissues)
KIDNEY STONES
Paralysis
Rheumatism (chronic)
Scurvy
URINARY PROBLEMS

HYSSOP (Hyssopus officinalis)
A.K.A.,: NONE

BODILY INFLUENCE: Anti-inflammatory, Anti-spasmodic, Anti-viral, Aromatic, Carminative, Cathartic, Diaphoretic, Expectorant, Hepatic, Nervine, Parasiticide, Pectoral, Sedative, Stimulant, Stomachic, Tonic, Vulnerary.
PART USED: The whole plant.

Hyssop has been used since Biblical times as a cathartic. There has been a recent revival of the herb. An extract of Hyssop has been shown to have anti-viral activities used to combat the Herpes Simplex virus. The word "Hyssop" is of Greek origin and means "holy herb." Psalms 51:7 states: "Purge me with Hyssop, and I shall be clean; wash me and I shall be whiter than snow." It was believed to be used for cleansing and purifying the body.

Culpepper says, "Mixed with honey will kill worms of the belly."

Because of its strong camphor-like odor, Hyssop has a history of use as a cleansing herb. There is reference to the plant back into the seventh century, where it was strewn about the floors of sick-rooms and used to improve the smell of kitchens. During the seventeenth and eighteenth centuries, tinctures and teas of the flowers and leaves were used to reduce perspiration and to cure jaundice and dropsy.

The healing virtues of this plant are due to its volatile oil which is stimulative, carminative and sudorific in nature. Hyssop is used primarily for quinsy and other sore throat afflictions. Hyssop is excellent as a blood regulator, since it both increases the circulation and lowers the blood pressure.

• Hyssop is used to strengthen the immune system.

- Hyssop also helps the healing process by producing sweating (perspiration).
- Hyssop is an excellent blood regulator.
- Hyssop has a splendid effect on the mucus lining of the stomach and bowels.
- Hyssop is a good remedy for any eye trouble.
- Hyssop contains essential hormone oils to build resistance to infectious diseases.
- Hyssop has a multitude of specific curative powers from treating poor digestion to inflammation of the breast, to clearing phlegm from the bronchial area. It is good for treatment of coughs due to colds and is helpful in the treatment of nose and throat infection.
- It will help to free congestion in the intestinal tract due to an excess amount of mucus.

Amenorrhea (suppressd menstruation)	Hoarseness
	Jaundice
Asthma	Kidney problems
Blood pressure	Lice (external)
Bronchitis	Liver problems
Bruises	LUNG AILMENTS
CATARRH (CHRONIC)	Mucus (intestinal)
Colds	PHLEGM (HARD)
CONGESTION	PLEURISY
COUGHS (IRRITABLE)	Rheumatism (muscular, external)
Cuts (external)	Spleen problems
Dropsy	SORE THROAT
Dyspepsia	Viruses
Ear ailments	WHEEZING
Epilepsy	WORMS
Fevers	

ICELAND MOSS (Cetraria islandica)
A.K.A.,: Eryngo-leaved liverwort, Iceland Lichen.

BODILY INFLUENCE: Anti-emetic, Demulcent, Expectorant, Mucilant, Nutritive, Pectoral, Tonic.
PART USED: The whole plant. (It is a Lichen)

Iceland Moss is a cure for all kinds of chest ailments. It is a member of the animal kingdom (it is a Lichen), found on rocks. It nourishes children, invalids and aged persons that tend to be lacking strength and are anemic. It was said to cure tuberculosis. Iceland Moss and Irish Moss contain some of the same properties. The vitamin and mineral contents are about the same as Irish Moss.

Iceland Moss is soothing because of it high mucilage content. It has been useful in the treatment of gastritis and to soothe the stomach in cases of vomiting, dyspepsia and heartburn. It is very effective anywhere that mucous membranes are irritated.
It helps to soothe respiratory membranes in the case of dry coughs and consumptive lung diseases.

ANEMIA
BRONCHITIS
CATARRH
CONGESTION
COUGHS
Diarrhea
DIGESTIVE PROBLEMS
Dysentery
Dyspepsia

Fevers
Gastritis
Hoarseness
Lactation
LUNG PROBLEMS
Respiratory catarrh
Thyroid
TUBERCULOSIS

IRISH MOSS (Chondrus crispus)
A.K.A.,: Carrageenin, Red-Sea Weed, Chondrus.

BODILY INFLUENCE: Alterative, Anti-tussive, Demulcent, Emollient, Laxative-mild, Mucilant, Nutritive, Tonic.
PART USED: The Whole Plant, dried plant.

This plant is a seaweed. Irish Moss's most important ingredient is a pectin called carrageenin which is similar to agar agar. Its mucilage content makes this plant useful in any treatment of the skin or the mucous membranes. However, its main use is in respiratory problems such as bronchitis, because of its ability to absorb liquid and eliminate it from the body. It finds a use in cosmetics as a skin softener, because it has moisture absorbing qualities.
• Irish Moss is useful as a reducing aid by eliminating extra body fluids.
• It's mucilaginous in nature, so it absorbs toxins from the bowel.
• Irish Moss provides bulk to the stool and soothes inflamed tissues.
• Irish Moss helps to pull radiation poison from the body.
• It reduces appetite by virtue of its ability to absorb moisture, thus increasing its volume, filling the intestinal tract with a muclinginous bulking type material, aiding the body in its elimination process by increasing in the discharge of tissue waste through the G.I. tract.
• Due to its high iodine content, Irish Moss supplies iodine through the intestinal tract in the interplay of fluids between the intestinal content and the bloodstream by way of the intestinal villi.

Bladder problems
BRONCHITIS (CHRONIC)
Cancer (Parathyroid)
Catarrh
Convulsions
Cough
Diarrhea
Digestive problems
Dysentery
GLANDS
GOITER
Halitosis (bad breath)

Intestinal problems
LUNG PROBLEMS
Parathyroid
Peptic ulcers
Pneumonia
Radiation poisoning
Swollen joints
THYROID PROBLEMS
Tuberculosis
Tumors
Varicose veins
WEIGHT REDUCTION

JOJOBA   (See Oils Section)

JUNIPER   (Juniperus spp.,)
A.K.A.,: Dwarf Juniper, Ground Juniper.

BODILY INFLUENCE: Anodyne, Anti-fungal, Anti-rheumatic, Urinary Antiseptic, Anti-spasmodic, Aromatic, Astringent, Carminative, Diuretic, Emmenagogue, Lithotriptic, Parasiticide, Stimulant, Stomachic, Digestive Tonic.
PART USED: Berries.

The scent of Juniper was believed to ward off the plague in ancient Europe. Juniper Berries have a long history of use as a diuretic. Its in the volatile oil where the active diuretic principles of Juniper berries reside. The American Indians believed in Juniper's cleansing and healing powers and used it to keep away infection, relieve arthritis and cure various wounds and illnesses. Being a moderate circulatory stimulant, it has on occasions served well in certain types of rheumatic disorders when these were due to diminished circulation and general toxicity. Being an excellent antiseptic, Juniper berries, when used in a combination, is very helpful with conditions such as cystitis to remove acid and toxic wastes. The berries can improve impaired digestion and strengthen weak stomachs.
• Juniper in a formula, is beneficial in helping to dissolve kidney stones and prostate sediment, as well as in the treatment of water retention.
• Juniper works well to increase the flow of urine.
• When uric acid has been retained in the system, Juniper has been found to be very beneficial by preventing the crystalization of uric acid in the kidney thus, retaining it in solution to be passed in the urine.

- Juniper cleans the blood so well that it tones the system helping to reduce the bodies. susceptibility to disease.
- Juniper is naturally high in producing usable insulin aiding in the healing effect on the entire body where there is an insulin deficiency.
- Juniper is used as an excellent blood cleanser, having the ability to tone the pancreas providing that the congestive conditions or other deleterious lymphatic damage has not progressed beyond its ability to repair.
- As a poultice, Juniper may be applied directly onto wounds to prevent infection. Internally, Juniper, because of its blood cleaning properties, will effect similar control of infection.
- If kidney disease is suspected, Juniper berries may over-stimulate the kidneys and adrenals, so it should be avoided. Marshmallow and Cornsilk are more soothing herbs that may be substituted.
- Glomeruli filtration is vastly increased by the action of Juniper berries on the kidneys increasing the urine flow and promoting the blood purification process.

NOTE: Avoid during pregnancy, as it has a strong vaso-dilating, diuretic effect.

Abrasions
Acne
ADRENAL GLANDS
Adrenal weakness
Allergies
Arthritis
Arteriosclerosis
BEDWETTING
BLADDER PROBLEMS
    (GENERAL)
BLEEDING
Blood
Boils
Bright's disease
Bursitis
Catarrhal conditions
COLDS
Colic
Contagious diseases
Coughs
Cramps
Cystic fibrosis
DIABETES
DROPSY
Dysentery

Dyspepsia
FUNGAL INFECTIONS
Gargle
Gas
Gonorrhea
Gout
Gums (bleeding)
Hair loss
Hayfever
HYPOGLYCEMIA
Incontinence
INFECTIONS
Insect bites (poisonous)
KIDNEY INFECTIONS
KIDNEY STONES
Mouth sores
Mucus
NEPHRITIS
OPTIC NERVE WEAKNESS
PANCREAS
Pimples
Prostate gland
Rheumatism
Scurvy
Snakebites

Stomach
URIC ACID (BUILD-UP)
Urination (burning)
URINARY PROBLEMS

Vaginal discharge
WATER RETENTION
Worms

KAVA KAVA (Piper methysticum)
A.K.A.,: Kawa.

BODILY INFLUENCE: Analgesic, Anesthetic, Anodyne, Antiseptic, Anti-spasmodic, Aphrodisiac (female), Bitter, Diuretic, Nervine, Relaxant, Sedative, Stimulant, Tonic.
PART USED: Root.

Captain Cook discovered Kava Kava and gave the plant the name, 'intoxicating pepper.'

Kava Kava, as an analgesic sedative is used to relieve pain in rheumatic complaints, alleviate insomnia and calm nervousness. It was used by the ancient Tahitians to create a "stupefying" drink. They used Kava Kava as a tonic and stimulant in small doses.

Kava Kava root is also known as one of the most powerful of the herbal muscle relaxants. Kava Kava is helpful in increasing flexibility influencing the motor units of the nervous system, relaxing muscle tension and aiding with structural alignment.

In the urinary system, it produces a relaxing effect which has been used to calm bladder infections, to treat gonorrhea and because of its antiseptic qualities, it can be used as a douche for vaginitis. Being a potent analgesic, it can be applied directly to a painful wound or may be taken internally.

Anxiety
Asthma
Bronchitis
Fatigue
GONORRHEA
Gout
INSOMNIA

NERVOUSNESS
Pain
Rheumatism
Spasms
Urinary tract infections
Vaginitis

KELP   (Fucus vesiculosus)
A.K.A.,: Sea Weed, Bladderwrack.

BODILY INFLUENCE: Alterative, Anti-rheumatic, Demulcent, Diuretic, Emollient, Expectorant, Mucilant, Nutritive, Stimulant, Tonic.
PART USED: The Whole Plant.

Kelp is a plant of the sea and is harvested off the coast of many of the oceans of the world, in places such as California, Norway and many others. As a product of the ocean, it contains many of the numerous elements that the oceans contain. Since the seas are water, they can dissolve into solutions the many elemental products that the land under the seas contain and thus, transmit these elements to the many plants that grow in the seas.

Kelp is one of those plants that is readily available and useable to mankind for many purposes and nutrition is one of them. Among the many elements in Kelp are the minerals to include Iodine, bromine, alginic acid, alginates and their organic salts, especially sodium alginate. These effect such organs as the thyroid gland which has very vital functions to perform in the body in the way of controls over many important functions, such as the endocrine system.

Japanese's studies show a direct relationship between the ingestion of the Algin contained in Kelp and the prevention of breast cancer and have concluded that Algin is responsible. This is both a mechanical (due to the fiber content of Kelp) and biochemical action to enhance immune system function. It is reasoned that the alginates effect the T-cells.

Kelp, a 'Gift from the sea' provides its treasured iodine, which is needed by the thyroid to healthfully function. Due to its unique ingredients acquired from the rich supply of nutrients from the sea, Kelp has the buffering ability to neutralize wastes from the body fluids to be more easily discharged from the body.

Kelp also helps soothe an irritated throat and mucous membranes. Kelp's action soothes coughs, dissolves firm masses, such as tumors, treats enlarged thyroids, lymph node enlargement, swollen and painful testes and reduces edema, all of which can be caused by the malfunction of the thyroid gland.

• Iodine is important for thyroid disorders, whether underactive or overactive and obesity.

• Iodine feeds the thyroid which controls metabolism. For this reason, Kelp has been used for a long time in weight loss formulas.

• Sodium alginate is known to reduce strontium absorption (radiation).

• Kelp is effective as a diet aid, thyroid stimulant and glandular balancer.

• Kelp aids in a cleansing regimen, since it can bind radioactive strontium, barium, and cadmium in the gastrointestinal tract, preventing their absorption into the body.

- Kelp may reduce the risk of poisoning from environmental pollution by providing fiber that increases fecal bulk and reducing cholesterol levels through the retardation of bile acid absorption.
- Kelp, by its normalizing effect on the thyroid gland has effectively accelerated the burning of excess calories by regulating the body's metabolism.
- Kelp contains all of the minerals and vitamins and the high nutritive qualities of iodine and cell salts considered vital to health, in a concentrated form necessary to life, thus it stimulates the metabolism, strengthening the body system and could well be used by everyone.
- Kelp would be especially useful for the ailing and convalescent patient and during pregnancy.
- It promotes the healthy growth of hair, skin and nails, it helps to balance the effects of stress, guards against sickness, aids digestion and respiration and generally promotes a healthy functioning balanced system.
- Kelp provides nutritional support to the nervous system and heart and is important in herbal combinations used for improving mental alertness.
- Kelp also supplies hypotensive and serum cholesterol lowering principles which have a sparing effect on cardiac and neural tissues saving them from unnecessary stress and prolonging their effective lifetime, increasing their efficiency.
- Uric acid contributes to rheumatic pain and Kelp has those elements that help handle uric acid and eliminate it from the body system. Acidity and lack of essential nutrients for nerves and their insulating sheaths leads to inflammation and neuritis. Iodine acts as a tranquilizer and interrupts the disease chain, "disease-to-pain-to-aggravation-more-disease-more pain and so on."
- Kelp is used by Asian peoples to treat genito-urinary tract problems, including the kidney, bladder, prostate and uterus. Clinical documentation shows that taking Kelp daily reduces enlarged prostates in older men and urination becomes painless.`

ACNE (THYROID IMBALANCE)
ADRENAL GLAND
  (WEAKNESS)
Anemia
ARTERIES (CLEANS)
Arthritis
BIRTH DEFECTS (PREVENTION
  OF)
Bursitis
Cancer

COLITIS
COMPLEXION
Debility
Diabetes
Digestion (poor)
ECZEMA
ENDOCRINE GLANDS
ENERGY
Fatigue (low thyroid)
FINGERNAILS

Gallbladder
Gas
Glands (enlarged)
GOITER
HAIR LOSS
Headaches
Heart disease
Hypothyroidism
INFECTION
Kidneys
Lead poisoning
Leg cramps
MENOPAUSE
MORNING SICKNESS
NAILS (PROBLEMS WITH)
OBESITY
Pancreas
PITUITARY GLAND
PREGNANCY
Prostate gland (tones)
Psoriasis
RADIATION POISONING
THYROID (LOW)
TUMORS
Vitality (low)
Water retention

KELP, NORWEGIAN   (Fucus Vesiculosis)
A.K.A.,: Sea Weed.

Many herbalist's consider Norwegian Kelp to be a cleaner source of Kelp as it comes from the cold North Sea which is supposedly freer of pollution than other sources.

LADY'S SLIPPER   (Cypripedium pubescens)
A.K.A.,: American Valerian, Moccasin Flower, Nerve Root, Noah's Ark.

BODILY INFLUENCE: Anti-periodic, Anti-spasmodic, Astringent, Carminative, Diaphoretic, Hypnotic, Nervine, Relaxant, Sedative, Tonic.
PART USED: Root.

Lady's Slipper popularity as a bouquet flower has lessened its availability as a healing herb. Lady's Slipper, found in health food stores have to be commercially grown specifically for that market. Lady's Slipper's historical use has been as a sedative, mild hypnotic and used for relief of spasms. In the treatment of female organs, it has been effective. The root of Lady's Slipper is "Nature's Tranquilizer". It is able to enhance calming and easing of one's mind. Lady's Slipper is an effective nervine for all stress, tension and anxiety states. Lady's Slipper has been used in cases of chronic insomnia and anxiety and when "the brain just won't shut off" and allow sleep. It has been used with good results for reflex functional disorders, nervous headaches, low fevers and nervous depression associated with stomach ailments.
• Lady's Slipper makes a good tonic for the exhausted nervous system, has a sedative effect on and relieves muscle spasms and makes an effective remedy for recurring headaches.
• Lady's Slipper's beneficial nervine calming action, reduces the

problems with twitching muscles, crawling skin and other nervous conditions.
- Its nervine action is so safe that Lady's Slipper may be used to calm hyperactive children.

Abdominal pain	Hypochondria
After pains	HYSTERIA
Anxiety	INSOMNIA
Bell's Palsy	Menstruation (painful)
CHOREA	Muscle spasms
Colic	NERVOUSNESS
Cramps	Neuralgia
Cystic fibrosis	PAIN
Depression	RESTLESSNESS
Epilepsy	Tremors
Headaches (nervous)	Typhoid fever

LEMON GRASS (Cymbopogon citracus)
A.K.A.,: Oil Grass, Fever-grass.

BODILY INFLUENCE: Astringent, Carminative, Expectorant, Febrifuge.
PART USED: Leaves.

In China, Lemon Grass is used for colds, pain resulting from headaches, stomach problems, abdominal cramps and rheumatic conditions.
- Lemon Grass has been found to be an excellent remedy for those suffering from cramps, headaches, dizziness or for people under stress.
- Lemon Grass is an excellent blood cleanser and can be very beneficial when used as part of a periodic cleansing program.
- Lemon Grass is used to treat colds with fevers.
- Lemon is reputed to slow the discharge of mucus, as well as, reduce mucus discharge in respiratory conditions, due in part to its astringent properties.

Anxiety	Headaches
Asthma	Indigestion
Bladder	Insect bites
Boils (warm poultice)	Kidneys
Bronchitis	Liver
COLDS	Menstruation (suppressed)
Colic	Nausea
DIGESTION	Nervousness
FEVERS	Respiratory problems
Flu	Spleen
Gas	Vomiting

LICORICE (Glycyrrhiza glabra)
A.K.A.,: Licorice Root, Sweet Wood.

BODILY INFLUENCE: Adaptogen, Alterative, Anti-inflammatory, Aperient, Aphrodisiac, Demulcent, Diuretic, Emollient, Expectorant, Hormonal-Adrenal, Hypertensive, Laxative (mild), Pectoral, Sialogogue, Stimulant (slightly), Tonic-Glandular, Sugar Substitute.
PART USED: Root.

Glycyrrhizic acid is the chief active principle in Licorice. Glycyrrhizic acid is 50 times sweeter than sugar cane, but will not increase the thirst. Actually, Licorice will alleviate thirst. Glycyrrhiza, is derived from the Greek root words glukus, meaning "sweet", and riza meaning "root" and refers to the fact that the dried roots, because of their sweet flavor can be chewed like candy. Alexander the Great supplied his troops with rations that included Licorice sticks, so they could chew on them in battle which alleviated thirst and kept their energy up which helped to win the battles.

• Licorice root possesses substantial anti-arthritic activity. Glycyrrhizinic acid provides the anti-inflammatory effects found in Licorice which is related to a release of corticoids from the adrenals and can then be helpful for people with arthritis.

• Licorice root normalizes ovulation in women experiencing infrequent menstruation. Licorice stimulates the production of interferon, that is said to be the key to preventing and treating immune-response deficiency diseases.

• Licorice was recommended for soothing throats and quenching thirsts.

• Licorice root effects the concentrations of blood salts and stimulates and sustains adrenal function, yet protects the liver which is the body.s detoxification plant insuring its purity from liver diseases, such as cirrhosis and hepatitis.

• Licorice contains a natural hormone that will replace cortisone. It induces the adrenal cortex to produce larger amounts of cortisone and aldosterone. Licorice root acts in the body like the cortin hormone and assists in helping the body handle the stress, allowing blood sugar levels to remain normal giving a general feeling of well-being. Glycyrrhizin, one of the compounds found in Licorice, has a chemical structure similar to that of human steroid hormones. It helps to raise blood sugar levels to normal.

• Licorice stimulates adrenal function without depleting them.

• Perhaps the most common medicinal use is in cough syrups and cough drops. Licorice soothes the chest and helps to bring up phlegm.

• It soothes and heals inflamed mucous membranes of the respiratory tract.

NOTE: In very large doses, it induces sodium retention and potassium depletion and can lead to hypertension and edema. Occasionally, Licorice root elevates blood pressure. Use Licorice root with Potassium if high blood pressure is a problem.

Abscesses
ADDISON.S DISEASE
ADRENAL GLAND
    (EXHAUSTION)
Age spots
Allergies
Arteriosclerosis
Arthritis (natural cortisone)
Asthma
BLOOD CLEANSER
Bronchitis
Chills
CIRCULATION (POOR)
COLDS
Constipation
COUGHS (SOOTHE THROAT)
Cushing's disease
DIABETES (RAISES BLOOD
    SUGAR)
Dizziness
Dropsy
DRUG WITHDRAWAL
Duodenal ulcers
EAR INFECTIONS

Edema
Emphysema
ENDURANCE (LACK OF)
ENERGY
Estrogen (low)
Fatigue
FEMALE PROBLEMS
Food poisoning
Herpes
HOARSENESS
HYPERGLYCEMIA
HYPOGLYCEMIA
Longevity
LUNG PROBLEMS
Menopause
PHLEGM (EXPELS)
SEXUAL STIMULANT
Sores
SORE THROAT
TONIC
Ulcers
VITALITY
VOICE

LILY OF THE VALLEY (Convallaria majalis)
A.K.A.,: May Lily, Our Lady's Tears, Jacob's Ladder, Ladder-to-Heaven.

BODILY INFLUENCE: Anti-spasmodic, Cardiac tonic, Diuretic.
PART USED: The whole plant.

From the Middle Ages, Lily of the Valley was esteemed as a heart medicine, but when the more potent digitalis, derived from foxglove, came into use 200 years ago, it fell into disuse. After many years of using digitalis as a heart medicine, we have come to know some of its side effects. Digitalis is cumulative - it remains in the heart muscle for a long time. It is evident that treatment may do serious damage. Whereas Lily of the Valley, with its active glycoside substance, is broken down by the body within four hours and its medicinal effect continues much longer has little or no cumulative effect and is considered safe for medicinal use.

- Lily of the Valley has properties similar but milder and much less accumulative than digitalis.
- Lily of the Valley's diuretic action also stops edema which is often associated with heart problems.
- During World War I, Lily of the Valley was used extensively for gas poisoning.
- Lily of the Valley strengthens both the heart muscle and the blood vessels. Measured against the same dose of digitalis, its action is gentler and has none of the side effects produced by accumulation of the herb in the tissues.

ARRYTHMIAS	Epilepsy
EDEMA	HEART DISEASE

LOBELIA (Lobelia inflata)
A.K.A.,: Bladderpod, Indian Tobacco, Asthma Weed, Pukeweed.

BODILY INFLUENCE: Analgesic, Anodyne, Anti-spasmodic, Astringent, Cathartic, Counter-irritant, Decongestant, Diaphoretic, Diuretic, Emetic, Emmenagogue, Expectorant, Nervine, Sedative.
PART USED: The whole plant.

Many authorities consider Lobelia to be the most important of all the herbs! Medically, Lobelia is used in the treatment of bronchitis and asthma. Lobelia is a specific in anti-smoking preparations due to the cross-tolerance seen between its major alkaloid (lobeline) and nicotine. The action closely resembles that of nicotine, but is milder. It thus decreases the desire for tobacco. Its the Lobeline salts used as a tobacco substitute in the body, that make nicotine taste terrible when its smoked.

The basic physiological action of Lobelia is stimulation of the autonomic ganglia followed by depression. Lobelia depresses the vasomotor center and peripheral vagus nerve resulting in dilation of the bronchioles by means of relaxation of the bronchial muscles.

In the digestive tract, Lobelia has a role as a gastrointestinal inhibitor/stimulant and appetite suppressant. Lobelia will generally induce vomiting when taken in very large doses over a very short period of time. Capsicum is generally added with this regime for flushing the poisons from the stomach and the bowels.

Samuel Thomson, an herbalist-physician of the early nineteenth century, recommended Lobelia as a muscle relaxant during childbirth and as a poultice for healing abscesses. Given in the right amount, it opens the bronchioles. Dr. Thomson said that there is no herb more powerful in removing disease and promoting health than Lobelia. It has healing powers with the ability to remove congestion within the body, especially the blood vessels.

Dr. Thomson said that, .If I can get to a person soon enough, I can always save them. He would first instruct that a fire be built in the fireplace. He would use hot water from the fireplace, giving them a high enema, cleansing the toxins from the bowel. On first arriving, he would give them large doses of Lobelia to produce an emetic/vomiting situation, continuing with Lobelia in large doses over a short period of time until he had achieved the cleansing of the body from this method. He then would wrap them in blankets taking hot bricks from the fireplace, packing the bricks around them creating a sweating situation just as they did in the Indian sweat lodges. This purifies the lymph system. It has a genuine effect on the whole system. Lobelia is a special herb for bronchial spasms.

* Copious amounts of water need to be taken with Lobelia so as to aid the body in the elimination of body and drug-induced toxin waste.
* Lobelia is known to be a powerful relaxant, effecting the nervous system. It is considered the strongest relaxant in the herb kingdom.
* Lobelia increases urine flow, perspiration and helps to reduce fever.
* A poultice of Lobelia is very soothing for inflammations, rheumatism and boils.
* There has never been a study done anywhere in the world that has proven that Lobelia is a poison.
* Lobelia in a poultice with Slippery Elm and soap can be used to bring abscesses or boils to a head.
* As a powerful anti-spasmodic, Lobelia is effective in causing immediate relaxation and expansion of the contracted parts of the respiratory system. This allows the .breath of life. to flow freely to the exhausted tissues.

NOTE: LOBELIA HELPS TO RELAX THE MOTHER DURING DELIVERY AND SPEEDS UP THE DELIVERY OF THE PLACENTA.

ALLERGIES
Angina
ARTHRITIS
ASTHMA (ACUTE ATTACK)
Bites/Stings (apply externally)
Blood poisoning
BLOOD VESSELS
Boils
Bronchial asthma
Bronchial spasms
BRONCHITIS
Bruises

Bursitis
CANKER SORES
CATARRH
CHICKEN POX
CHILDHOOD DISEASES
COLDS (EXPECTORANT)
Colic
CONGESTION (GENERAL)
CONTAGIOUS DISEASES
CONVULSIONS
COUGHS
CROUP

Delirium
Digestive disorders
EARACHE
EAR INFECTIONS
EMPHYSEMA
EPILEPSY
FEVERS
FOOD POISONING
Hayfever
HEADACHES
Heart
Heart palpitations
HEPATITIS
HYPERACTIVITY
INSOMNIA
LOCK JAW
LUNG PROBLEMS
Meningitis
MIGRAINE HEADACHES
MISCARRIAGE
Mucous membranes
MUMPS
NERVE RELAXANT
PAIN

Palsy
PLEURISY
PNEUMONIA
Poison ivy
Rheumatic fever
Rheumatism
Respiratory stimulant
Ringworm
Scarlet fever
SEIZURES
Shock
Sleep (promotes)
Small intestines
Smoking (stops)
SPASMS
Sprains
St. Vitus' Dance
TEETHING
TOOTHACHES
Tumors
WHOOPING COUGH
WORMS
Wounds (open)

MA HUANG   (Ephedra sinica)
A.K.A.,: Ephedra, Yellow River, General of Respiration.

BODILY INFLUENCE: Astringent,Y Bronchiodilator, Decongestant, Diaphoretic,Y Diuretic, Expectorant,Y Nervine, Sedative, Stimulant,Y Tonic, Vasoconstrictor.
PART USED: Whole herb.

Ma Huang, the common Chinese name for Ephedra, is one of the most powerful of medicinal plants. It is highly regarded in Chinese herbology, where it has been used for over 5,000 years to treat colds, coughs, fevers (including malaria), headaches and skin eruptions.

The first known record concerning the medicinal uses of herbs was by the Chinese in the Divine Husbandman's Classic of Materia Medica, 220 B.C. In it, is recorded the use of Ma Huang as being a part of Chinese Medicine. Ephedra sinica, use was only mentioned in the Western World relatively recently.

Several Ephedra species that contain no ephedrine were used extensively by the Indian tribes of the Southwest. Modern man has extracted out of Ma Huang, the active ingredient Ephedrine. Man, has made it synthetically as Epinephrine or Extracted it from as Ephedrine, and when used in this form, there are danger warnings given regarding its use. This warning is not as necessary when the whole herb is used.

Ephedrine as extracted from (Ma Huang) is a bronchial and blood vessels relaxant, warming to the body for all "cold" conditions of the chest. Reduces the allergic response in a wide range of conditions. Ephedrine is used as a bronchiodilator and is a life-saving herb in extreme cases of chronic asthma. Ephedrine stimulates the sympathetic nervous system, depresses smooth muscle function and subdues cardiac muscle action, demonstrating similar results to those of epinephrine. The outstanding difference with epinephrine is that Ephedrine is not altered in the GI tract or upon absorption into the blood vascular system, thus giving it a longer lasting effect.

Ephedrine stimulates the heart muscles, constricts the blood vessels, increasing circulation and blood pressure. This increased blood pressure, in turn, forces more blood to the extremities head, arms, hands, legs and feet and provides a stimulant action on the brain and nerve centers, reducing fatigue and weariness.

This principle makes Ephedra (Ma Huang) a popular herb in diet formulas. When blood is diverted from the organs of digestion to the extremities, the digestive organs do not function properly and hunger is decreased. However this effect is more beneficial when Ephedra (Ma Huang) is taken on an empty stomach. It should be understood that when there is food in the digestive tract and digestion is in progress and the blood is then diverted from the organs of digestion, to the extremities by the action of Ephedra(Ma Huang), digestion ceases and indigestion occurs.

Ma Huang (Ephedra) can be used effectively when combined with other herbs to create Thermogenesis in the body, "thermo" meaning, 'heat' and genesis. meaning, 'life of the cell'. Such formulas are used to create heat and increase metabolism, this increases heat, burning off the excess body weight.

University studies have shown that if you raise normal body temperature by one degree above normal (98.6 degrees - normal body temperature) and hold that for one whole year and if you exercise no more or no less or eat no more or less, you should have lost an average of 30 plus pounds.

Ephedrine in the Ephedra (Ma Huang) is known to raise blood pressure and as such should be avoided by those who are hypertensive and already have an increased blood pressure.

- Ma Huang has been used for bronchial and chest congestion.
- Ma Huang gives you the effects similar to adrenaline.
- In Russia, they have used Ma Huang to treat rheumatism and syphilis.
- The ephedrine in Ma Huang is also known to dilate the pupils.

- Ephedra (Ma Huang) is a good decongestant, tonic, diuretic and fever and cold medication.
- Ma Huang (Ephedra) tea or cold preparations relieve congestion. Ephedra is a long-acting stimulant and should not be taken at bed time or by people who have high blood pressure.
- Ma Huang (Ephedra) is a long lasting central nervous system stimulant that calms the mind as it stimulates the body.
- Ma Huang (Ephedra) contains ephedrine and pseudo-ephedrine.
- Ma Huang (Ephedra) acts as an energy tonic to strengthen and restore body vitality. (excellent for mental energy during a long test or meditation).
- Ma Huang Ephedra is a strong, natural bronchio-dilator and decongestant for respiratory problems.
- Ma Huang (Ephedra) is used in many weight loss formulas for its ability to increase metabolism.
- Ma Huang (Ephedra) it is a cardiac stimulant and should be used with caution by anyone with high blood pressure.
- Ma Huang (Ephedra) is a desert herb known for its ability to increase blood pressure.
- Ma Huang (Ephedra) alleviates pain associated with arthritis and rheumatism. It increases nervousness and restlessness in some people.
- The Chinese species of Ma Huang (Ephedra) are believed to contain much more ephedrine than the American species, possibly due to older plants and more selective harvesting.
- Ma Huang (Ephedra) is successfully used in the treatment of Asthma and associated conditions because of its ability to relieve muscle spasms in the bronchial tubes.

The Ephedrine extracted from the Ephedra or Ma Huang or its synthetic copy epinephrine, are outside of the scope and expertise of this book, and as such we take no responsibility as to any advice or information concerning its use.

CAUTION: Ma Huang (Ephedra) is contraindicated in cases of heart problems and high blood pressure. Ephedra(Ma Huang) or the isolated Ephedrine should not be taken during pregnancy.

BRONCHIAL ASTHMA
Emphysema
Epilepsy

Hayfever
Malarial fevers
Myasthenia gravis

MALE FERN   (Dryopteris filix-mas)
A.K.A.,: Bear's Paw, Knotty Brake, Shield Fern.

BODILY INFLUENCE: Astringent, Cardiac depressant, Parasiticide, Tonic, Vulnerary.
PART USED: Roots.

The Male Fern got the name Bear's Paw from the rough, hairy appearance of its brown root and the genus name Dryopteris meaning 'oak-fern' in Greek, because the plant oftens grows in oak forests. The species name, filix-mas ('male fern') was given by botanists because of its vigorous nature.

Filicic acid is the main active principle of the Male Fern root. Taken internally, it is excellent for expelling intestinal parasites, specifically the tapeworm or hookworm.

Externally, Male Fern in an ointment form, is considered excellent for healing wounds and it has been known to treat cancerous tumors.

Aspidium, an ancient drug derived from the root of the Male Fern was used in the time of the Greek physician, Dioscorides in the 1st century A.D. to treat tapeworms (Taenia saginata, beef tapeworm). It still is used in some combinations in the treatment of intestinal worm infestations.

CAUTION: Avoid during pregnancy as it is too strong a parasiticide.

Hookworms
TAPEWORMS
Parasites

MANDRAKE   (Podophyllum peltatum)
A.K.A.,: May Apple, Raccoon Berry, Indian Apple, Duck's Foot.

BODILY INFLUENCE: Alterative, Anti-bilious, Cathartic, Cholagogue, Diaphoretic, Emetic, Hepatic, Hydrogogue, Parasiticide, Tonic.
PART USED: Root, Resin.

The Mandrake, like other nightshades, derives its reputation for magical power partly from its toxicity. Adding to the Mandrake's mystique is the appearance of its root. Thick and tuberous, it can be imagined to look like a little human being. It is a plant that phosphoresces which means, sometimes at night, chemical substances in its berries react with the dew to give a pale light, a phenomenon that today is explained by science our ancestors attributed to spirits and magical forces.

Mandrake is used mostly for bowel and liver complaints. It is very irritating to the GI tract, making small doses necessary. North American Indian tribes made use of Mandrake, as a tonic or as a cathartic.

Used as a cathartic agent, Mandrake is a slow reliable purgative. It has a long lasting effect that will continue far into the day after it is ingested. The main effect is on the duodenum and will increase intestinal secretion and bile flow. Mandrake being most effective taken in very small doses, makes it very functional in combinations. It may be combined with less active and corrective laxatives which allows the herbalist to tailor-make formulas to meet the patients needs. Mandrake has been used to retard the growth of warts, especially venereal warts.

• Mandrake regulates the bowels and is highly beneficial when used in chronic liver diseases, skin problems, digestion and eliminating obstructions. It has a powerful stimulating effect on the liver and increases bile flow.

• Mandrake has been known to dissolve and remove tumors.

• Mandrake is a strong glandular stimulant, acting as an appetite suppressant. It has been used as part of a formula to promote female gland activity and eradicate sterility.

• Due to Mandrake's potent action, it should be used in formulas with other herbs.

CAUTION: This herb is laxative in nature and should be used sparingly or in combinations during pregnancy as it causes cramping and stomach griping.

BOWELS (HELPS REGULATE)
CANCER
Colitis
CONSTIPATION
Diarrhea
Dyspepsia
FEVERS
GALLBLADDER
Gallstones

Headaches
INDIGESTION
Jaundice
Liver
Tumors (cancerous)
Uterine disease
Vomiting (bilious)
Warts (venereal)
WORMS (EXPELS)

MARIGOLD   (Calendula Officinale)
A.K.A.,: African Marigold
(SEE CALENDULA)

MARJORAM   (Origanum vulgare)
A.K.A.,: Mountain Mint, Wintersweet.

BODILY INFLUENCE: Antiseptic, Anti-spasmodic, Carminative, Diaphoretic, Emmenagogue, Expectorant, Rubefacient, Stimulant, Tonic.
PART USED: The Herb.

Marjoram has been used so long ago that there are even Greek legends about it. They called it "joy of the mountains". Wreaths and garlands were made of it for weddings and even funerals. They associated the Goddess of love with Marjoram, claiming that it is what made it so gentle as a healing balm. Medicinally, it was used to treat rheumatism and sprains and also to adorn grave sites. They believed that if you anointed yourself with it, you would dream of your future mate.

Healthwise, we find Marjoram to be a stimulating diaphoretic, promoting perspiration and helpful in relieving the symptoms of colds, flu and fevers. It has been found to be effective as a digestive aid for indigestion, sour stomach and to eliminate gas. Marjoram is excellent in the kitchen and is used as an herbal food flavor enhancer, especially in salad dressings made with lemon and olive oil. This is a very good way to use Marjoram and also gain its health-promoting benefits.

• For nausea associated with menstruation and for severe cases of abdominal cramps, Marjoram can be of benefit.

• Marjoram has been used as an antidote for poisoning as experienced with certain narcotics and has been effective in treating convulsions and water retention.

• It works well as a mouthwash and gargle for sore throats and irritated gums.

• It can be used as an antiseptic for cuts and wounds and the oil can be used externally to relieve aches and pains and also can be applied to toothaches.

ABDOMINAL CRAMPS
Asthma
Bedwetting
COLIC
Colds
Convulsions (violent)
COUGHS (VIOLENT)
Diarrhea
Dropsy
Fevers
Flu
GAS
Gastritis
HEADACHES (NERVOUS)

Indigestion
Measles
Narcotic poisoning
Nausea
Neuralgia
Nightmares
RESPIRATORY PROBLEMS
Seasickness
Toothaches (oil)
Tuberculosis
Vomiting
Water retention
Whooping cough

MARSHMALLOW (Althaea officinalis)
A.K.A.,: White Mallow, Mortification root, Sweetweed.

BODILY INFLUENCE: Astringent, Absorbent-soothing, Demulcent, Diuretic, Emollient, Galactagogue, Laxative, Lithotriptic, Mucilant, Nutritive, Tonic, Vulnerary.
PART USED: The whole plant.

The generic name, Althaea, is derived from the Greek, altho, meaning "to cure". The family name, Malvaceae, comes from the Greek word malake or "soft" with reference to the soft mucilaginous character of this herb. Marshmallow was advocated as a wound healer by the Greek Physician Hypocrites and has been used for hundreds of years in treating wounds with excellent results. The leaves are often used as poultices and fomentations and is excellent to draw out poisons, and or any debris that might be imbedded in an open wound. In this case, Marshmallow used as a poultice on an open wound of any sort will benefit and shorten the healing time of that wound due to its ability to cleanse the wound by its drawing abilities. Due to its drawing power, Marshmallow is added to many formulas.

Marshmallow is a unique plant that is very valuable in several categories of healing. As a demulcent, it is used as an excellent poultice for a variety of uses. Marshmallow is very soothing for any sore or inflamed part of the body. In fact, a poultice of Marshmallow powder can be used anytime a poultice is needed. Due to the high content of mucilage and starch, the powdered Marshmallow plant will draw out and absorb moisture from damp surfaces. If Marshmallow were used for no other purpose than as a poultice, it would be immeasurable valuable to mankind.

Marshmallow is a mucilaginous calcium-rich herb and can be used to soothe and heal mucous membranes such as the lungs, digestive tract and bowel. It has been used as a food from very ancient times of which many different mallow plants had been eaten. In the Bible, we find that Mallow was eaten in time of famine (Job30:3,4).

Marshmallow will enrich the milk of nursing mothers and at the same time increase milk flow. It is effective to combine Blessed Thistle and Marshmallow together as nutrient for enriching mothers milk. Marshmallow works as a natural fiber to regulate bowel activity and increase colonic flora. Marshmallow, being both mucilaginous and nutritive, is an excellent "coating" of the intestinal tract when the natural mucus of the intestine has been, scraped or rubbed off, whatever the cause may be.

Marshmallow's highest medicinal acclaim is as a demulcent. Internally, it has a soothing effect on inflammation and irritation of the alimentary canal and of the urinary and respiratory organs. It is said to ease the passage of kidney stones. Marshmallow is used in combination with other diuretic herbs during kidney treatments to assist in the release of stones and gravel. As a constituent of a diuretic formula, Marshmallow is of special value due to its non-astringent soothing effect. It is used externally for varicose veins and skin abscesses or dermatitis.

When eaten as food, Marshmallows' non-absorbable polysaccharides coat the mucous membranes of the digestive tract and absorb toxins. Tannins (acids) along with the volatile oils of Marshmallow are responsible for the Marshmallows' diuretic effects. Their presence irritates the mucous membranes of the urinary tract until mucous is secreted to isolate and neutralize the toxins. Marshmallow has factors allowing it to combine with and eliminate toxins, aiding the body to cleanse. This ability to combine with body toxins makes Marshmallow excellent when added to other formulas to help neutralize toxins that are the causative factors of arthritis.

- Marshmallow is anti-inflammatory in nature and also works as an anti-irritant making it a soothing treatment for the gastro-intestinal tract.
- Marshmallow is very soothing for any sore or inflamed parts of the body.
- Marshmallow works well for urinary problems.
- Scientific evidence discloses that Marshmallow contains 286,000 units of vitamin A per pound.
- Because Marshmallow is an anti-irritant, it may be used effectively in treating soreness associated with diarrhea or that of dysentery.
- When Marshmallow is used as a poultice with Cayenne, it has been discovered as an effective treatment for cleaning infections such as blood poisoning, gangrene and to help the healing of bruises, burns and wounds. Its power in the decoction form for arresting mortification or putrefaction has been so great that it has been popularly called the 'mortification root.'
- Marshmallow is one of the best mucilage agents, giving off about 35% each of the vegetable mucus and starch which accounts for its demulcent effects on the digestive tract.

Allergies	Constipation
ASTHMA	Coughs (dry)
BEDWETTING	Cystitis
BLADDER	Diabetes
BLEEDING (URINARY)	Diarrhea (soothing)
BOILS	Dysentery
Bowels	EMPHYSEMA
BREAST MILK (INCREASES & ENRICHES)	Enteritis
	Eyes (inflammation of)
BRONCHIAL INFECTIONS	Gangrene
Burns (acid or fire)	Gonorrhea
Catarrh	Gravel

Inflammation
KIDNEY PROBLEMS
KIDNEY STONES
LACTATION
LUNGS
Mouth infections (gargle)
Mucous membranes
NERVOUS CONDITIONS
PNEUMONIA
Septicemia

Sore throat
Stomach problems
Teething
URINARY TRACT -
   (INFLAMMATION)
Urination (painful)
Vagina (irritated)
Voice loss
WHOOPING COUGH
WOUNDS (INFECTED)

MILK THISTLE (Silybum marianum)
A.K.A.,: Marian Thistle, Our Lady's Thistle.

BODILY INFLUENCE: Cholagogue, Demulcent, Galactogogue, Hepatic, Nervine, Stimulant, Tonic.
PART USED: Ripe Seeds.

In 1597, A prominent herbalist named Gerard, wrote that Milk Thistle was the best remedy that grows against all melancholy diseases. The word melancholy is taken from the Greek, 'black bile,' and in Gerard's day referred to any liver or biliary derangement. Milk Thistle was used by the Greek herbalist Dioscorides, to cure the poison of snakebites. It has been used for the elimination of obstructions in the liver and spleen.

It has been observed in practice that, when Milk Thistle extract has been given, an exciting reversal in symptoms of both acute and chronic liver problems, ranging from viral hepatitis to cirrhosis, has occurred. There is significant antioxidant and free radical scavenger action properties in Milk Thistle. This is due to its rich bioflavonoid content which acts in the body to increase membrane strength and reduce membrane permeability.

Milk Thistle is very beneficial for the liver, both protecting and rejuvenating it. It has also been shown to protect the kidneys, brain and other tissues from chemical toxins. Milk Thistle can help in rejuvenating the liver when overcoming alcohol toxicity, especially cirrhosis. Milk Thistle is a detoxifying, rebuilding herb for the liver and is specific for the gall bladder, with significant anti-oxidant properties to prevent free radical oxidation. Milk Thistle has been helpful in alcohol-induced fatty liver disorders, chronic hepatitis (inflammation of the liver), chemically induced fatty liver disorders, cholangitis (inflammation of the bile ducts resulting in decreased flow of bile), cholestasis (suppression of bile flow), cirrhosis or hardening of the liver and hepatic organ damage and psoriasis.

The active ingredient in Milk Thistle is Silymarin. Silymarin increases protein synthesis in liver cells, by increasing the activity of ribosomal RNA. Silymarin also induces an alteration of liver cellular membranes to stop absorption of many toxins.

Milk Thistle (Silymarin) is known to stop the toxicity of Amanita mushroom poisoning and common dry-cleaning fluid (carbon tetrachlorid poisoning). It has appeared more effective than any other known substance. Milk Thistle extract reduces the effect of many toxins on the liver. One such toxin is cadmium, which often causes problems.

- Milk Thistle accelerates protein synthesis by the liver cells. It stimulates the liver to produce SOD, a potent free radical scavenger. It prevents depletion of glutathione (takes part in oxidation-reduction processes) in the liver.
- The liver is your toxic waste disposal plant.
- Researchers have shown that Milk Thistle stimulates the synthesis of RNA (an important molecule that helps carry out and control protein synthesis).
- Milk Thistle contains some of the most potent life-giver protecting substances known.
- Milk Thistle also protects kidneys and is beneficial to those with psoriasis.
- As an anti-oxidant, it has been discovered that Milk Thistle will act to inhibit free radical scavengers.
- Milk Thistle has been found to maintain the basic function of the liver, thereby keeping the blood vascular system clean which has an overall effect of maintaining health and well-being to the entire body.
- Milk Thistle blocks allergic and inflammatory reactions.
- Milk Thistle is mucilaginous in nature and increases immune response, eradicates infection and soothes inflamed tissues.
- Milk Thistle aids immune response by increasing the production of T-lymphocytes and soluble proteins (interferon).

Alcoholism
Appetite stimulant
Blood pressure (high)
Boils
Chemotherapy (protects against)
Cholera
CIRRHOSIS
Convulsions
Delirium
Depression
Epilepsy
Fatty deposits
Gallbladder
Gas
Heartburn
Heart problems
Hemorrhage

HEPATITIS
Hypoglycemia
Indigestion
JAUNDICE
KIDNEY CONGESTION
Lactation (promotes)
LIVER CONGESTION
LIVER DAMAGE
Menstruation (suppresses)
Nervous conditions
Poisons (toxic)
Radiation
Skin diseases
Snake bites
Spleen congestion
Varicose veins

MISTLETOE   (Viscum flavescens-American Mistletoe)
(Viscum album-European Mistletoe) (Phoradendron flavacens)
A.K.A.,: American Mistletoe, Birdlime, Golden Bough.

BODILY INFLUENCE: Anti-spasmodic, Cardiac depressant, Diuretic, Emetic, Emmenagogue, Hypotensive, Nervine, Sedative, Stimulant, Tonic.
PART USED: The Leaves.

By 1682, in France, herbalists prescribed Mistletoe remedies for epilepsy, nervous disorders and St. Vitus' dance (spasms). Elsewhere, it was used for apoplexy and giddiness, to stimulate glandular activity, to serve as a heart tonic and to aid digestion, It is helpful for headaches with dizziness, is beneficial in a formula for migraine headaches and helps with high blood pressure.

Mistletoe can stimulate the heartbeat, increasing cardiac output. It can suppress abnormal rhythms in any heart chamber, correcting unnecessary "flutters." Mistletoe is a powerful nervine and cardiac depressant that acts on the vagus nerve.

Mistletoe was often used as a folk remedy for cancer, but was rejected by the so-called regular physician. At long last, the latest research indicates that it may be useful in tumor therapy.

Mistletoe will quiet, soothe and tone the nerves and lessen cerebral excitement.

• Mistletoe acts on the nervous system to quiet any excitement.
• Mistletoe also relieves spasms.
• Mistletoe is an emmenagogue that causes uterine contractions.
• Because Mistletoe acts upon the nervous system as a sedative, it will still the mental activity of the brain, allowing the body to rest.

CAUTION: Avoid during pregnancy as it is an emmenagogue that causes uterine contractions. The berries are considered to be poisonous. Mistletoe acts on the nervous system.

Arteriosclerosis	Delirium
Arthritis	EPILEPSY
Asthma	Gallbladder
Bedwetting	Heart trouble
Blood cleanser	HEMORRHAGES (INTERNAL)
Blood poisoning	Hypertension
BLOOD PRESSURE (HIGH)	Hypoglycemia
Cholera	Hysteria
CHOREA	Infections
CIRCULATION (STIMULATES)	Mental disturbance
CONVULSIONS	MENSTRUATION

(SUPPRESSES)
Migraine headaches
NERVOUSNESS
Neuralgia
Rheumatism

Skin (inflammatory conditions)
SPLEEN
St. Vitus' Dance
Tumors
Wounds

MORMON TEA (SEE Ma Huang)

MUGWORT (Artemisia vulgaris)
A.K.A.,: St. Johns Plant.

BODILY INFLUENCE: Anti-spasmodic, Aromatic, Diaphoretic, Diuretic, Emmenagogue, Hemostatic, Narcotic (mild), Nervine, Parasiticide, Stimulant, Stomachic, Tonic (bitter).
PART USED: The whole plant.

Mugwort has been used in cases of internal bleeding, worms and bad breath. It is as an antidote for many poisonous mushrooms. Mugwort has nervine qualities that are excellent for treating uncontrollable shaking, nervousness and insomnia. Mugwort is toxic in large doses. Herbalists have used it internally, to tone digestion, strengthen the liver and gall bladder and for travel sickness. Externally, it has been used as the active substance in a liniment for sprains, bruises and lumbago.
•   Mugwort is a bitter tonic and can be used for digestion and liver function improvement.
•   Mugwort is an invigorating, aromatic herb that has antiseptic qualities and is capable of expelling worms and other parasites.
•   Mugwort has been useful for all complaints of the digestive system such as constipation and indigestion. It is useful in stimulating sweating in dry fevers and for stomach acidity.
•   Mugwort is effective in promoting menstruation, has a stimulating effect on uterine circulation and also helping with cramps.
•   Mugwort is best used in small quantities and for short periods of time.
•   Mugwort is rarely given to children. It has been used externally and internally to check falling out of hair and baldness.
•   The bitter herb, Mugwort has long been used as an insect repellent.
•   For centuries, Mugwort has been used as a worming medicine for men and animals.
•   Mugwort has similar properties to Wormwood and can be taken when traveling to tropical countries to prevent malaria.

CAUTION: Avoid during pregnancy, as it stimulates uterine contractions and can be toxic taken in large doses.

Appetite	Gas
Arthritis	Gout
Back pain (lower)	Indigestion
Boils	Insect repellent
Breath (bad)	JAUNDICE
Bruises	Kidney problems
Childbirth	Labor (pain relief)
Circulation (blood)	LIVER PROBLEMS
CONSTIPATION	Lumbago
CRAMPS (MENSTRUAL)	MENSTRUATION (PROMOTES)
DEBILITY	Morning sickness
Diarrhea	Nausea
DIGESTIVE AID	Obesity
Dropsy	Poisons
Earaches	Rheumatism
Eczema	Sprains
Female disorders	STOMACH PROBLEMS
Fever	Swelling
Gallbladder	WORMS (EXPELS)

MULLEIN   (Verbascum thapsus)
A.K.A.,: Bunny Ears, Jacob's-staff, Flannel Flower, Velvet Leaf.

BODILY INFLUENCE: Anodyne, Anti-spasmodic, Anti-tussive, Astringent, Demulcent, Diuretic, Emollient, Expectorant, Vulnerary.
PART USED: Leaves, flowers.

During the Civil War, the Confederates turned to Mullein to treat respiratory problems when their conventional medical supplies ran out.

Mullein is used to relieve pain. It has numerous uses, but the main one is in the treatment of lung disease, coughs, consumption and hemorrhage of the respiratory organs. Mullein has narcotic properties that do not induce euphoria. It quiets inflamed and irritated nerves, relieves pain and is soothing to any inflammation.

It is helpful in chest ailments by clearing the lungs and relieving spasms. Mullein is also used to treat lymphatic congestion and as an anti-spasmodic and astringent herb, it is effective for a wide range of respiratory problems and swollen membrane conditions.

The oil of Mullein is used as an excellent remedy for ear infections.
• The dry leaves and stems, make excellent tinder. They will readily ignite if exposed to the slightest spark.
• Mullein is soothing to any inflammation and relieves pain.
• Mullein soothes inflamed tissues, and increases the flow of

urine.
- Mullein strengthens sinuses and allows for free breathing.
- Mullein is very effective in relieving swollen joints.
- Mullein has the effect of calming the nerves; therefore, is effective in treating agitated or inflamed conditions of the nervous system which are caused by such things as coughs or spasms due to cramping.
- Excess mucus will be moved out of the body by doses of Mullein.
- Mullein provides mucilaginous protection to mucous surfaces, inhibiting the absorption of allergens through mucous membranes.
- Mullein a demulcent and a bacteriostatic has been used to treat tuberculosis for centuries.

ALLERGIES (RESPIRATORY)
Asthma
Baby rashes
BLEEDING (BOWELS & LUNGS)
Boils
Breathing problems
BRONCHITIS
Bruises
Colds
Constipation
COUGHS
CROUP
Diaper rash
DIARRHEA
Dropsy
DYSENTERY
Dysuria
EARACHES (OIL)
EMPHYSEMA
Eyes (sore)
Gargle
GLANDS (SWOLLEN)
Hayfever
HEMORRHAGE
INSOMNIA

JOINTS (SWOLLEN)
LUNG PROBLEMS
LUNGS (BLEEDING)
LYMPHATIC CONGESTION
MUCOUS MEMBRANES
Mumps
Nephritis
NERVOUSNESS
PAIN RELIEVER
PLEURISY
Pneumonia
PULMONARY DISEASES
Poison ivy
RESPIRATORY
SINUS PROBLEMS
Skin disorders
Sore throat
SORES
Tonsillitis
Toothache
Tumors
TUBERCULOSIS
Ulcers
Warts

MUSHROOMS

There are several general classes of mushroom of which there are two types that are consistent with proven benefits. They are the Reishi and Shiitake mushrooms.

These mushrooms contain elements that simulate the immune system, hinder blood clotting and slow the development of cancer.

These Mushrooms thin the blood, lower blood cholesterol, prevent cancer, stimulate the immune system and inactivate viruses.

REISHI   (Ganoderma lucidum)
AKA: Ling-zhi.

BODILY INFLUENCE: Adaptogen, Alterative, Anti-allergenic, Anti-tumor, Anti-viral, Nervine, Relaxant, Stimulant, Immune tonic.
PARTS USED: Body and Stem.

In new research, use of the Reishi Mushroom is showing success against chronic fatigue syndrome by the noticeable increase of vitality after its administration. In addition, it has been found that the Reishi helps regenerate the liver, lowers cholesterol and triglycerides, reduces coronary symptoms and high blood pressure and alleviates allergy symptoms.

Studies have confirmed that this mushroom has a strong anti-histamine action that can help control allergies. Reishi can lower cholesterol and help prevent blood clots. Reishi, or ganoderma has tonic activity that increases vitality, enhances immunity and prolongs a healthy life.

Reishi protects against several varieties of cancer, increases vitality and strengthens internal organs, relieves neurasthenia (fatigue due to exhaustion of the nervous system), improves conditions of viral hepatitis, protects the liver against chemical damage, helps to normalize body functions, relieves insomnia by enhancing muscle relaxation, improves the coronary arteries and reduces excessive levels of cholesterol in the blood, thus improving circulation.

• Reishi is used to alleviate the effects of stress, strengthens the heart, protects the liver, soothes the nerves, normalizes blood pressure, inhibits the release of histamine, thus relieving the allergic inflammatory response, supports adrenal function, stimulates the immune system, slows the aging process and is anti-carcinogenic and anti-bacterial in nature.

• Reishi is a powerful immune stimulating agent, with particular effectiveness against wasting and degenerative diseases such as cancer and AIDS.

• Reishi is a specific in a formula to stimulate T-cell activity and inhibit replication of the HIV virus.

• Reishi bolsters the immune system, stimulates health and improves or prevents allergenic conditions.

• Reishi is an anti-oxidant, used therapeutically for a wide range of serious conditions, including anti-tumor and anti-

hepatitis activity.
- Reishi helps reduce the side effects of chemotherapy for cancer.
- Reishi also calms the nervous system and relieves insomnia.
- Some people have observed dizziness, sore bones, itchy skin, increased bowel movements, hardened feces, and/or pimple-like eruptions, during the initial intake period. Body toxins that are excreted by the Reishi are considered to be normal signs that its working. These disturbances vary from person to person and will disappear when intake continues.
- It can be used as an antidote in mushroom poisoning.

AIDS	Dizziness
Allergies	Fatigue
Angina	Hepatitis
Blood pressure (high)	Insomnia
Bronchial asthma	Longevity (enhances)
Cancer	Mushroom poisoning (antidote)
Cholesterol (high)	Nervousness
Coronary heart disease	Pneumonia
Diabetes	Stomach diseases

SHIITAKE   (Lentinus edodes)
AKA: Forest mushroom.

BODY INFLUENCE: Adaptogen, Immuno-stimulant.
PARTS USED: Stems and Caps.

Shiitake is used in Oriental medicine to prevent high blood pressure and heart disease and to reduce cholesterol. The Shiitake Mushroom is adaptogenic in nature promoting vitality and longevity and is useful in increasing the production of interferon, thus reducing the possibility of tumor development. It is an anti-viral, which helps the body excrete excess cholesterol and as such, helps prevent heart disease. Studies suggest that these mushrooms may work by enhancing the immune system's ability to fight against infection.
- The Shiitake Mushroom is a large brown, beefy mushroom which is good for soup stock. Before eating, remove the woody stems. Shiitake needs a longer cooking time than other mushrooms due to its toughness.
- The Shiitake Mushroom contains an anti-viral substance, known as lentinan, that stimulates the immune system, as well as activating the T-helper cells and the macrophages.
- Japanese experiments have found lentinan to be more powerful than the prescription anti-viral drug, Amantadine

hydrochloride.
- The Shiitake stimulates the immune system to produce more interferon, a natural compound that fights viruses.
- The Shiitake mushroom originated in the Orient and is now cultivated commercially in America.
- The Shiitake mushroom in Japan and China is used as a cancer preventer and in its treatment.

MUSTARD   (Brassica nigra-Black mustard) (Sinapis alba-White mustard)
A.K.A.,: Black mustard, White mustard.

BODILY INFLUENCE: Alterative, Analgesic, Carminative, Diuretic, Emetic-in large doses, Expectorant, Irritant, Rubafacient, Stimulant.
PART USED: Seeds.

Mustard has been used to relieve digestive problems by early herbalists and applied externally to encourage blood flow. The English herbalist John Parkinson recommended the seeds for epileptic seizures and Nicholas Culpepper, another English herbalist, thought it useful for toothaches and many other ailments.

Mustard plasters since ancient times have been used as a cure for chest congestion. It makes the skin feel warm and clears the lungs to make breathing easier. Mustard plasters, made from the powdered seeds of black mustard or the milder species, is also used to relieve arthritis, rheumatism, and many other areas of complaints such as soreness and stiffness.

Mustard seeds powdered and mixed with water, reacts to form the essential oil. To make the Mustard plaster, depending on the size of the area to be treated, take a portion of Mustard seed powder and mix with sufficient water to form a thick paste and wrap this in a clean thin cloth. It is best to place this Mustard plaster on another sheet of cloth already placed on the skin. Remove the poultice as soon as it becomes uncomfortable. Wash the skin thoroughly to be sure no mustard paste remains. The pure powder or oil should not be applied directly to the skin. Some herbalists suggest applying castor oil or olive oil over sensitive skin before applying the plaster or using in a poultice.
- Mustard dispels phlegm, stops coughs and alleviates body and joint pain.
- Mustard is used in congestive areas of the body to help reduce menses.
- Mustard is very important to have on hand for narcotic overdoses.
- Mustard is used as an emetic, specifically to treat drug

poisoning and is valuable, because it works to empty the stomach without causing convulsions to the system.

• Mustard is used to draw poison from the body, as in a Mustard pack application and can be used to treat sore and stiff muscles.

MYRRH (Balsamodendron myrrha, Commiphora myrrha, C. molmol)
A.K.A.,: Gum Myrrh.

BODILY INFLUENCE: Alterative, Antibiotic, Anti-Catarrh, Antiseptic, Anti-spasmodic, Astringent, Cardiac, Carminative, Disinfectant, Emmenagogue, Expectorant, Stimulant, Tonic, Vulnerary.
PART USED: Resin.

The aromatic resin of Myrrh was of value over 2,000 years before Christ. Gold, Frankincense, and Myrrh were the gifts of the wise men given to the child Jesus, at the dawn of the Christian era.

Myrrh has the characteristic of stimulating the body to discharge mucus which makes it useful in many chest afflictions, such as colds, asthma and tuberculosis. Myrrh is effective as an antibiotic and disinfectant in that it causes the body to increase white blood corpuscles up to four fold their regular number. The tincture or the powder has often been applied to the umbilical cord after birth to promote healing.

Myrrh acts as a stimulant when taken as an infusion increasing the flow of blood to the capillaries.

• Myrrh used as a natural antiseptic is good for bathing open sores.

• Myrrh is a stimulant and where necessary, promotes menstruation.

• Where low blood sugar is a problem, Myrrh can be used in place of Golden Seal.

• Taken internally, Myrrh cleans the colon and brings order to the digestive system.

• Myrrh used as a gargle, removes bad breath, has been called the herbal breath freshener and can be used as a topical application for mouth and gum sores, denture-irritated gums, canker sores and pyorrhea.

• Myrrh can be used as an ear oil, as anti-fungal immune stimulant for thrush or Candida yeast infections or as a specific oil for repelling fleas and harmful 'kissing bugs.'

• Chronic sinus problems have improved with the use of Myrrh.

• Myrrh has been used as a stimulating tonic to promote peristalsis. It contains constituents that stimulate gastric secretions and relax the smooth muscles.

- Myrrh has antiseptic properties and has been used with Golden Seal to make a healing antiseptic salve. Myrrh is useful for the treatment of hemorrhoids, bedsores and wounds.
- Myrrh has been proven to be one of the finest anti-bacterial and anti-viral agents making it good for uterus and vaginal infections and dysentery.
- Myrrh destroys putrefaction in the intestines and prevents blood absorption of toxins.

ANTIBIOTIC
ANTISEPTIC
Arthritis
ASTHMA
Boils
BREATH FRESHENER
BRONCHITIS
Canker sores
CATARRH (CHRONIC)
Cavities
COLDS
COLITIS
COLON (CLEANS)
Coughs
CUTS
DIGESTION
Diphtheria
EMPHYSEMA
GANGRENE
GARGLE
GUMS
Halitosis
Healing (general)
HEMORRHOIDS
HERPES
HYPOGLYCEMIA

Indigestion
INFECTIONS
LUNG DISEASES
Menstruation
MOUTH SORES
Nervous conditions
Nipples (sores)
Phlegm (reduces)
PYORRHEA
Rheumatism
Scarlet fever
Shock
SINUS PROBLEMS
SKIN SORES
SORE THROAT
SORES (POULTICE)
STOMACH (CLEANS)
Thyroid
TONSILLITIS
TOOTHACHE
Tuberculosis
ULCERS (LEG)
VAGINAL DISCHARGE
WOUNDS
Yeast infections

NETTLE   (Urtica dioica)
A.K.A.,: Great Stinging Nettle.

BODILY INFLUENCE: Alterative, Antiseptic, Astringent, Diuretic, Expectorant, Galactagogue, Hemostatic, Nutritive, Tonic.
PART USED: Leaves (hairs on leaf).

Stinging Nettle was cultivated in Scotland for the fibers in the stalks, to make a durable linen-like cloth. This use goes back to the Bronze Age. The very name Nettle comes from words meaning 'textile plant.'

Stinging Nettle was popular as an agent that, by irritating the skin of an inflamed area, caused increased blood flow to the area, thereby reducing the inflammation. In Scotland, victims of gout and rheumatism allowed themselves to be scourged with Nettle in the dubious belief that this would alleviate their sufferings.

Nettle neutralizes uric acid, prevents its crystallization aiding in its elimination from the system, thus relieving gout and arthritis. Nettle as an astringent helps to stop bleeding. The Nettle 'sting' is from histamine and formic acid in the hairs that trigger allergic response.

- Nettle is good to use for anemic children as a tea, due to its nutritive value as an herb and its high in iron, silicon and potassium.
- Nettle is an alkalizing herb and is useful as a rich source of minerals.
- Nettle aids with diarrhea and dysentery and is good for inflammatory skin conditions.
- Nettle increases the flow of urine, shrinks inflamed tissues, helps blood circulation and purifies the blood.
- Nettle is a most excellent remedy for dandruff and will bring back the natural color of hair.
- Nettle helps to reduce menses flow.
- Nettle can also be used as a tincture for hypothyroid conditions to increase thyroid function.
- Nettle it also cleanses the digestive tract and helps with stomach problems.
- Nettle functions much like a mild Cayenne by opening the vessels, thus increasing circulation and uplifting a weary body relieving fatigue and exhaustion.
- Nettle can alleviate allergic symptoms such as teary eyes and a runny nose.

NOTE: This herb is beneficial during pregnancy. It is a mineral rich nutritive herb with vitamin K to guard against excessive bleeding. It improves kidney function and helps prevent hemorrhoids.

Arthritis
Asthma
Baldness
BLEEDING (INTERNAL &
  EXTERNAL)
BLOOD PRESSURE (HIGH)
BLOOD PURIFIER
Breast milk
BRONCHITIS
CATARRHAL CONDITIONS
Circulation (poor)
DIARRHEA
DYSENTERY
Gout
Hemorrhoids (bleeding)

Hives
Infections
Kidneys (inflamed)
MENSTRUATION (EXCESSIVE)
Mouth sores
Neuralgia
Nosebleeds
Respiratory tract infections
RHEUMATISM
Scalp infection
Skin conditions (inflammatory)
Tendenitis
Urinary tract infections
Vaginitis

OATSTRAW   (Avena sativa)
A.K.A.,: Common Oat, Groats.

BODILY INFLUENCE: Anti-depressant, Anti-spasmodic,
Demulcent, Nervine, Nutritive, Stimulant, Tonic.
PART USED: Stems, Seeds, Flowers.

Dr. Johnson, a writer of an English Dictionary fame,
dispraised Oats by referring to it as a grain, which it seems, in
England is given to horses, while in Scotland, it is for people.
Johnson may have found the Scots' appetite coarse, but it showed
their good sense, because oats are indeed a very nutritious food
that is rich in nutrients and healthful fiber.

The straw of the oats has many elements that have antiseptic
properties and is said to be a natural preventative for contagious
diseases when taken frequently as a food. Oatstraw has also been
found to be an excellent toner for the whole system. It is used for
both physical and nervous fatigue and is helpful for depression.
Oatstraw is useful for thyroid and estrogen deficiency, for multiple
sclerosis, colds and chills and to encourage sweating. Extract of
Oats strengthens yet calms the nerves in nervous prostration and
insomnia. As an anti-spasmodic, Oatstraw quickly relieves spasms
of the ureter and bladder.
• Oatstraw has a calming effect on the nerves and is a strong
nutritive nervine for depression.
• Oatstraw helps hold calcium in the body and is very high in
silica.
• Oatstraw is a stimulant and is rich in body-building materials.
• When used a food on a frequent basis, Oatstraw will provide
the body with its many elements that work to maintain body
balance, off-setting degenerative disease.

- Oats is very good for convalescing patients being an easily digestible food.
- A facial pack of oatmeal is helpful for slowing down wrinkles and an external pack can be used for psoriasis and other skin disorders.
- Oatbran and oatmeal, help to reduce high blood pressure by reducing cholesterol levels, thus increasing circulation, its benefits being directed to the brain and body. It works especially well for weak nerves and is used as a nerve tonic to help recover from disease.
- Oatbran is especially effective for ovarian and uterine disorders.
- Oatstraw is helpful for treating depression, eases menopausal problems and helps lessen the problems associated with drug withdrawal.

APPETITE (IMPROVES)
ARTHRITIS
BEDWETTING
Bladder problems
Boils
Bones (brittle)
Bursitis
Constipation
Eyes
FINGERNAILS
Frostbite
Gallbladder
Gall stones
Gout
HAIR

HEART (STRENGTHENS)
INDIGESTION
INSOMNIA
Kidney problems
Kidney stones
Liver disorders
Lungs
NERVOUS CONDITIONS
Pancreas
Paralysis
Rheumatism
Shingles
Skin problems
URINARY ORGANS
Wounds

OREGON GRAPE (Berberis aquifolium)
A.K.A.,: Mountain Grape.

BODILY INFLUENCE: Alterative, Anti-scorbutic, Antiseptic, Anti-syphilitic, Blood purifier, Cholagogue, Depurative, Hepatic, Laxative, Tonic.
PART USED: Root.

Oregon Grape is known in the Spanish-American tradition as Yerba de la Sangre, 'herb of the blood', indicating its widespread use as a blood purifier.
Tonics made from the Oregon Grape were first introduced in the late 1800's, when the herb was listed in official pharmacopoeias. It is considered an excellent blood purifier. Oregon Grape, a good source of berberine which is one of the

active principles in Golden Seal, has an anti-inflammatory effect, is a bitter and stimulates the production of hydrochloric acid in the stomach, as well as the production of digestive and liver secretions. It stimulates bile secretions, promotes liver function and also is a purifier of the blood, spleen and lymphatics.

Oregon Grape aids in the assimilation of nutrients, with its cleansing properties. It is a tonic for all the glands and can be substituted for Golden Seal.

• Oregon Grape is an excellent liver organ cleanser, with the ability to release stored iron into the bloodstream to help maintain a good supply of hemoglobin in the blood to maintain its healthy function and to maintain a healthy immune system. Because of its ability to release iron stored in the liver, it works very similar to Yellow Dock in treating anemia, but this is not because of its significant presence of iron in the plant as in Yellow Dock.

• Herbalists have rightly held that pure blood will maintain disease free living.

• It influences the kidneys with its antiseptic qualities and can also be used as a douche.

• As a stimulator of the liver and gallbladder, Oregon Grape helps to overcome constipation.

• Oregon Grape root is very similar to Barberry in its action, but it also has a stimulating effect on the thyroid.

• Unlike any other herb known, Oregon Grape has what seems like an almost direct effect on the skin. It has been used to restore the complexion of the skin to a smooth, clear velvet-like texture, following any kind of skin disease or other illness that may have dried out the skin or produced sores.

• Because Oregon Grape works to cleanse the blood vascular system, it is beneficial as a tonic for all glands.

ACNE
Anemia
APPETITE STIMULANT
Arthritis (rheumatoid)
BLOOD CONDITIONS
BLOOD PURIFIER
Bowels
Bronchial congestion
Bronchitis
Cancer
Crohn's disease
Constipation (chronic)
Diabetes
DIGESTION (PROMOTES)
ECZEMA
Hepatitis

Herpes
JAUNDICE
Kidneys
LIVER PROBLEMS
Lymphatic congestion
Menstrual irregularities
Mononucleosis
PSORIASIS
Rheumatism
Scrofula
SKIN DISEASES
STAPH INFECTIONS
Strength (increases)
Syphilis
Uterine diseases
Vaginitis (douche)

PAN PIEN LIEN (Ban Bian Lian, Lobelia chinensis)
A.K.A.,: Chinese Lobelia.

BODILY INFLUENCE: Analgesic, Anodyne, Anti-spasmodic, Astringent, Cathartic, Counter-irritant, Decongestant, Diaphoretic, Diuretic, Emetic, Emmenagogue, Expectorant, Nervine, Sedative.
PART USED: Leaves.

Pan Pien Lien, with its calming quality, is being used by herbalists in combinations to enhance and balance the effect of other herbs. Pan Pien Lien has been reported to contain the chemical component, Lobeline, which is also the major alkaloid in Lobelia. The action of Lobeline closely resembles that of nicotine, but is milder. It thus decreases the desire for tobacco. Its the Lobeline salts used as a tobacco substitute in the body that makes nicotine taste terrible when it is smoked.
- It aids in all respiratory problems.
- It is known to be a relaxant.
(SEE LOBELIA)

PAPAYA (Carica papaya)
A.K.A.,: Medicine Tree, Melon Tree, Custard Apple, Pawpaw.

BODILY INFLUENCE: Anti-inflammatory, Cardiac, Digestant, Embryo-toxic, Expectorant, Nutritive, Parasiticide, Stomachic.
PART USED: Fruit, seeds and leaves.

On one of his many journeys to the West, Columbus, in observing the eating habits of the natives of the Caribbean, noticed when they ate exceptionally heavy meals of fish and meat, and when the meal was followed by Papaya, there was no apparent indigestion. In modern times, we have discovered that the unripe Papaya contains, in its milky juice, a protein-digesting enzyme known as papain, which greatly resembles the animal enzyme pepsin, in its digestive action. Today the papain of the Papaya is used in various preparations for indigestion and in the manufacture of meat tenderizers.

The native Central American Indians use the juice of the plant (from unripened fruit) to remove warts, tumors and corns. The seeds were used as a parasiticide.

The unusual quality of papain, unlike other enzymes which can only digest protein in an acid or an alkaline medium, is that it acts in all three, neutral, alkaline or acid. The Papaya apparently has other digestive qualities that include the rest of the food groups, which are fats and carbohydrates.

It could be reasoned that, all stomach problems stem from the lost ability of the stomach to digest food. As such, the digestive enzymes in Papayas, to include the green Papaya and its leaves, are most beneficial to improve the digestive process.

Papaya is also known to have another important quality in that it is helps to prevent ulcers and helps to heal them after they have developed. Papaya has shown the ability to increase the bloods. coagulation properties and at the same time, reduce acid secretion, which could account for the beneficial action that it has on stomach ulcers.

In areas where Papayas grow, the natives have treated ulcerations of the skin and open wounds by wrapping fresh Papaya leaves around them. Other medicinal uses of Papaya have been in the use of the papain in surgery, especially in spinal disk ruptures. Instead of surgically removing the problem, they have injected the papain directly into the area to be removed which digests the decaying injured substance, thus relieving the problem. By this use and other surgical uses, papain has come to be known as "nature's scalpel," demonstrating its ability to digest dead tissue without effecting live tissue.

The use of Papaya's alkaloid, carpine, has been shown to decrease the heart rate and also decrease central nervous system activity. In addition to the use of papain as a digestive enzyme, it is known to be a powerful abortive agent in India.

In Wholistic Healing, the use of Papaya for healing purposes is on going and new uses are yet being discovered. The use of Papaya as a nutritive protein digestant is well documented and farther reaching enzyme therapy, properties and uses for Papaya for serious diseases, are being persued.

• Papain, one of the Papayas' enzymes, is, due to its health promoting properties, a cancer preventive.

• Papaya contains all the enzymes needed for digestion of food, thus it relieves gas and a sour stomach.

• Papaya helps prevent ulcers and is effective at stopping internal bleeding.

Allergies
Belching
COLON
Diarrhea (chronic)
DIGESTIVE DISORDERS
Diverticulitis
GAS
Hemorrhage
INSECT BITES
INTESTINAL TRACT
Paralysis
Stomach (sour)
Worms (expels)
Wounds

PARSLEY (Petroselinum sativum)
A.K.A.,: Garden Parsley, Rock Parsley.

BODILY INFLUENCE: Anti-rheumatic, Antiseptic, Antispasmodic, Aperient, Calcium solvent, Carminative (slightly), Diuretic, Emmenagogue, Expectorant, Lithotriptic, Nervine, Parasiticide, Stimulant, Tonic.
PART USED: Leaves, roots and seeds.

The ancient Greeks and Romans used the leaves as a flavoring and garnish for foods. Today, Parsley has the misfortune of being a token herb on plates at restaurants. That resilient sprig used for color is really edible and its high Chlorophyll content makes it a natural breath sweetener.

By the Middle Ages, Parsley had made its appearance in herbal medicines. It has been given credit for curing a great range of human ills, especially those having to do with the kidneys and liver. Parsley is an ancient remedy for kidney stones and gallstones. Culpeper.s writings showed that he thought of Parsley as the herb "par excellance" for the treatment of kidney and bladder disturbances.

One of the main medicinal uses of Parsley is to provide a toxic kidney with essential nutrients that aid in its cleansing, so that it might persue the necessary bodily function of filtering the blood. Parsley, as a blood purifier, provides the healthful nutritional material necessary for tissue maintenance of the urinary system. Parsley is a healing balm to the urinary tract making difficult urination, easier. Parsley has been shown to be a slow and gentle diuretic.

Parsley directly inhibits salt reabsorption by body tissues and in this manner, is able to increase diuretic activity by the kidneys. It is well to know that Parsley is the diuretic of choice and can be taken to improve urination when it is painful and incomplete, due to an enlarged prostate that is squeezing the urethra so as to make urination difficult.

There is information that shows that Parsley, in comparison with citrus juices has three times more vitamin C, gram for gram. Parsley has been shown to have a higher content of iron than other leafy greens and is rich in potassium and other essential elements. Parsley roots are more potent acting than the leaves. Preparations made from Parsley roots have their major influence on the liver and spleen. Clinical physicians for the last 100 years have stated that Parsley root has been effective for treating liver diseases. Parsley has been used to dissolve and help pass gallstones and kidney stones, if they're not too large.

The roots and leaves of Parsley are used in cases of low blood sugar if there is adrenal malfunction. Fresh Parsley juice helps heal conjunctivitis and blepharitis, an inflammation of the eyelid.

The roots and leaves work to normalize delayed menstruation, has a uterine toning effect and also effects the prostate in men.

Parsley can be used during pregnancy, but not in high doses, as it tends to induce labor pains. Parsley has a drying up effect on mother's milk and can be used to help in the weaning process, but nursing mothers should avoid using it in large quanities. While mild doses of Parsley have a strong diuretic effect, large doses are known to cause congestion of the uterus membrane causing irritation and discomfort, so it is recommended that Parsley be only used in moderation during pregnancy.

- Parsley has been used as a cancer preventative.
- The generous use of Parsley can lower blood pressure and increase the depth of respiratory movement.
- Parsley acts as a gentle laxative and increases the flow of urine.
- Parsley has been used for ailments of the liver and is a good tonic for blood vessels, capillaries and arterioles.

ADRENAL GLAND WEAKNESS
Allergies
Amenorrhea
Appetite (stimulates)
Arthritis
Asthma
BEDWETTING
BLADDER INFECTIONS
BLOOD BUILDER
BLOOD CLEANSER
Blood pressure (low)
Breath (bad)
Breath freshener
Bronchitis
Bruises
CANCER PREVENTION
Colds
Coughs
Digestive disorders
DROPSY
Dysmenorrhea
Dyspepsia
Dysuria
EDEMA
Eyes
Fevers

Gallbladder problems
GALLSTONES
Gas
Gout
HALITOSIS (CHEW)
Hayfever
Indigestion
Insect bites/Stings
JAUNDICE
KIDNEY PROBLEMS (TO PREVENT)
KIDNEY STONES
Liver
Menstrual difficulties
Mucus (respiratory)
Nephritis
NURSING (CESSATION)
PITUITARY GLAND
PROSTATE GLAND
Spleen
Thyroid
Tumors
URINARY PROBLEMS
Venereal diseases
WATER RETENTION

PARTHENIUM   (Parthenium integrifolium)
A.K.A.,: Wild Quinine, Prairie Dock, Missouri Snakeroot.

BODILY INFLUENCES: Anti-venomous, Diuretic, Mucilant.
PARTS USED: Root.

Parthenium root bears "an uncanny resemblance," to Echinacea, but does not possess Echinacea's distinctive flavor or fragrance. Parthenium also weighs four to five times more than Echinacea purpurea. While the roots resemble each other, the tops are distinctly different. The tops of the Parthenium plant possess a 'quinine-like' bitterness and has been used to treat intermittent fevers. This explains one of the plants common names, 'wild quinine.' Parthenium root has been used historically, as a diuretic and has been useful for kidneys and bladder diseases.

Parthenium's common name, Missouri snakeroot, suggests it has been used for snakebites, bringing one to believe that it might have blood purifying and liver stimulating properties. Both Echinacea and Parthenium belong to the Sunflower family as do such herbs as Burdock, Milk Thistle and Boneset, all of which are credited with having a strong affinity for the digestive system, the liver and the kidneys.

Medicinally, a poultice can be made from Parthenium leaves for treating burns. Parthenium has been used for treating malaria-type intermittent fevers.

Ague (malaria)
ACNE
BITES/STINGS
    (INTERNAL/EXTERNAL)
BLOOD POISONING
BOILS
Bladder problems
ECZEMA
Emphysema
GANGRENE
Kidney problems
Liver problems
Lymphatic congestion
Wounds

PASSION FLOWER   (Passiflora incarnata)
A.K.A.,: Passion Vine, Maypops, Purple Passion Flower.

BODILY INFLUENCE: Anodyne, Antispasmodic, Diaphoretic, Hypotensive, Nervine, Sedative(mild).
PART USED: The Leaves and Fruit.

Passion Flower gets its name from the finely cut corona found in the center of the flower blossom. It resembles the Crown of Thorns given to Jesus of Nazareth. Passion Flower, the symbol of the crucifixation during the early seventeenth century, was professed to be seen by the early Jesuit priests and other explorers from Spain and Italy and interpreted this as a sign of divine assurance for the success of their efforts to convert the natives to Catholicism.

• Passion Flower was used by North American Indian tribes and was applied to earaches, boils and other inflammations. In the Yucatan, Mexico, it was introduced by the Mayan Indians who used it to treat insomnia, hysteria and convulsions in children

• In Italy, Passion Flower has been used to treat hyperactive children.

• Passion Flower can best be used in nervous problems with children such as muscle twitching and irritability and is also helpful with problems of concentration in school children.

• Passion Flower has been used primarily as a motor nerve depressant, to lowers motor nerve activity. It can also be used for increasing the rate of respiration and produces a temporary reduction of blood pressure. It helps to vitalize the sympathetic nervous system in weakened conditions improving circulation and nutrition of the nerve centers.

• In elderly people, it is good for sciatica and general nerve debility.

• Passion Flower can be used to calm nerves that get on edge during the periods of hormonal adjustment common to most women.

• Passion Flower is quieting and soothing to the nervous system and yet there are no side effects of depression nor disorientation.

• Passion Flower is rich in flavonoids. It is effective in combinations to overcome alcohol abuse without the accompanying narcotic hangover.

• Passion Flower has been found to possess analgesic (pain-killing) and anti-inflammatory properties, to aid, without side effects, sleeplessness caused by brain inflammations.

• Passion Flower can be helpful for people who do not want to continue dependence on synthetic sleeping pills and tranquilizers.

• It has been noted that Passion Flower kills the bacteria that is said to causes eye irritations. A claim is made that in some cases it surpasses in results to commercial products that are given for inflamed eyes and weakness of vision.

ALCOHOLISM
Anxiety
BLOOD PRESSURE (HIGH)
BRONCHIAL ASTHMA
Convulsions
Depression (severe)
Diarrhea
Dysentery
Dysmenorrhea
EPILEPSY

EYE INFECTIONS
Eye strain
EYE TENSION
Fevers
HEADACHES
HEART BEAT (IRREGULAR)
HEART WEAKNESS
Hemorrhoids
HOT FLASHES
Hypertension (caused by mental —

attitude)
HYSTERIA
INSOMNIA (CHRONIC)
MENOPAUSE
Menstruation (painful)
Muscle spasms
Nervous breakdown
NERVOUS DISORDERS

Nervous tension
NEURALGIA
Parkinson's disease
Restlessness
Seizures
Shingles
Sleeplessness
Vision (dimness)

PAU D' ARCO (Tabebuia heptaphylla)
(A.K.A., Taheebo, Lapacho, Ipe Roxo)

BODILY INFLUENCE: Alterative, Analgesic, Anodyne, Antibacterial, Antibiotic, Anti-diabetic, Anti-dotal, Anti-fungal, Anti-inflammatory, Anti-microbial, Anti-neoplastic, Antiseptic, Anti-tumor, Anti-viral, Astringent, Bitter tonic, Blood purifier, Digestive, Diuretic, Fungicide, Hypotensive, Parasiticide.
PART USED: Inner Bark.

Pau D'Arco was valued by the ancient Incas who noted that when other flora disappeared in the hot and humid conditions of the Amazon jungle, it still remained. It is being used today among the Callaway tribe in South America.

The best Pau D'Arco, which grows mainly in Argentina is the violet-flowered Tabebuia heptaphylla. Lapacho is a tropical tree, yet it may start out as a vine which, when mature, resembles a tree, because of its size. In the Brazilian jungles, the tree is known to reach great heights. Lapacho (Pau D'Arco) has significant anti-fungal properties making it useful for vaginal douches, suppositories or tampons soaked in the tea for vaginitis. Its anti-fungal effect is matched by its anti-viral action. Several studies have tested Lapacho's (Pau D'Arco) successful effectiveness for treating cancer in patients.

South American Indians brought the healing use of Pau D'Arco to the attention of the early Portuguese, to treat the disease called Schistosomiasis. The trematode (flatworm) Schistosoma mansoni, the causative agent of the common tropical disease (Schistomiasis), has been prevented from penetration into the body by the use of Lapacho (Pau D'Arco).

Pau D'Arco is an effective blood purifier and is successful against many blood toxicity conditions such as dermatitis, eczema and psoriasis. It also is a blood purifier and blood builder in leukemia and pernicious anemia and as a primary immune enhancer against viruses such as the flu, herpes and hepatitis. It has also been part of a treatment to eradicate environmentally produced allergies and asthma.

- Pau D'Arco is a protector for the liver and helps to neutralize poisons that involve the liver.
- Some hospitals in South America have used it on cancer patients with great success. Pau D. Arco seeems to have the ability to stop the destructive process of cancer when taken with chemotherapy. Chemotherapy is known to destroy the liver and kidneys. Pau D'Arco also has the ability to help stop the pain of cancer.
- Pau D'Arco is a an anti-fungal agent discouraging Candida Albicans and Herpes Simplex and at the same time, strengthens the immune system.
- Pau D'Arco seems to have the ability to reduce tumors of all kinds by dissolving them.
- Pau D'Arco is given free by the Argentina government to cancer and leukemia patients.
- Pau D'Arco has been used in cases of diabetes in lowering dependence on insulin injections.
- Pau D'Arco has a natural anodyne (pain-relieving) effect helping to relieve the pain of arthritis and cancer pain.
- Lapacho is credited with eliminating the pain caused by disease and then multipling the numbers of red corpuscles.
- Pau D'Arco has helped many types of liver ailments including reducing aging spots.
- Pau D'Arco is used with Licorice by hypoglycemics.
- Pau D'Arco has anti-fungal properties which is seen when the trees never mold or mildew after beng chopped down.
- Pau D'Arco exhibits anti-tumor activity, especially in certain blood and skin cancers.
- Pau D'Arco aids in blood purification, supplies anti-mutagenic properties, provides antibiotic, anti-viral and anti-fungal support in combating yeast infections and functions as an excellent disease preventive.
- One of the properties peculiar to Pau D'Arco is that it is high in iron, which makes it effective in aiding in the natural assimilation of nutrients. This encourages improved elimination through the intestinal tract.

AGE SPOTS
AIDS
Allergies
Anemia
ANTIBIOTICS (SIDE EFFECTS OF)
Arteriosclerosis
ARTHRITIS
Asthma
BLOOD PURIFIER
Boils

Bronchitis
CANCER (IMMUNE BOOSTER)
CANDIDA ALBICANS
Circulation (poor)
Colitis
Constipation
Cystitis
DIABETES
Diarrhea
Dysentery
ECZEMA

Esophagus
Fevers
Fistulas
Gastritis
Gonorrhea
Hemorrhages
HERPES
HODGKIN'S DISEASE
IMMUNE DEFICIENCY
Infections
Intestines
JAUNDICE
LEUKEMIA
Leukorrhea
LIVER CONDITIONS
Lungs
Lupus
Nephritis
Osteomyletis
PAIN (RELIEVES CANCER)
Paralysis (of eyelids)
PARASITES
Parkinson's disease
Pharyngitis

POLYPS (INTESTINAL)
PROSTATE PROBLEMS
PROSTATITIS
Psoriasis
Respiratory problems
RHEUMATISM
Ringworm
Scabies
SKIN CANCER
Skin diseases
Snake bites
Sores (external)
Syphilis
TONIC
TOXEMIA
TOXIC BLOOD
TUMORS
Ulcers (stomach/duodenal)
Urinary tract (inflammation)
Varicose (ulcers)
VENEREAL DISEASES
Wounds
YEAST INFECTIONS

PEACH BARK   (Prunus persica)
A.K.A.,: NONE

BODILY INFLUENCE: Alterative, Antibiotic, Anti-cancer, Antiseptic, Anti-spasmodic, Astringent, Carminative, Demulcent, Diuretic, Emmenagogue, Expectorant, Laxative, Nervine, Parasiticide, Sedative, Stomachic.
PART USED: Bark, Leaves, Seed and Flower.

The Peach tree has a long history of usage dating back to 25 B.C. in China. The Peach contains cyanide with the highest concentration being in the seed. Some feel the amount of cyanide is low enough for the plant to be used therapeutically and not be toxic.   In this regard, it has been used extensively for cancer patients.

Peach Bark is one of the stronger blood-moving herbs and therefore is useful in reducing tumors.

Peach Bark is given in cases of delayed menses and congested blood especially in the lower pelvic cavity.

• Peach Bark relieves inflammation particularly in the bladder, it acts as a mild laxative and also has a soothing effect on the nerves.

- Peach Bark is excellent for bladder problems such as burning urine and urine retention by stimulating the flow of urine.
- The noted Herbalist, Jethro Kloss wrote that the bark of Peach has a quinine effect upon the system.
- Peach Bark is strengthening for the nervous system, has mild sedative qualities and has helped in chronic bronchitis and lung problems due to it's mucus releasing (expectorant) qualities in the lungs.
- Peach Bark has qualities that relieve irritations of the throat and windpipe, help to overcome chest pains, relieve stomach and intestinal spasms and acts as an anti-spasmodic for convulsions.

NOTE: The cyanide in the peach plant could be harmful in large concentrated doses. The derivative of the cyanide in peach and apricot pits (B17 or laetrile) has become famous as an anti-cancer remedy. The seed of the Apricot has been found to contain higher cyanide amounts than Peach seeds and are considered superior therapeutically.

Abdominal inflammation	MORNING SICKNESS
BLADDER	NAUSEA
Blood cleanser	Nephritis
BRONCHITIS	NERVOUS CONDITIONS
CANCER	Parasites
Constipation	Stomach problems
DIURETIC	Urinary problems
Dysentery	Uterine troubles
Dyspepsia	VOMITING
Hair loss	WATER RETENTION
Insomnia	Whooping cough
Jaundice	WORMS
KIDNEY PROBLEMS	Wounds
LUNG CONGESTION	

PENNYROYAL (Mentha pulegium, Hedeoma pulegiodes)

A.K.A.,: European Pennyroyal/American Pennyroyal, respectively
AKA.,: Euorpean - Pudding Grass, American - Squaw Mint.

BODILY INFLUENCE: Anti-spasmodic, Anti-venomous, Aromatic, Carminative, Diaphoretic, Diuretic, Emmenagogue, Nervine, Parasiticide, Sedative(mild), Stimulant, Stomachic, Tonic, Vulnerary.
PART USED: The whole plant.

European Pennyroyal and American Pennyroyal have similar properties. The difference being that the European Pennyroyal is much more potent.

The Indians of North America taught the white settlers how to use the leaves of Pennyroyal. It will repel insects by rubbing the leaves into the skin. The Chickasaws soaked the plant in water and placed it on the forehead to relieve itchy and watery eyes. The Mohicans drank Pennyroyal tea to soothe the stomach and the Katawbas used the herb to relieve colds.

Pennyroyal has been used effectively to treat delayed menstruation. In feverish conditions, Pennyroyal has a noticeable, increased beneficial effect due to its diaphoretic and stimulant properties. It is most effective when used as a vapour bath. It is also effective for gas, intestinal spasms, colic, pain and restlessness in children. It has been used to purify water and in times past, it was hung in the sleeping room to induce sleep and retard insects.

The oil of Pennyroyal is an abortifacient by its abilities to irritate the kidneys and bladder during excretion and exciting uterine contractions reflexively. This oil is also known to be a CNS depressant. It has been used for spasms and hysteria.

• Pennyroyal is a spicy smelling herb that promotes perspiration in colds and flus. Pennyroyal aids in expeling intestinal gas. It has a sedative, calming effect on the nerves.

• Pennyroyal is useful in lung problems, helps with toothaches, brings on perspiration allowing for improved circulation, is helpful in skin diseases and has had good results in gout.

CAUTION: Avoid during pregnancy in first two trimesters, as it can cause an abortion, but may be used in final (5) weeks.

BRONCHITIS
CHILDBIRTH
COLDS
COLIC
Convulsions
Coughs
CRAMPS
Delirium
Fainting
FEMALE PROBLEMS
FEVERS
Flu
GAS
Gout
Insect bites
Insect repellent
Intestinal pain
LUNG INFECTIONS
Measles

MENSTRUATION (PROMOTES)
Migraine headaches
Morning sickness
Mucus
Nausea
NERVES
PERSPIRATION (PROMOTES)
Phlegm (expels)
Pleurisy
Pneumonia
Smallpox
Sunstroke
SWEATING (INDUCES)
Toothache
Tuberculosis
Ulcers
Uterus
Vertigo

Peppermint is much stronger in action than Spearmint and is more of a stimulant. Spearmint is more of a diaphoretic.
SEE SPEARMINT

PEPPERMINT (Mentha piperita)
A.K.A.,: Brandy mint, Balm mint, Curled mint.

BODILY INFLUENCE: Alterative(mild), Analgesic, Anodyne, Anti-bacterial, Anti-microbial, Anti-nauseate, Antiseptic, Anti-spasmodic, Anti-viral, Aromatic, Astringent, Calmative, Carminative, Diaphoretic, Digestive, Febrifuge, Nervine, Rubefacient, Sedative, Stimulant(gastric), Stomachic, Tonic, Rubefacient, Stimulant, Sudorific.
PART USED: Leaves, stem, Oil.

Peppermint is one of the oldest household remedies. Peppermint has been noted in Chinese medical literature since the Tang pen tsao period, 659 A.D. Peppermint has been in use since the dawn of recorded history in every known society. The American Indian used Peppermint for bowel eliminations, tonification, colds and to control fever.

Peppermint Oil is a relaxant for the lower sphincter muscle of the esophagus, is used as a digestive aid and eases gas and burping and the bloat after a meal.

• Peppermint is good for spasms and convulsions in infants. It may also be used for griping pain in the intestines.

• Peppermint as a gastric stimulant, tends to stimulate the flow of stomach digestive fluid so necessary to healthy digestion and as a stomachic and tonic, it strengthens and tones the stomach. This spicy, pleasant smelling herb is used primarily to alleviate stomach and intestinal problems.

• Peppermint in enemas can be helpful for colon problems.

• Peppermint makes a stimulating tea, aids in digestion and is a catalyst for other herbs.

• Peppermint is an energizer oxygenating the bloodstream and encouraging digestive fluid production.

• As a nerve stimulant the oil of Peppermint increases the functions of respiration increasing the oxygen supply to the blood, which cleans the blood resulting in strengthening the body systems.

• Peppermint is used as a specific in almost every digestive, colon cleansing and bowel combination, to control gas, flatulence, nausea, diarrhea, ulcerative colitis and Crohn's disease. The oil is a specific for irritable bowel syndrome.

NOTE: Peppermint is beneficial during pregnancy and may be used after the 1st trimester to help digestion, to soothe the stomach and overcome nausea. Peppermint is an over-all body strengthener and cleanser.

APPETITE
Boils
BRONCHITIS
CHILLS
Cholera
COLDS
COLIC
COLITIS
Constipation
Convulsions
Coughs
Cramps (stomach)
Depression
DIARRHEA
DIGESTION (AIDS)
Diverticulitis
Dizziness
DYSENTERY
DYSPEPSIA
FAINTING
FEVERS
FLU
Gallbladder
GAS
HEADACHES

HEART
HEARTBURN
HEART PALPITATIONS
Herpes simplex
Hysteria
Insomnia
Measles
Menstruation pain
Migraine headaches
Morning sickness
Motion sickness
Mouth sores
Mouthwash
Muscle spasms
NAUSEA
NERVES
Neuralgia
NIGHTMARES
Seasickness
Shingles
SHOCK
Sore throats
STOMACH SPASMS
Toothaches
VOMITING

PERIWINKLE (Vinca major, V. Minor)
(Catharanthus roseus)
A.K.A.,: (Greater Periwinkle, Hundred Eyes)(Common Periwinkle, Myrtle) respectively, (Madagascar Periwinkle)

BODILY INFLUENCE: Anti-neoplastic, Astringent, Hemostatic, Nervine, Sedative.
PART USED: The whole plant.

Periwinkle has been used as a healing herb in many places and countries and for many different uses. India used Periwinkle to treat wasp stings with the juice from the leaves. In Hawaii, Periwinkle was boiled and an extract was made to stop bleeding. In South America, a gargle is made to ease sore throats and chest ailments.

Madagascar Periwinkle has two anti-cancer alkaloids, Vincristine and Vinblastine that inhibit the growth of tumors and are effective in treating childhood leukemia, testicular cancer and Hodgkin.s disease (cancer of the lymphatic system). Like many drugs used in chemotherapy, both alkaloids produce such side effects as nausea and hair loss.

In addition to their anti-neoplastic (combats tumorous growths) qualities, Vincristine and Vinblastine carry more oxygen to the brain than any other herbal substance known, save Capsicum and act as a liquid 'sponge' causing the blood to absorb more oxygen than normally is the case. This is the method by which leukemia is stopped and by the same principle is the brain nourished and fed.

Vinblastine is showing promising results for treating choriocarcinoma and Hodgkin's disease. Periwinkle, as an effective astringent, is used to control excessive menstrual bleeding and uterine discharge, colitis, diarrhea, hemorrhoids and bleeding gums. It can be ingested or used as a douche. Periwinkle has proven effective, thus far, in the treatment of various types of cancer. It is being further researched for treatment of cancer of the lung, liver, kidney and others.

Lesser Periwinkle has been used by herbalists as an agent to stop the flow of blood. Other uses for Periwinkle in addition to its anti-hemorrhaging qualities, has been as an astringent, a remedy for 'nervous disorders' and for high blood pressure. Periwinkle can be used as a sugar-balancing agent in diabetics.

- The tea is used for nervous conditions.
- Periwinkle also makes a good remedy for diarrhea.

NOTE: Periwinkle has powerful drug-like actions resembling that of medically prescribed drugs.

Bleeding	Hysteria
Blood pressure (high)	Leukemia
CANCER	Menstrual flow (excessive)
Colitis	Mucus
Cramps	NERVOUSNESS
Dandruff	Nightmares
DIABETES	Skin disorders
Diarrhea (chronic)	Sores
Fits	Toothache
Hemorrhages (internal)	Ulcers
HEMORRHOIDS (BLEEDING)	Wounds
Hodgkin's disease	

PINE TREE BARK   (Pinus maritima)
A.K.A.,: French Maritime Pine Tree, (Pycnogenol-Trademark).

BODILY INFLUENCES: Anti-inflammatory, Anti-oxidant, Stimulant.
PARTS USED: Bark.

Jacques Cartier, in his book, "Voyages to Canada" (1534-5), credited a tea made from the needles and bark of the Anneda Tree, a Canadian pine tree, with saving the lives of his crew when they were stranded by ice on the St. Lawrence River. The French explorer Jacques Cartier attempted, in the beginning of winter, to sail up what is now known as the St. Lawrence River in Canada. The river froze, trapping his ship. Cartier and his crew tried to subsist on biscuits and salted meat. They later landed on the Quebec Peninsula to hunt and trap for food as their provisions were dwindling, but lacking fresh fruit and vegetables, his crew fell victim to the dreaded scurvy. Some 25 crew members of the 110 man crew died. Another 50 were seriously ill and the remainder of the crew were too weak to even bury the dead before Cartier and his crew were rescued by friendly Quebec Indians. Being experts on the medicinal properties of plants and trees, the Indians told the Frenchmen of a tea prepared from the needles and bark of pine trees growing in the area (the Anneda Tree) and taught them how to harvest and prepare this life-saving concoction from the pine tree for themselves. They first tried this tea on two of the sickest members of the crew, who improved so much that within a week, he gave the tea to all the surviving members of his crew. This tea saved their lives.

The end result was that Cartier and his crew returned home safely with the recorded account of this miraculous cure. Cartier later wrote his book on his voyage and included the account of this experience. Four hundred years later, Professor Jacques Masquelier while a visiting professor at the Quebec University was doing research on flavonols in pine bark, grape skins and several nut shells. When pursuing his research in the University library, he came across the records of Cartier's experience. He came to the logical conclusion, which directed his research to the bark of the pine tree and later, while back in France found the Maritime Pine grows in abundance along the southern coast of France.

The Maritime Pine was found to contain the richest available supply of the assorted bioflavonoids. Research has found that the Maritime Pine Bark contained a blend of flavonols called proanthocyanidins which he later patented under the name Pycnogenol.

The pine tree needles contained vitamin C and the pine bark was a source of flavonoids, which enhances the vital functions of the vitamin C.   These are the nutrients that are lacking in a diet lacking in fresh food, fruits and vegetables which can result in scurvy.

Pycnogenol (Maritime Pine Tree Bark) is a blend of special bioflavonoids, called proanthocyanidins.   Another good source of proanthocyanidins has been found in the Grape seed. Proanthocyanidin, a powerful anti-oxidant,   reduces free-radical caused tissue damage, is many times more effective than vitamin E, C, Carotene, Selenium or any other known source of flavonols. Pycnogenol brings out the health-giving effects of vitamin C and protects brain and nerve tissue with its unique ability to penetrate the blood-brain barrier and protect the brain cells.

Free radicals are toxic by-products of the body's natural metabolic processes that cause oxidative damage to cells and tissues. In addition, environmental factors add to our free-radical burden.   These include: alcohol, cigarette smoke, air and water pollutants, pesticides used in gardening, fried foods, household cleaners, radiation, anesthetics, physical or emotional stress, coffee, ultra-violet rays from tanning lamps, microwave ovens, electro-magnetic fields and power lines.

Always keep in mind that anything that improves health in one area, improves the health of the entire body by way of the blood vascular system due to the improved quality of the blood. The blood must contain all of the necessary life-giving and life-sustaining properties. The blood traverses through the body in from two to four minutes. Thus, a rich supply of proanthocyanidins can reach every cell in our bodies to do their life-saving and life sustaining duties.

Pycnogenol (Proanthocyanidin) has been found to reduce inflammation while improving circulation of the blood.   This makes it effective as an aid to treat arthritis. It can be useful in the treatment of those suffering from pain due to diabetes.

Pycnogenol works to reduce inflammation of the lymphatic system, thereby making it useful in improving the blood vascular system.   The result of this, is improved conditions resulting in lessening distress due to arthritis and diabetes. Bioflavonoids have the ability to provide the substance of life that will help rebuild the system by supplying the anti-oxidants that reduce free radical scavengers that cause aging, which result in an improved condition that may avoid problems that often lead to strokes or other cardiovascular problems or eventually cancer.

Pycnogenol has cosmetic value due to its ability of attacking free radicals, which makes it an anti-aging tonic. It has been said to function as an oral cosmetic.

• All plants have pigments (color). Pigments are primarily the result of Bioflavonoids. The brilliant red and purple colors are due to Proanthocyanidins.

• For the absorption of vitamin C in the intestinal tract, it is essential that bioflavonoids be present. One of the function of bioflavonoids is to assist vitamin C in maintaining collagen which is the binder that holds cells intact in a natural condition.

• It is essential for anti-oxidants to be present, in order to keep vitamin C and adrenaline from being oxidized.

• Bioflavonoids have a natural chelate process, which can remove, for example, such heavy metals as copper from the blood.

• Weak capillary cells will leak blood fluid out rather than allow it to be selectively processed back into the blood vascular system. Pycnogenol improves the quality of tissue, thereby maintaining the system to resist leakage.

• Pycnogenol will remain active in the system for about three days. Within that period, what is diffused into the blood by osmotic action, is circulated into the body fluids and is retained by the collagen (the framework of the tissue). It is further dissipated during this period through the lymphatics, perspiration, kidneys and urine.

• Pycnogenol has a low pH and is therefore acidic. The pH of a normal healthy stomach is acidic. When food is introduced into the system, it is usually neutral, with a pH around 7.0 and the system works to reduce the food intake and return the stomach to its original acidic state.

• Dr. J. Masquelier of the University of Bordeaux isolated and identified Proanthocyanidin and characterized the product called Pycnogenol. He, in fact, invented the name Pycnogenol to denote the highly bio available, water soluble, class of bioflavonoids which he had discovered.

• Pycnogenol inhibits the natural enzymes of the body. All cells in the human body are glued together with collagen. By restoring collagen, Pycnogenol helps return flexibility to skin, joints, arteries, capillaries and other tissues.

• An important function of Pycnogenol is that it inhibits inflammation caused by free radical enzymes. It helps maintain the arterial tissue by reducing histamine production. The effect is that mutagens are resisted, improving the elasticity of the arteries; thus, cardiovascular degeneration may be arrested and with an intake of the vital nutrients, regeneration of tissue takes place.

• One of the primary constituents of Pycnogenol is catechin, which is well known for its anti-oxidant properties. Catechin helps support collagen.

• Another quality of Pycnogenol is that it helps maintain circulation, which improves nourishment necessary for tissue health. This makes it valuable for those who suffer from diabetic problems, stroke victims and helps alleviate congestion resultant from smoking or other substances like drugs.

• Pycnogenol helps rebuild tissue cross-links to reverse some of the damage done over the years by injury and free radical attacks.

• Pycnogenol strengthens the entire arterial system and

improves circulation. It reduces capillary fragility and develops skin smoothness and elasticity.
• Pycnogenol stimulates collagen-rich connective tissue against atheroscleroisis and helps joint flexibility in arthritis.
• Pycnogenol has been used successfully for diabetic retinopathy, varicose veins, and hemorrhoids. It is one of the few dietary anti-oxidants that readily crosses the blood-brain barrier to directly protect brain cells and aid memory.

ALLERGIES
ARTHRITIS
ATHEROSCLEROSIS
BRAIN DYSFUNCTION
CANCER
CIRCULATORY PROBLEMS
Edema
DIABETIC RETINOPATHY
Hayfever
HEART DISEASE

Memory
Osteoarthritis
Phlebitis
Rheumatoid arthritis
Skin eruptions
SPORTS INJURIES
STRESS
Varicose veins
Viruses

PLANTAIN   (Plantago spp.,)
A.K.A.,: Common Plantain, Ripple Grass, White manfoot, Cuckoo's bread.

BODILY INFLUENCE: Alterative, Anti-inflammatory, Antiseptic, Anti-spasmodic, Anti-syphilitic, Anti-venomous, Aperient, Astringent(mildly), Demulcent, Deobstruent, Depurant, Diuretic, Emollient, Expectorant, Mucilant, Parasiticide, Refrigerant, Styptic, Vulnerary.
PART USED: The whole plant.

Plantain was known as the "Mother of Herbs," by the Anglo-Saxons, by the English herbalists as "All-Heal,, and by the native American Indians, the Navahos, as "Life Medicine". Plantain is among the most common plants in the world. The action of Plantain is it tonifies mucous membranes, reduces phlegm and is good for topical healing.
A characteristic of Plantain is that the outer layer of the seed contains mucilage which swells up when exposed to moisture, making the seed valuable in controlling cholesterol levels. The seeds and leaves have the effect of reducing the intestinal absorption of the bile acids. Where Plantain is used as an appetite suppressant, it has been found that the cholesterol levels are lowered. This moisture absorbing ability of the Plantain seed, when ingested, will swell and fill the intestinal tract, as does Psyllium seed hulls and by the mucilage mixing with and adhering

to the intestinal contents, helps prevent cholesterol absorption.

Plantain mucilage added to the diet significantly lowers serum cholesterol levels. Taken before meals, Plantain causes a marked decrease in triglycerides and beta cholesterol (bad guys) with a related balanced increase of serum levels of alpha cholesterol (good guys). It has been conjectured that Plantain works by filling and coating the stomach thus, reducing the appetite, which limits caloric intake by reducing the absorption of fats.

In herbal combinations, Plantain adds superior mucilaginous qualities that provide healing properties not possessed by other mucilaginous herbs. There have been reported some miraculous results in the treatment of poison ivy and poison oak dermatitis. When applying the crushed Plantain leaves on the effected areas, the itching stopping almost immediately and did not return. It provides a soothing mucilage, beneficial for internal problems symptomatic of the urinary tract and for external relief of inflamed and painful mucous membranes. Plantain is the cooling balm to balance astringent actions of the other herbs in the particular compounds.

The use of Plantain was a favorite of early American physicians in treating skin problems and is still being used successfully today. Chronic bronchitis has been treated with Plantain today with good results, symptomatic relief of pain, coughing, wheezing and irritation, being obtained.

As an independent single herb, Plantain is helpful in treating female disorders with fluent discharges. It is used to treat hemorrhoids, snakebites and coughs. Plantain is an excellent remedy in kidney and bladder problems and an effective remedy for poisonous bites and stings. The poison of fresh stings is extracted rapidly (often within an hour's time) by the use of a Plantain poultice.

Plantain is also an excellent herb for treating blood poisoning, as it reduces the swelling and completely heals, as in cases where dangerous poison seems to have made amputation imminent. Plantain is known to ease pain and facilitates the healing of problems in the lower intestinal tract. The actions of the main glycoside of Plantain, aucubin, helps heal bladder infections and stomach ulcers. An important constituent of the leaves in the Plantago genus is tannin and is an astringent which tightens tissues.

The herb Plantain is not to be confused with the cooking banana, Plantain. The plantain banana gets its name from the Spanish platano, meaning 'plant tree' or 'banana tree.'

- Plantain is helpful for incontinence in children and the aged.
- Plantain's astringent properties make it useful to stop bleeding and to promote the healing of wounds and injuries.
- It is an excellent poultice for wounds, burns and skin irritations.

- It absorbs toxins from the bowel, soothes inflamed tissues and promotes normal bowel function.
- Plantain herb is an excellent remedy for cuts, skin infections and chronic skin problems.
- It is useful for infections, including such ailments as hemorrhoids and inflammations.
- The New England Journal of Medicine printed an account of the successful use of crushed Plantain leaves to stop the itching of poison ivy.
- The root can be chewed to ease the pain of a toothache.
- Plantain works to rid the body of poisons, or excess body fluids such as mucus.

Back pain (lower)
BEDWETTING
BLADDER INFECTIONS
BLEEDING
BLOOD POISONING
Blood purifier
Boils
Bronchitis
BURNS
Cholesterol (reduces)
Colitis
Coughs (dry)
Cuts
Cystitis
DIARRHEA
Douches
Dysentery
Edema
Epilepsy
Eyes (sore)
Female problems
Gas
HEMORRHAGES (EXTERNAL)
Hemorrhoids
Incontinence (children)
Infections
Insect bites/stings

Jaundice
KIDNEYS
Leucorrhea
Lungs
Menstruation (excess)
NEURALGIA
Pain
Phlegm (reduces)
Poisoning
Respiratory problems
Scalds
Skin infections
Skin irritations
SNAKE BITES (NON-POISONOUS)
SORES (OPEN)
Stomach problems (chronic)
Toothache
Toxins
Ulcers (stomach)
Urinary tract infections
Uterine infections
Vagina
Venereal disease
Wheezing
Worms
WOUNDS (CHRONIC)

PLEURISY ROOT   (Asclepias tuberosa)
A.K.A.,: Butterfly Weed, Wind Root, Colic root, Silkweed.

BODILY INFLUENCE: Anodyne, Anti-spasmodic, Carminative(mildly), Cathartic(mildly-large doses), Diaphoretic, Diuretic, Emetic(large doses), Expectorant, Nervine (slightly sedative), Stimulant, Tonic.

PART USED: Root.

Pleurisy root was in use before the Europeans arrived on this continent. It was used primarily for its special benefits in regard to the lungs hence, the name Pleurisy. Pleurisy root is used in treating lungs, to include such conditions as pleurisy, pains in breathing (mostly any intercostal muscle congestion (intercostal neuralgia) or an inflamation of the pleural cavity, the common cold, flu, pneumonia, acute bronchitis and chest congestion with thick mucus and fevers accompanied by a tight chest conditions.

Pleurisy root, often known as butterfly weed because monarchs, swallowtails and other butterflies are especially attracted to the plant when it is in flower.

Pleurisy root was held in high esteem by the North American Indians as one of the best gifts to the children of nature by the Great White Father, due to its wonderful powers to bring about healing of the lungs.

As mentioned earlier, Pleurisy root has a powerful diaphoretic action which first increases the body temperature which in turn, opens the pores and sweating follows. Pleurisy root opens up the lung capillaries, which action helps release any thick mucus, thinning it for easier discharge of the congested material and also allows for some reabsorption back into the blood vascular system to be better discharged through the normal avenues of elimination, which is the skin, kidneys and bowels. Due to its lung circulatory improvement, it eases chest congestion which reduces painful breathing.

In all cases of lung disease such as lung congestion and pneumonia, there is a great danger of so filling up the lungs with body fluid waste (pneumonia) as to literally drown the patient in their own fluids that is a result of the bodies. need to cleanse itself of this debris, thus the need of Pleurisy root and common sense treatment, such as colonics or numerous high enemas, hot baths etc. to help aid in the elimination of these excess body toxins.

A good treatment plan well should include the:
1. high intake of liquids,
2. the taking of high enemas
3. artificial sweat baths to increase body temperature and to induce free perspiration to rid the body of any excess fluid material with their accompanying body toxins.

4.Along with taking Pleurisy root, taking several grams of vitamin C with bioflavonoids daily and other vitamins and necessary herbs would be most helpful.

Specific action on the lungs by Pleurisy root, subdues inflammation, loosens phlegm and exerts a mild tonic effect on the system relieving the pain and the difficulty of breathing.
Due to its relaxing diaphoretic action, Pleurisy roots use should not be for those with a weak pulse and cold skin. Yarrow would be the herb of choice to use, due to its more stimulating diaphoretic action.

Pleurisy root stimulates expectoration and with a large increased use of liquid, it subdues inflammation, bringing about some reabsorption of fluids from the lungs. It has a tonic effect on the whole system.
• Pleurisy root is useful for calming spasms and relaxing the body.
• Pleurisy root increases urine secretions and perspiration.
• Pleurisy root is effective in the treatment of bronchial and respiratory ailments, to break up congestion due to colds, flu, chest congestion etc.
• Pleurisy root is an effective pulmonary catarrhal expectorant which clears the lung tissue to improve oxygen intake when breathing is difficult and relieving difficult pain of breathing.

ASTHMA
BRONCHITIS
Circulation
Colds
Colic
Contagious diseases
Coughs
Croup
Diarrhea
DYSENTERY (ACUTE)
EMPHYSEMA
FEVERS
Flu
Kidneys

LUNG CONGESTION
Measles
Mucus
Perspiration
PLEURISY
PNEUMONIA
Poisoning
Rheumatism (acute)
Scarlet fever
TUBERCULOSIS
Typhoid fever
Typhus
Water retention

POKE   (Phytolacca decandra)
A.K.A.,: Pokeroot.

BODILY INFLUENCE: Alterative, Anodyne, Antibiotic, Anti-inflammatory, Anti-rheumatic, Anti-scorbutic, Anti-syphilitic, Anti-tumor, Cathartic, Emetic, Parasiticide.
PART USED: Root and berries.

   Poke root demands a strong statment as to it use.   In the first place, there is the attractive due to its great variety of uses of achieving quick popularity.   It is beneficial only if used in a very precise manner.   The fact of the matter is that in review of the the positive beneficial uses that it has been accredited it, one could easily come to an erronous conclusion and that is, that this herb could be used for almost anything and should be.   This is not the case due to the very powerful potency that the herb possesses and great care is demanded when considering its use.
   Poke root is a powerful emetic and purgative.   Only small amounts should ever be used and mainly in combination with other herbs. Poke root's preparation in the drying process requires special expertise.
   According to some herbalists, Poke is considered to be a good blood and lymphatic purifying herb. It is said to be excellent for the treatment of cancer, tumors, arthritis and degenerative diseases, but, should be used with respect and preferably in combinations with other herbs and in a formula with the proper herbs, that will combine to tone down its powerful effects and blend its stimulative detoxifying qualities.
   Poke root is highly regarded by herbalists for its cleansing and stimulating effects upon the glandular system and is used for a variety of glandular ailments, from swollen, inflamed and congested glands to disorders of the breast, including cysts and tumors.
•   The herb comes from the root of the Poke plant.   It has cleansing and healing qualities that will effect the whole body.
•   The Poke plant is especially good for dissolving tumors by cleansing the tissues though the blood vascular and lymphatic systems. This will also result in the cleansing and removing of boils, sores, etc. It has been used to treat some venereal diseases with good effect also.
•   Poke root has a variety of uses basically due to its tonic effect upon the lymphatic system. By cleansing the lymphatic system, it works as a stimulant for the body to help remove collected waste material congested in the tissues throughout the body, while also improving lymphatic and blood vascular elasticity in such organs as the liver that has experienced hardening, due to its congested condition.
•   Poke root has been found useful in reducing inflammation,

making it helpful in the pain control of rheumatism.
- Poke root helps with fungal infections and is also helpful in removing the cause of scabies, eczema and acne internally, as well as to be used externally as a salve.
- Poke root is also useful as a poultice to treat abscess conditions such as boils and sores and to relieve difficult urination by using a poultice over the bladder area. It is also a useful poultice for breast tumors and caked breasts.
- This herb is used as a drastic measure and should not be used as the herb of choice when there is another milder acting herb that will meet the need.
- This herb does all the things that has been written here, but its action is far too harsh for anything less than a dire emergency and then should only be used as directed by a highly experienced herbalist or knowledgeable Health Professional.

CAUTION: This plant is very powerful in its action and should only be used in very small amounts, in herbal combinations and in a knowledgeable fashion, under professional supervision.

ARTHRITIS
Back pain (lower)
Blood cleanser
Boils
BREASTS
Bursitis
CANCER
CATARRH (CHRONIC)
COLDS
ECZEMA
GLANDS
Goiter
Hemorrhoids
INFLAMMATION
Laryngitis
LYMPH GLANDS
MUCUS
Mumps
PAIN
Parasites (skin)
Psoriasis
Respiratory problems
RHEUMATISM
Scrofula
Skin diseases
Tonsillitis
Wounds

PRICKLY ASH   (Zanthoxylum americanum)
A.K.A., Toothache bark, Angelica Tree, Yellow Wood.

BODILY INFLUENCE: Alterative, Antiseptic, Antispasmodic(mildly), Astringent, Carminative, Deobstruent, Diaphoretic, Diuretic, Emmenagogue, Nervine, Rubefacient, Sialagogue, Stimulant(cardiac), Tonic.
PART USED: Root, Bark, Berries.

As with so many of the healing herbs, there are similarities in their uses with some being more powerful in their results but being used for the same complaints. So it is with the Prickly Ash. Prickly Ash is best used in combination with other herbs.

In 1849-50, there was an outbreak in America of a serious epidemic called Asian Cholera. It was discovered, at this time, that there was an herb out there that could reverse the symptoms of this disease. That herb was Prickly Ash Bark. Prickly Ash bark is in use today, being the main ingredient in the Hoxsey formula for cancer. Prickly Ash bark has also been used in treating syphilis.

The berries of the Chinese variety of Prickly Ash are known as brown peppercorns or Szechuan peppers which is used in Szechuan cooking. American Indian tribes from the northeast used Prickly Ash as an expectorant, cold remedy, toothache remedy and all-round panacea.

Prickly Ash is an excellent herb to use for increasing the general circulation. This lends it to being used in a great many problem areas, due to the fact that everything is dependent on good circulation. It has been used with success to increase peripheral lymphatic and blood vascular circulation and used to treat paralytic conditions.

Prickly Ash has a mild central nervous system stimulating effect which aids it in improving circulation. It helps with leg cramping which is due to deficient blood and lymphatic circulation, also helping with varicose veins. It is used externally and internally for rheumatism, stomach pain and even skin diseases. Further, due to its circulation enhancing qualities, it is used for joint problems and rheumatic complaints, due to tissue accumulations, usually uric acid.

Prickly Ash can be helpful in a great many conditions such as stimulating saliva, relieving toothaches and is a booster for convalescing patients. It is good as a blood purifier and as such, helps improve the healing of slow healing wounds. Prickly Ash has been found useful in treating skin diseases. It helps improve weak digestion, colic and stomach cramps by warming the stomach through improved circulation.

It is said that the stimulatory action of Prickly Ash is slower than Capsicum but has a longer lasting action and is more permanent. It is effective in opening up obstructed areas in all parts of the body and has helped with rheumatic fever.

Prickly Ash bark promotes general perspiration, invigorates the stomach and strengthens a sluggish digestive system. Prickly Ash is good to combine with other remedies when trying to break fevers. Powdered Prickly Ash bark is used successfully as an application on slow healing ulcers and old wounds. It has a drawing action that stimulates and cleanses the wound, dries it up and allows it to heal.

• Prickly Ash increases blood circulation throughout the body. It is beneficial where poor circulation causes soreness or pain to

the bones or joints.
- Prickly Ash can be applied as a poultice which will improve the healing of wounds, removing infected debris as it cures.
- Prickly Ash is known to help increase the flow of saliva. It will help to eliminate dryness of the mouth and tongue, when such conditions are caused by liver malfunctions.
- Prickly Ash is also useful in paralysis of the tongue and mouth.

Arthritis
Asthma
Blood purifier
Cholera
CIRCULATION (POOR)
Colic
Cramps
Digestion (weak)
Diarrhea
Dropsy
Female problems
FEVERS

Gas
Lethargy
Liver problems
MOUTH SORES
PARALYSIS
Rheumatism (chronic)
Scrofula
Skin diseases
Syphilis
Typhoid
ULCERS
WOUNDS

PSYLLIUM   (Plantago psyllium, P. ovata, Psyllium ovata)
A.K.A.,: Fleaseed, Fleawort.

BODILY INFLUENCE: Absorbent, Demulcent, Lubricating Bulk Laxative, Mucilant. (The outer husks are used as a bulk-fiber laxative and are not as irritating as the seeds while the whole seed is a lubricating laxative.)
PARTS USED: Seeds and Husks(Hulls).

Psyllium comes from the Greek word 'psylla' meaning a flea, because the seed resembles a flea.

Psyllium is a bulk laxative that increases the volume of the intestinal contents. The major component of Psyllium is mucilage. The seeds and the husk are hydrophilic bulking agents which swell several times greater than their original size in water. This increased bulk creates a stretching action on the wall of the intestine that stimulates peristaltic activity in the bowel.

The indigestible mucilage (active principle) is found both in the whole seed and the husk and swells when it comes in contact with water. This property has been used in diet aids to fill the stomach and intestines, as a bulk laxative and also works in diarrhea by forming a bulk that will slow down rapid, loose stools. Its drawing action makes it a good base for an internal poultice.

When Psyllium is taken with water or liquids and when six

cups or more of fluid are taken with Psyllium in a day, the Psyllium acts as a bulking laxative by swelling in the intestinal tract. This aids in standardizing the habitual bowel movement, preferably a bowel movement with each normal sized meal.

If less fluid is taken in, the Psyllium will have to draw moisture from the gastrointestinal (GI) tract and its tissues, thus becoming astringent in action, which will further (block) constipate an already (blocked) constipated condition.

The mechanism involved is this procedure is that each seed of Psyllium has a husk (a thin, white translucent membrane). These husks are tasteless and without any odor, but when soaked in water, increase to 8 to 14 times their original size. This is due to the presence of mucilage, a complex carbohydrate that attracts and retains water.

Psyllium seeds are composed of from 10 to 30 per cent of their total weight as mucilage, which is present mainly in the husk. When used in this manner, Psyllium is a form of dietary fiber taken purposefully to add bulk to the intestinal tract. It should not be consumed by any persons while they are in a constipated state.

An important purpose of the normal functioning of the large bowel is to reabsorb moisture from the loose stool as it traverses the colon and delivers it to be discharged from the system in a semi-formed or a formed stool. The longer the contents of the colon are in the colon the drier they get and thus constipation results.

When used in this manner as a dietary bulking agent in the intestinal tract, Psyllium acts like both a soluble fiber, preventing cholesterol absorption and an insoluble fiber, a scrubbing, clinging substance going through the intestines and adhering to and cleaning out old putrified waste material.

In this process, the husks are most often employed since the seed germ contains oils and tannins which are undesirable in bulk laxative preparations. These preparations are often compounded with other agents that aid in this process and are designed not to spoil, but to have an extended shelf life. The whole ground psyllium seed, once the protective hull is broken, would spoil and the oils would become rancid due to the enzyme present in the whole raw seed.

The special asset of this compound or the raw hull is that, being a vegetable substance, it has a purely mechanical action, lubricating and cleansing the intestines simultaneously. Thus, there are no harmful side effects, either physiological or chemical.

This whole process is only safe to start after the bowels have had a thorough cleansing and start out open and mostly empty. Then it is to be remembered that at least two quarts of water (8 glasses) must be taken along with the Psyllium hulls, daily.

The Psyllium husks are a lubricating, mucilaginous, fibrous

herb with drawing, cleansing, laxative properties. The Psyllium husks acts as a "colon broom" for those suffering with chronic constipation. This process of the use, made by an intake of Psyllium seed hull, is effective for inflammatory diverticulitis, as a lubricant for ulcerous mucosal lining tissue, a balancer and regulator for digestive enzymes and colon bacteria.

To sum it all up again, taken properly internally, Psyllium helps overcome chronic constipation. Taken externally, Psyllium can, when using the whole psyllium seed, either whole or whole ground, and specially prepared, relieve skin irritations. Psyllium used as a poultice will draw out pus from boils, carbuncles and sores when used as a drawing agent, as an external poultice applications.

Psyllium has a unique action in the bowels as it can act as a demulcent or emollient, it can be used to either stop diarrhea or to do away with constipation, depending on the technique used. These hydrophilic bulking qualities have made it popular for weight loss programs as it fills the gastrointestinal tract with a bulk that is mostly calorie free, thus doing away with the urge to eat and helping to reduce excess weight.

In India, Psyllium has been used as a diuretic, and in China, related herbal combinations are used to treat bloody urine, coughing and high blood pressure, etc. These get results due to the healing abilities of the body when the colon waste is removed and the body is allowed to gain better health, which in turn aids in all bodily areas.

Psyllium used in the above described manner will relieve a physical condition described as autointoxication, in which the body due to an indecent intake of wrong foods and food combinations and other unhealthful habits, poisons itself by producing and reabsorbing an excess of intestinal waste products. The proper use of Psyllium, as described above, helps over a period of time to remove the offending substances. Health and well-being are the result of properly following these described procedures.

• Psyllium used in a proper manner, is an excellent cleanser for the intestines and colon. It also acts to lubricate, moisten and heal the intestinal tract.

• Psyllium is very moisture absorbing, so it is essential always to take over 8 glasses of water daily with it, as it expands, and it would be advantageous, even essential, to use an herbal laxative with it.

• Psyllium's soluble fibers prevent cholesterol absorption, It has insoluble fibers that have a scrubbing action as they pass through the intestines ridding it of old excess intestinal debris.

• Psyllium removes putrifactive toxins from the intestines, and adds bulk to the stool which absorbs toxins, soothes inflamed tissues, promotes the growth of friendly colon bacteria and

reduces transit time through the colon.
- Psyllium serves as a lubricant to the intestinal tract.
- Psyllium can be useful to promote elimination of material that is putrefying the colon and thus the body. It will absorb bile (which is liver waste) and move it through the intestines, removing toxicity which if left in the system promotes disease.
- Psyllium, when taken in a proper manner, lowers bowel transit time, it absorbs toxins from the bowel, it regulates colonic bacteria, it adds a demulcent(soothing, coating) to the digestive tract.
- The whole seed meal can be applied to the surface of the skin as a poultice to help relieve and heal skin irritations such as boils, swollen irritated areas etc..
- There has never been any record that can establish Psyllium seed as being toxic in any manner; however, problems could occur if a person has not received proper instructions on how to properly use it.

COLITIS
COLON CLEANSER
CONSTIPATION (PREVENTIVE)
Cystitis
Diarrhea (chronic)
DIVERTICULITIS
Dysentery

Gonorrhea
Hemorrhage
Intestinal tract
Irritable Bowel Syndrome (IBS)
Ulcers
Urinary tract

PUMPKIN   (Cucurbita pepo)
A.K.A.,: Pumpkin seeds, Field Pumpkin.

BODILY INFLUENCE: Demulcent, Diuretic(mild), Laxative, Nutritive, Parasiticide, Taenifuge, Vermifuge.
PART USED: Seeds.

The pumpkin in China, is a symbol of prosperity and health and is known as the "Emperor of the Garden". Pumpkin received its name from the Greek word pepon, meaning 'cooked in the sun.'
Intestinal parasitic worms have a strong dislike for pulverized Pumpkin seeds. Pumpkin seeds are effective when used as a treatment for tapeworm and round worm. It appears that the active principle is in the bitter and resinous envelope immediately encircling the embryo that is the most effective part in ridding the body of the intestinal worms. Pumpkin seeds can be eaten raw to be effective. Squash seeds are also helpful in eradicating intestinal parasites, but are not as effective as the Pumpkin seeds. Pumpkin seeds have a revitalizing effect upon the prostate gland

and acts as a stimulant to male hormone production.

Pumpkin seeds have a soothing effect in basic cystic inflammations resulting in irritating, scalding urination. The Pumpkin seed is a soothing diuretic and is effective as a treatment for an enlarged prostate. Pumpkin seeds have been known to be effective in alleviating nausea, motion sickness and are used as a 'male' tonic.

Pumpkin seeds are a rich natural source of Zinc and Magnesium. Magnesium has been successfully used by French doctors in the treatment of enlarged prostate glands.

The use of pumpkin seeds is partly due to a rare amino acid called myosin which is only found in the seeds of certain Cucurbita species. Myosin, which is the primary protein constituent of nearly all muscles in the body is important in the chemistry of muscular contraction.

• With the use of parasiticides such as Pumpkin or other similar functioning herbs, by removing the cause of problems in the particular organs involved (with the removal of the parasite), normal function of the organ can be restored if there has not been permanent damage. Parasites can cause problems and symptoms in the liver as well as cause problems in the pancreas, if invaded there. They can retard function, for example: if the pancreas is invaded, insulin production possibly could be impaired causing a diabetic situation. Removing the cause will restore the organ to normal function, if there has not been permanent damage.

• As a nutrient, Pumpkin seed contains nearly 4 times more beta-carotene than carrots.

• Pumpkin seed contains amino acids that are valuable to muscle action.

• Pumpkin seed is an excellent parasiticide.

Burns	TAPEWORM
Nausea	Urinary problems
Prostate problems	WORMS
Round worms	Wounds
Stomach problems	

PYGEUM (Prunus africana)
A.K.A.,: Pygeum Africanum.

BODILY INFLUENCE: Anti-inflammatory, Diuretic, Hormonal.
PART USED: Bark.

Pygeum is from the bark of a South African evergreen tree and is commonly used for prostate problems both in Africa and in Europe. Pygeum contains chemical compounds to include, plant-type steroids which reduce swelling and inflammation of the prostate.

The mode of function of Pygeum is that it blocks the entry and breakdown of cholesterol in the prostate, this tends to encourage the production of certain prostaglandins, which exhibits an anti-inflammatory action. Pygeum is the prescription of choice given by European doctors in cases of benign prostatic hyperplasia (BPH), which is the common prostate problem among American men. This is a condition that involves a congested, enlarged and inflamed prostate accompanied by diminished urine flow and an increase frequency of urination, especially at night.

Results in Europe have been very good and noticeable improvement has been achieved in as short as a few days, but can take several months of consistent faithful use. Pygeum can also be taken as a preventative (prophylactic).

Pygeum Africanum can be taken alone or in combination with Saw Palmetto and/or with many other suitable herbs that are known to be helpful in treating prostate problems. Pygeum is used as part of a combination to dissolve uric acid sedimentary formation and to prevent further sedimentation in the prostate. Improved circulation is always helpful to improve total body health and this is so, especially in the case of uric acid retention in the cellular tissue which causes arthritic calcification in the bodily and prostatic tissue.

PROSTATE GLAND (INFLAMMATION)

QUEEN OF THE MEADOW
(Eupatorium purpureum)
A.K.A., Gravel root, Joe-Pye Weed, Kidney Root.

BODILY INFLUENCE: Antibiotic(mildly), Antiseptic, Anti-lithic, Anti-rheumatic, Astringent, Carminative, Diuretic, Lithotropic(dissolves stones), Nervine, Relaxant, Stimulant, Tonic.
PART USED; Leaves, Root.

Gravel Root (Queen of the Meadow) was a remedy of choice among many Indian tribes. The common name of "Joe-Pye" was given in honor of a New England Indian healer who used it to induc profuse sweating and cured typhus.

Queen of the Meadow is a soothing herb for the urinary mucous membranes, it is a diuretic herb with the ability to dissolve stones and sediment, to help dissolve the systemic inorganic crystalline deposits in gout, rheumatism and arthritis.

Queen of the Meadow, due to its astringent tonic effect on the cystitic mucosa, is beneficial in cystitis that is associated with a heavy mucus formation.

Queen of the Meadow does not dissolve urinary calculi but does prevents the precipitation of uric acid crystals and as a diuretic stimulates their free elimination.

Queen of the Meadow is used for many urinary tract problems, especially those of a chronic nature including gravel or stone like substances in the urine, hematuria(blood in the urine) and frequent and nighttime urination. Gravel root (Queen of the Meadow) is also helps eliminate uric acid deposits in the joints and for edema.

Gravel Root or Queen of the Meadow is used as a therapeutic agent for the urinary-genital areas, it works on the kidneys, liver, bladder, prostate gland and uterus. It relaxes, stimulates, tones the pelvic viscera and mucous membranes (aiding in casting off any sediments settled on surfaces.

Queen of the Meadow is said to influence the whole sympathetic nervous system due to its nervine quallities Queen of the Meadow is used for rheumatism and gout. It increases the elimination of solids in the urine. Queen of the Meadow is used for edema and helps relieves lower back pain caused by kidney inflamation.

• Queen of the Meadow's common name, Gravel root, so named because of its effectiveness in loosening, dissolving and eliminating gravely sediment in the kidneys passageways.

• Queen of the Meadow has been shown to be an effective herb for rheumatic and gouty conditions caused by uric acid deposits in the joints. It is also beneficial im many other forms of inflammatory diseases.

• Queen of the Meadow influences chronic renal and cystic problems, where uric acid levels are high. As an anti inflamatory Queen of the Meadow encourages a reliable urine flow in cases where the urge is there, but the flow is not.

• In women, Queen of the Meadow (effects and affects the central nervous system to relieve any pain in the uterus during the menses. In India they use a related herb to treat diseases of the uterus and cancer of the womb.

Back pain (lower)	GRAVEL
BLADDER INFECTIONS	Headaches
BLADDER STONES	KIDNEY INFECTIONS
BURSITIS	Kidney stones
Childbirth (eases)	Menstruation (irregularities & pain)
Diabetes	Nervous conditions
Dropsy	NEURALGIA
Edema	Prostate problems
GALLSTONES	RHEUMATISM
GOUT	RINGWORM

Typhus
URINARY PROBLEMS
Uterine disease

Vagina
Water retention

RED CLOVER (Trifolium pratense)
A.K.A.,: Purple Clover, Wild Clover, Trefoil, Cow Grass.

BODILY INFLUENCE: Alterative, Antibiotic(mild), Anti-inflammatory, Anti-viral, Anti-fungal, Anti-microbial, Anti-neoplastic, Anti-spasmodic, Anti-tumor, Blood Purifier, Depurant, Diuretic, Expectorant, Female Tonic, Laxative, Nutritive, Sedative Stimulant(mild).
PART USED: Flowers, Leaves, Blossoms.

Red Clover has a long history of uses other than as a medicinal herb. Red Clover is valuable as fodder (food) and grazing for cattle, it is used as a soil-improving cover crop to restore and rebuild the soil and it is a source of nectar for honeybees. As with Alfalfa, Red Clover sends roots far into the ground. This makes possible for it to draw upon an abundance of nitrogen and minerals. Red Clover is also the State Flower of Vermont.

Medicinally, the elements of Red Clover contain one of the best mucus clearing sources in nature. Red Clover is an outstanding herb, beneficial for all varieties of cancer anywhere in the body. It has been known to be useful for both esophageal and breast cancer.

Nutritional scientists have discovered that Red Clover blossoms contain the trace element Molybdenum, that is now beginning to be recognized as a very essential nutrient in relatively minute quantities. Molybdenum plays an important role involving the discharge of nitrogen from our bodies. Molybdenum's essential trace accumulations are in the liver, kidneys, bone and skin. The Molybdenum, in Red Clover tops, helps the system to discharge nitrogenous waste, aids in cleansing the system of impurities and helps retard the spread of infection. Molybdenum affects the mammary glands by helping with lactation in nursing mothers. Chaparral also is known to contain trace amounts of Molybdenum. It is noted that when Molybdenum is added to iron supplements, it produces a more rapid hemoglobin formation than iron administered alone in people suffering from anemia. Molybdenum and iron possess the ability to form special antibodies of protection from rattlesnake, scorpion or any kind of bites or stings.

Red Clover, for over a 100 years in Europe and America, has been used to treat and prevent cancer, as sedative for whooping cough, as a diuretic to treat gout and as an expectorant. Red

Clover is a highly nutritious plant that has provided, as a dependable source, many vital nutrients, vitamins and minerals and is a dependable source of nutritive supplements for all forms of degenerative diseases. Red Clover's antibiotic qualities have shown it useful against several bacteria, including the tubercular bacilli.

Red Clover is an alterative agent for counter-acting scrofulous and skin diseases and as an external wash for boils, sores and acne. Red Clover an effective and reliable remedy for wasting-type diseases of weakly and delicate children. Fomentations and poultices of Red Clover have been used for cancerous growths. Dr. Harry Hoxsey, N.D., who started the first cancer clinic in Mexico, used Red Clover in his treatments. Red Clover is a liver stimulant and it activates the gall bladder. It also has a slight laxative effect on the system.

It is often used in bronchitis and it can best be taken as a warm infusion which helps cleanse and soothe bronchial nerves. Red Clover when used alone, has been known to ease arthritic pain by its ability to help rid the system of uric acid, which is considered by some as the main cause of arthritis.

- Red Clover is an excellent blood purifier and is beneficial for bathing sores in its tea.
- Red Clover has been used extensively in the treatment of cancer.
- Red Clover is the principal ingredient of the Hoxsey cancer formula.
- Red Clover mixed with Chaparral and Dong quai has also been effective in the treatment of cancer.
- Red Clover, due to its high content of several important nutrients, including vitamins and minerals, has become a dependable nutritive supplement in all forms of degenerative diseases.
- Red Clover is a tonic for nerves acting as a calmer for nervous exhaustion. It will strengthen the systems of delicate children. It is beneficial in wasting diseases, especially rickets, spasmodic affections and whooping cough, weak chests, wheezing, bronchitis, lack of vitality and nervous energy.

ACNE
AIDS
ANTI-CANCER
Arthritis (rheumatoid)
Appetite suppressant
Athletes foot poultice
BLADDER PROBLEMS
BLOOD CLEANSER
BLOOD PURIFIER

BOILS
BRONCHITIS
Burns
CANCER
Childhood diseases
Colds
Constipation
Coughs
Digestive

Eyewash
Flu
Gallbladder
Gout
Inflamed lungs
Kidney problems
LEUKEMIA
LIVER CONGESTION
Lymphatic congestion
Muscle cramps
NERVOUS CONDITIONS
Ovaries (strengthens)
PSORIASIS
Rectal irritation

Rheumatism
Scarlet fever
SKIN DISORDERS
Sores
SPASMS
Syphilis
TOXINS
Tuberculosis
TUMORS
Ulcers (skin)
Urinary problems
Vaginal irritation
Whooping cough
Wounds (fresh)

RED RASPBERRY (Rubus idaeus)
A.K.A.,: Garden Raspberry.

BODILY INFLUENCE: Alterative(mild), Anti-abortive, Anti-emetic, Anti-spasmodic, Astringent, Cardiac, Diaphoretic, Emmenagogue, Hemostatic, Laxative, Oxytocic, Parturient, Refrigerant, Stimulant, Stomachic, Tonic.
PART USED: Leaves, Fruit.

Red Raspberry, where mothers and babies are concerned, is an herb made in heaven. It can be taken throughout the pregnancy with good results. It builds tissue to the extent that it prevents tearing of the cervix of the uterus during birth. During childbirth, hemorrhaging is prevented, the contraction of the uterine muscles are regulated during delivery and it also reduces false labor pains prior to birth.

Red Raspberry leaves are high in iron and enrich early colostrum found in mother's milk. It also cleanses and prepares breasts for a pure milk supply for the nursing infant by cleansing and purifying the blood.

Red Raspberry was used by American Indians as an astringent. They used an infusion, of the root bark and applied it to the sore eyes. The fresh fruit of Red Raspberry was used for dissolving tartar on the teeth.

Red Raspberry can be used for children's stomachaches, diarrhea, dysentery, bleeding gums, mouth sores, as a sore throat gargle, an astringent for the flu and vomiting and as an effective eyewash for swelling or inflammation.

For centuries, crude raspberry leaves have been used to aid in morning sickness, and to ease many menstrual problems. It is also very useful for ridding the body of mucus. In cases of diarrhea, Red Raspberry, as an astringent, helps to control the bowels.

Raspberry leaves have been used to clean cankerous conditions of the mucous membranes throughout the body. Raspberry has been a long-established remedy for dysentery and diarrhea, especially in infants.

- Raspberry helps to promote painless and bloodless childbirth. It helps quiet nausea and acts to stop diarrhea, especially in children.
- Raspberry leaf can be taken throughout pregnancy.
- Red Raspberry leaves have a manganese content double that of any other herb, that would make it one of the richest sources of herbal manganese.
- Raspberry strengthens the walls of the uterus and the entire female reproductive system.
- Raspberry decreases profuse menstrual flow.
- Drinking Raspberry leaf tea helps relieve painful menstruation and regulates the flow.
- Raspberry leaf is a preventative for hemorrhaging during labor. It reduces false labor pains, makes delivery easier and relieves after-pains.
- Raspberry leaf tea increases and enriches milk for lactation.
- Raspberry leaf is soothing to the stomach and bowels and cankerous conditions of mucous membranes in the alimentary canal.
- Raspberry leaf is an excellent herb for children to use for cleansing colds, slowing diarrhea, easing colic and fevers.

NOTE: Red Raspberry has been used as a preventative for hemorrhaging during and after labor, reduces false labor pains, assists labor by stimulating contractions and relieves after-pains. Can be taken throughout the pregnancy.

AFTER-BIRTH PAINS
BOWEL PROBLEMS
Breast feeding (discomfort)
Bronchitis
Canker sores
CHILDBIRTH (PAINLESS)
Cholera
COLDS
Constipation
Coughs
Cystitis
Diabetes
DIARRHEA
DIGESTIVE DISORDERS
Dysentery
Eyewash
FEMALE ORGANS

FEVERS
FLU
GAS
HEART
Hemorrhoids
Indigestion
LABOR PAINS
LACTATION
Leucorrhea
Measles
MENSTRUAL IRREGULARITIES
MISCARRIAGE
MORNING SICKNESS
MOUTH SORES
MUCOUS MEMBRANES
NAUSEA
Nervous conditions

PREGNANCY
Prostate gland
Rheumatism
Sore throat
Stomach
Teething

Ulcers
Urinary problems
UTERUS (STRENGTHENS &
TONES)
VOMITING
Wounds

REISHI   (See Mushrooms)

RHUBARB   (Rheum palmatum, R. officinale)
A.K.A. Chinese rhubarb, Da huang, Turkey rhubarb.

BODILY INFLUENCE: Alterative, Anti-bacterial, Antibiotic, Anti-inflammatory(extract), Anti-microbial (extract), Anti-tumor, Astringent, Cathartic, Diuretic, Hypotensive (extract), Laxative, Digestive aid (small doses), Parasiticide, Sialagogue, Stomachic, Tonic, Vulnerary.
PART USED: Root, Stems.

Rhubarb, was imported from Europe to treat constipation, where its use as a laxative was the standard. Experience taught that due to Rhubarb's powerful action as a laxative, the amounts used should be carefully monitored and avoided by those with old intestinal problems, such as colitis. In China, it is the root known as da huang, which means 'big yellow' which is the the color of Rhubarb's tinctures and decoctions.

Rhubarb's effectiveness is controlled by the amount taken. When taken in small doses, it has a tonic effect as a blood builder and blood cleanser. Rhubarb can be used as a treatment for chronic blood diseases. It increases salivary and gastric flow, improves appetite and cleanses the liver by encouraging bile flow.

In large doses, Rhubarb is can be used for emptying the bowels thoroughly. Rhubarb supports the colon as a laxative in constipation and as an astringent in case of diarrhea.
• Rhubarb can be a gentle laxative, strengthens the gastrointestinal tract, and tones and tightens bodily tissues.
• Rhubarb is ideal for disorders of the colon, spleen and liver.
• Rhubarb is helpful to prevent and to eliminate hemorrhoids.
• Rhubarb, by its cleansing action, encourages the healing process of duodenal ulcers and enhances gallbladder function.

NOTE: This herb is laxative in nature and should be used sparingly or in combinations. It is not to be taken alone during pregnancy as it causes cramping and stomach griping.   Do not use the leaves as they are potentially toxic.

Amenorrhea	Headaches
Anemia	Hemorrhages (internal)
Boils	Hepatitis
Colitis	Jaundice
CONSTIPATION	LIVER PROBLEMS
DIARRHEA	Menstruation (promotes)
Digestion (aid)	Skin eruptions (boils/pustules)
Dysentery	Stomach
Dysmenorrhea	Ulcers (duodenal)
Gallbladder	Worms (ring/pin/thread)

ROSE HIPS   (Rosa canina)
A.K.A.,: Hip Tree, Wild Brier, Dog Brier.

BODILY INFLUENCE: Anti-microbial, Anti-pyretic, Antiseptic, Anti-scorbutic, Anti-spasmodic, Astringent(mild), Diuretic(mild), Laxative(mild), Nutritive, Stomachic, Tonic.
PART USED: Fruit.

"Rosa" originally comes from the Greek word "Roden" or red. It seems that the roses in ancient Greece were deep crimson.

For those alive and old enough to remember World War II, it should be no surprise to learn that there was a shortage of citrus fruit in England, due to the German submarine blockade of the British Isles. To offset the loss of Vitamin C, the British Government organized the country to harvest all the Rose Hips in England to be made into a Vitamin C syrup for the people, so as to prevent scurvy. This was the start of the use of Rose Hips as a therapeutic entity.

While the use of citrus has been the base of our knowledge on the subject of vitamin C, investigations have revealed that there are many other sources of that vitamin. It seems that one of the richest sources available today of vitamin C is Rose Hips.

It reportedly has 60 times more vitamin C than citrus fruit. As a matter of explanation, Rose Hip is the fruit of the rose which develops after the peddles have fallen off the blossom, as with any other fruit. Capsicum ranks well with Rose Hips in vitamin C content. Most of us are familiar with Linus Pauling and his vitamin C beliefs and his campaign to popularize it. He investigated its beneficial use in the treatment of disease and its essential use to maintain optimum health.

Large quantities of vitamin C can be most useful for a great many of the common diseases that we have today to include the common cold, flu, pneumonia and many other common complaints. Another good use of vitamin C can be as a cleansing, so as to avoid a disease problem before it happen by using a prophylactic dosage on a daily basis.

Vitamin C is related with bio-flavonoids and that it is most vital for them to be used together. Natural vitamin C and flavonoids are combined in nature. Rose Hips is rich in the bio-flavonoids and in vitamin C. The bio-flavonoids are vital to build and strengthen body tissues and are especially important in the building and maintaining of a good blood vascular system to include, preventing and healing of fragile capillaries.

Vitamin C is vitally necessary for every cell in our bodies, without which we could not maintain life for even one hour. Vitamin C is especially useful in herbal combinations designed for a variety of uses, such as general debility, exhaustion, gallbladder dysfunction, for kidney health, for tissue tone and balance, as a strengthening part of a diuretic formula and more. How wonderful that nature has provided these vital elements, vitamin C and the flavonoids, in so great an abundance in Rose Hips.

Rose Hips with its Bio-flavonoids and vitamin C combined together enhances the body.s ability to absorb vitamin C in those having difficulty in absorbing it.

Most of us understand the necessity of vitamin C, especially in regard to its anti-Scurvy properties and how the administration of the common lime (vitamin C) did away with the scurvy among the sailors of the British Navy and Marine services.

• Indians are reported to have used Rose Hips to treat muscle cramps. Vitamin C and bio-flavonoids, as in Rose Hips, could be used with good results for almost every named or unnamed disease or condition that there is.

• Rose Hips is the highest herb in vitamin C and contains the entire vitamin C complex to include bio-flavonoids.

• Rose Hips helps in preventing and in treating infections and helps to curb stress.

• Rose Hips has 60 times the vitamin C than is found in lemons.

• It has been reported by researchers that arteriosclerosis is a deficiency disease of vitamin C.

• Large doses of vitamin C from Rose Hips, have been known to cure cancer and in smaller doses has been a preventative in cancer.

ADRENAL GLANDS
ARTERIOSCLEROSIS
Bites
BRUISES
Bladder conditions
BLOOD PURIFIER
CANCER
CIRCULATION
COLDS
Colic
Constipation
CONTAGIOUS DISEASES
Coughs
CRAMPS
Diarrhea
Dizziness
Earaches
Emphysema
EXHAUSTION
FEVERS

FLU
Gastritis
MIGRAINE HEADACHES
Heart
Hemorrhoids
INFECTIONS
Jaundice
Kidneys
Kidney stones
Mouth sores

Nerves
NERVOUSNESS
PMS
Psoriasis
SORE THROAT
SORES
Stings
STRESS
Thirst

ROSEMARY   (Rosmarinus officinalis)
A.K.A.,: Compass-weed, Poplar Plant, Old Man.

BODILY INFLUENCE: Analgesic(mild), Anodyne, Anti-inflammatory, Anti-pyretic, Antiseptic, Anti-spasmodic, Aromatic, Astringent, Carminative, Diaphoretic, Nervine, Stimulant, Stomachic, Tonic.
PART USED: The whole plant.

During World War II, a mixture of Rosemary leaves and Juniper berries was burned in the hospitals of France to kill germs. The botanical name for Rosemary is from the Latin ros (dew) and marinus (of the sea), as the plant grows in great abundance near the seashore.

In ancient Greece, Rosemary was believed to strengthen the memory.   Due to this memory enhancement belief, it became popular for students of the time to wear sprigs of Rosemary in their hair while they studied. Thus to the Greeks, Rosemary became a symbol of remembrance.

Rosemary leaf is effectively used in Europe and in distant China to treat headaches, stomach pains, as an analgesic, smooth muscle stimulant, and is anti-malarial.

In the Middle Ages, in Europe, Rosemary was used to clear vision, to sharpen the senses, to help weak memory and to alleviate nervous ailments.   Rosemary tea is a long-standing folk remedy for nervous headaches. Rosemary stimulates capillary circulation bringing more blood to the cells, making Rosemary helpful in healing colds, sore throat and sluggish liver.

Rosemary tea can be used as a mouthwash to freshen the mouth. When mixed with Myrrh, it is good for bleeding gums. Rosemary is used to calm and soothe irritated nerves, upset stomachs and calms strenuous anxiety.

It has been found to be effective for digestive problems, is specific in headache and tension relief formulas, counteracts depression, is a specific nervine combinations that eases neuralgia, neuritis, tendinitis and muscle pain.

Rosemary is used in hair rinses to darken and retain original hair color and in shampoos or oils to control premature balding or as part of a sleep pillow to alleviate insomnia and restless sleep. Bees are particularly fond of Rosemary. Rosemary is an anti-oxidant herb and a strong brain and memory stimulant. Rosemary has been found to be effective as a circulatory conditioning agent and nervine in stress, tension and depression.

• Hair loss caused by oil and acid attacking the hair follicles can be prevented by a Rosemary rinse used after washing.

• Rosemary has been in use for many years as a heart strengthener that helps reduce high blood pressure.

• Rosemary can be used in any female problems and helps regulate the menses.

• Rosemary is a blood cleaner and an antiseptic. This makes it useful for treating pains in the uterus when bleeding excessively.

• When taken as a tonic, Rosemary will help to soothe the nerves and strengthen the nervous system.

• Rosemary is a good treatment for sores around the mouth.

• Rosemary tea has been effective as a mouth wash and an eye wash to clean eyes that are sore due to allergic irritation.

BALDNESS
BLOOD PRESSURE (HIGH)
BREATH (BAD)
Bruises
Circulation (improves)
COLDS
Colic
Convulsions
Coughs
Eczema
Edema
Eyewash
Female problems
Food poisoning
Gallbladder
Gas
Gout
Hair growth
HEADACHES(NERVOUS/
    MIGRAINE)

HEART TONIC
Hysteria
Indigestion
Infections
Insomnia
Joint inflammation
Liver
Memory
Menstrual problems
Nervous disorders
Prostate
Restlessness
Rheumatism
Scalp
Sores (open)
SPASMS (MUSCLE)
Sprains
Stings
STOMACH DISORDERS
Wounds (external salve)

SAFFLOWER   (Carthamus tinctorius)
A.K.A.,: American Saffron, False Saffron.

BODILY INFLUENCE: Alterative(mild), Analgesic, Anti-inflammatory, Carminative, Diaphoretic(mild), Digestive, Diuretic, Emmenagogue, Laxative.
PARTS USED: Flowers.

There are records in history of the medicinal use of Safflower dating back into the Middle Ages. A tonic of Safflower seed juice mixed with chicken stock or sweetened water was said to have been taken for constipation or respiratory problems. Safflower made up into a tea is used as a treatment for colds, flu and fevers. When it is taken as a hot tea it increases perspiration. It has also been found to have calming effect on hysteria.

Of recent times, the Oil of the Safflower has come into prominence as being one of the vegetable oils with the lowest cholesterol content. Research has established that an intake of polyunsaturated oils in man's diet lowers the level of blood cholesterol which reduces heart disease. Since it was discovered that animal fats in the diet raise the cholesterol blood level, a search was made among the vegetable oils, for the best oils to replace the animal fats in the diet and Safflower oil was found to have one of the highest percentage levels of polyunsaturated fatty acids of the oils tested.

Past history records that the Safflower plant was valued for its red and yellow dyes. It was used in rouge for centuries and also for dyeing silks.

Safflower flowers properly aged and with the oxygen exposure of the air combined with the volatile properties in the plant, develop a sugar-like compound that stimulates the production of adrenaline by the adrenal gland and also stimulates the pancreas to produce more insulin. This can be a life-saving event.

However, I'd like to add a word of caution here. If there is a problem with the pancreas to produce sufficient insulin for life's necessities and also with the adrenal gland in producing sufficient adrenaline and both can be stimulated to increase their present production, this can only be a temporary improvement, as these original symptoms are indicative of an insufficient supply of nutrients present in the blood to maintain the proper function of these organs.

The increase in the production of insulin and adrenaline by this herb indicates only a temporary increased production of insulin and adrenaline, (like sparking an almost dead battery). This extra time of improvement should be used to re-supply the blood's levels of these lacking necessary nutrients, so as to build up the health of the organs effected.   In this manner, herbs can be very beneficial in buying extra time to aid in restoring a healthy system.

- Safflower is used as part of an arthritis, gout or kidney stone formula to indirectly neutralize and dissolve uric acid deposits.
- Safflower is a bitter herb which helps digestion, improves colon function and helps with blood vascular cleansing.
- Combined in herbal formulas for women, Safflower helps stimulate congested, thick or obstructed blood flow in menses.
- Safflower was used as an effective wash for measles rash.
- Safflower is a part of a cholesterol lowering formula to remove plaque, and is used to help reduce blood cholesterol.
- It is beneficial as a mild and gentle bladder and bowel cleanser.
- Safflower is a soothing digestive tract healant for heartburn, diverticulitis and ulcer lesions.
- Safflower is used as part of a sports formula to reduce lactic acid build-up.
- Safflower is beneficial in treating and reversing a condition involving congested and stagnant blood, (poor blood circulation), blood clots and lower abdominal pains caused by blood congestion in women.
- Safflower helps to increase bowel functions and increase the flow of urine.
- Safflower produces perspiration and also can be used to promote menstruation and relieve gas.
- Safflower is the food the body uses for production of hydrochloric acid and to help eliminate uric and lactic acid from the system.
- For children's complaints such as eruptive diseases and fevers, Safflower has been found to be beneficial.
- Safflower removes phlegm from the system and clears the lungs, thus helping in pulmonary tuberculosis.
- Safflower increases the production and release of bile and is an excellent herbal source of unsaturated fatty acids.

Appetite (stimulates)
Arthritis
Boils
Bronchitis
Chicken pox
DIGESTIVE DISORDERS
FEVERS
Gallbladder problems
Gas
GOUT
HEARTBURN
Heart (strengthens)
Hyperglycemia
Hypoglycemia
HYSTERIA
JAUNDICE

Lactic acid
LIVER PROBLEMS
Measles
Menstruation
Mumps
PERSPIRATION
PHLEGM
Poison ivy
Psoriasis
SCARLET FEVER
STOMACH (ACID)
SWEATING
Tuberculosis
URIC ACID
URINARY PROBLEMS

SAFFRON   (Crocus sativus)

A.K.A.,: Spanish Saffron, Autumn Crocus.

BODILY INFLUENCE: Alterative, Anti-spasmodic, Aphrodisiac, Carminative, Diaphoretic, Emmenagogue, Rejuvenative, Stimulant.

PART USED: Flowers (stigma), Seeds.

Safflower is much more available than is Saffron which keep its price down, so it has been used as a substitute for Saffron. To the ancients, Saffron's yellow powder was considered a luxury item. The Greeks made what has been referred to as, a royal dye color with Saffron, as did the Chinese. Medicinally, Saffron has been used by the Chinese for such emotional problems as depression, shock and fright.

Cost wise, Saffron is considered to be very expensive, as herbs go, but in light of its vital qualities, being one of the finest blood vitalizers known, this more than makes up for its extra expense.

Saffron counteracts inflammatory conditions while at the same time, powerfully stimulates the circulation and regulates the spleen, heart and liver. Saffron combined with food, will aid assimilation into the deeper tissues.

Saffron is helpful to take for acid-burning digestive problems. Saffron helps the body to regulate the lactic acid and also allows the body to digest and assimilate correctly, its use of oils.

After exhaustive muscle action which results in an acid burning sensation in the deep muscles from lactic acid build up, Saffron is of great benefit. Saffron is also helpful in cases where there is kidney break-down and uric acid begins to accumulate along with lactic acid in the tissues. These are the conditions that lead up to the building of kidney stones. Gouty conditions are known to result from uric acid built up in the tissues. This happens more rapidly in a gouty or low blood sugar type individual and taking Saffron when eating meat temporarily stops the uric acid build-up. One who has this condition should look to changing their diet and learn how to better eat and live with out the use of any animal products.

In conditions of hypoglycemia and adrenal fatigue, there is a lack of the cortin hormone, there is a build up of lactic acid that results from fatiguing activities (over exercise).

Lactic acid build-up from over-exercise necessitates that the lactic acid in the muscles be removed or changed chemically. The usual route for this is that the lactic acid is picked up by the blood vascular system and transported to the liver where it is changed back into glycogen, (muscle sugar) to be used later for energy. The usual problem with lactic acid is that it accumulates in the muscles after strenuous activities and when the adrenals do not produce sufficient cortin hormone, this stops the nature's process and the lactic acid remains in the muscle tissues. Eventually, there is seepage into the abdominal cavity which is absorbed by stomach. This is not normal and digestion is interrupted resulting in an acid-burning stomach.

* Saffron has beneficial effects on the organs of digestion, the gallbladder and the liver.
* Saffron may be used interchangeably with Safflower, as an excellent blood purifier and builder and as an inflammatory reducer. It is a natural source of hydrochloric acid to help supply the needs of digestion as performed in the stomach. Saffron supplies necessary nutrients for improved blood sugar and fat metabolism.
* It can be used as a specific in a formula that acts as a blood and circulatory stimulant, that contains regulating benefits for the liver, spleen, kidneys and heart,
* Saffron is beneficial as a treatment for arthritis, gout, bursitis and kidney stone formulas.
* Saffron is used for its anti-inflammatory abilities and for better controlling an over supply of uric acid which binds organic calcium in the joints interfering with joint function.
* Saffron can be used as part of a sugar regulating formula for hypoglycemia, referring to its insulin balancing ability.
* It soothes and coats the membranes of the stomach and colon, it aids in chest congestion, relieves abdominal pain after childbirth, improves circulation, affects the heart and liver and promotes energy.
* Saffron is helpful in eliminating toxins through the skin, as it promotes perspiration.
* Saffron has been historically used for treating cancer.

Arthritis	MEASLES
Bronchitis	Menstruation (delayed)
Cancer	PERSPIRATION
Colds	PHLEGM
Conjunctivitis	Psoriasis
Coughs	RHEUMATISM
DIGESTIVE DISORDERS	SCARLET FEVER
FEVERS	Skin diseases
Gas	Smallpox
GOUT	STOMACH (ACID)
Headaches	SWEATING
Heartburn	Tuberculosis
Hyperglycemia	Ulcers (internal)
Hypoglycemia	URIC ACID
Insomnia	URINARY PROBLEMS
Jaundice	Uterine hemorrhages
Lactic acid	Water retention
LIVER PROBLEMS	Whooping cough

SAGE   (Salvia officinalis)
A.K.A.,: Garden Sage, Common Sage.

BODILY INFLUENCE: Anti-galactagogue (lactation inhibitor), Anti-pyretic, Antiseptic, Anti-spasmodic, Aromatic, Astringent, Carminative, Diaphoretic, Digestive, Parasiticide, Stimulant, Tonic(mild), Vulnerary.
PART USED: The whole plant.

As with many of the herbs that have been used in antiquity, Sage has its unique history. It was thought of as the herbal Saviour of mankind. As an indication of this, that has held over, is its Latin name "salvia" which means Saviour.   Sage's reputation from the past has also come with it. It is considered a memory strengthener and the promoter of the growth of wisdom. It has been thought of as associated with longevity and as restoring failing memories of the elderly.

Among its many uses has been its abilities to slow down the secretion of fluids which reduces excessive perspiration (night sweats) and excessive sweating of menopausal hot flashes. Sage is known to be useful for nervousness, trembling and depression.

Among the many uses of Sage is its ability to dry up mothers breast milk as practiced in some communities. It is used for dysmenorrhea, as a natural deodorizer, from the inside out, it is used in dyspepsia and as a gargle for sore throats. Sage lowers saliva flow by its astringent action causing a drying up of the mucus membranes of the throat.

Sage was used by the American Indians as a salve which they mixed with bear grease and used for healing skin sores.   They used its leaves to massage over their gums and teeth.   In their baths the Indians used it for rubdowns and as an infusion.

Sage in its many uses has been used by some for epilepsy, sleeping problems, dysentery, seasickness, colds, worms and a variety of simple things. If they had a problem, and there was nothing else to use, Sage being common was around so it got used for whatever it might be, and surprisingly many times it helped and so the word got out and others used it.

• The volatile oils and tannins in Sage no doubt account for its ability to dry up perspiration. The oils have antiseptic, astringent, and irritant properties. This is what makes Sage useful in treating a variety of problems such as sore throats, mouth irritations, cuts and bruises.

• Experiments in 1939 showed it had estrogenic properties, which may have some connection to the herb's reputed ability to dry up milk.

• Sage infusions have been used to color silver hair, and as a hair rinse to help return hair to its original color.

• It is also useful to quiet the nerves, relieve spasms and expel

worms from children and adults.
- Sage is credited with being a powerful antioxidant, it shrinks inflamed tissue and decrease perspiration, cleans old ulcers and sores.
- It is beneficial for mental exhaustion and strengthening the ability to concentrate. It improves memory and has been used to cure some types of insanity. As stated earlier, Sage was there, it was used and its reputation of abilities was enlarged.
- Sage is used as a lotion to heal sores and other skin eruptions. It will stop bleeding from wounds and may be useful as a poultice for tumors
- It has gained the reputation of promoting circulation to the heart.
- Sage is considered one of the best remedies for stomach troubles.
- Sage has even been employed as a spring cleaning, high mineral tonic herb, and as being effective to helping a weak digestion.
- It relieves the reaction to insect bites

BALDNESS
Bites
Bladder infections
Bleeding gums
Bleeding wounds
Blood infections
Brain (stimulates)
Bronchitis
Canker sores
Circulation
Colds
COUGHS
Cystitis
Dandruff
DIABETES
Diarrhea
DIGESTIVE DISORDERS
Dyspepsia
Epilepsy
FEVERS
Flu
Gas
GUMS (SORE)
HAIR TONIC
Headaches
Heart

Hoarseness
Insomnia
Kidney
LACTATION (STOPS)
Liver
Lung problems
Measles
MEMORY (IMPROVES)
Menstruation
Morning sickness
MOUTH SORES
NAUSEA
NERVOUS CONDITIONS
NIGHT SWEATS
Palsy
Pneumonia
Sex depressant
Skin disorders
SORES (CLEANS & HEALS)
SORE THROAT (GARGLE)
Stomach problems
Tongue (inflammation)
Tonsillitis
Ulcers (mouth & throat)
VOICE LOSS
WORMS (EXPELS)

ST. JOHNS WORT   (Hypericum perforatum)
A.K.A.,: Goatweed, Klamath Weed.

BODILY INFLUENCE: Alterative, Anti-bacterial, Anti-depressant, Anti-fungal, Anti-inflammatory, Anti-spasmodic, Anti-tumor, Anti-viral, Aromatic, Astringent, Diuretic, Expectorant, Nervine, Sedative, Vulnerary.
PARTS USED: The Herb, Tops, Flowers.

St. Johns Wort: According to legends surrounding St. Johnswort, it was espoused by St. John of Jerusalem who is said to have used it in the time of the Crusades as a battlefield balm for its abilities to clean and heal some terrible battle wounds. It is said to have worked so well that legends are built around it.

In accordance with the legend of wound healing during the Crusades, we find agreement in modern times. St. Johns Wort today has been found to be very beneficial in healing wounds and is especially good for dirty, septic wounds. St. Johns Wort has been used in cases of putrid leg ulcers, that nothing heals. Like the leach that was used not too many years ago for wound cleansing it does not destroy the healthy tissues and healthy cells but it cleans the dirt out of septic wounds. It helps reduce the inflammation in septic sores, in boils, in cellulite and lymphangitis.

The compound Hypericin was isolated from St. Johns Wort in 1942 and has been used as an anti-depressant for emotionally disturbed people. This tranquilizing quality from small quantities hypericin increase blood flow to stressed tissue. There is a reduced capillary fragility and enhanced uterine tone due to the increased Hypotensive blood flow.

The use of St. Johns Wort has been shown to demonstrate a side effect producing a photosensitivity. Hypericin is absorbed in the intestines and concentrates near the skin. An allergic reaction takes place when those with light fair skin are exposed to sunlight. That exposure causes tissue damage and in some cases death has resulted. While taking St. Johns Wort one should avoid strong sunlight whether the skin is dark or light. There is a photosensitizing substance produced under the skin by this exposure to sunlight that causes the skin to burn.

St. Johns Wort relieves pain, it has a sedative effect, it is used for treatment of neuralgia, anxiety and nervous tension. It can be applied as liniment or poultice to relieve pain, for treatment over the spine for relief of nervous diseases that are related to the spine, sciatica, neuralgia, rheumatic pains, as a lotion for pain relief, eases bruises.
• Among the uses for St. Johns Wort are a variety of conditions such as Chronic Fatigue Syndrome, and mental burnout.
• St. Johns Wort is used for control of viral infections, for

reduction and control of tumor growths, both malignant and benign.

• St. Johns Wort is also known to be useful for pulmonary complaints, bladder trouble, suppression of urine, dysentery, worms and nervous depression.

• St. Johns Wort acts to dissolve and remove tumors and also boils. It calms the nerves and increases the flow of urine.

• It is an excellent blood cleanser and blood purifier.

• St. Johns Wort is used to relieve phlegm obstructions in the chest and lungs. It is beneficial with bronchitis and is known to eliminate all signs of the ailment.

• It is known to be valuable for treating internal bleeding.

• St. Johns Wort is very good in chronic uterine problems and will correct irregular and painful menstruation.

• St. Johns Wort contains an alkaloid that is a heart and artery stimulant.

AFTER-BIRTH PAINS
Anemia
Anxiety
Appetite
BEDWETTING
Bites (insect)
Bleeding (internal)
Blood cleanser
Boils
BRONCHITIS
CANCER
Coughs
Depression
Diarrhea
Dysentery
Gallbladder
Gout
Headaches
Heart
Hemorrhage

Hysteria
Insomnia
Jaundice
Lower back spasms
LUNG CONGESTION
Melancholy
Menopause
MENSTRUATION (PAINFUL)
MENSTRUATION
   (REGULATES)
Nervous conditions
Palsy
Sciatica
Skin problems (external)
Spasms
TUMORS
URINATION (SUPPRESSED)
UTERINE CRAMPS
WORMS
Wounds

SARSAPARILLA   (Smilax officinalis)
A.K.A.,: Honduras Sarsaparilla.

BODILY INFLUENCE: Alterative, Antiseptic, Anti-syphilitic, Aromatic, Blood Purifier, Carminative, Diaphoretic, Diuretic, Hormonal, Tonic.
PART USED: Bark, Root.

The Sarsaparilla plant (Spanish zarza, 'bramble', and parilla, 'little vine') are native to the pacific coast of Mexico south to Peru.

Sarsaparilla alone or with sassafras are the herbs from which root beer is made. The flavor is the natural flavor of Sarsaparilla and its saponin content.

Heavy metallic contaminants form in the blood from the foul and corrupted air breathed in daily by millions of people in large metropolitan areas afflicted by smog.   Sarsaparilla is especially good for removing these heavy metals if taken properly.

Sarsaparilla bark and root aid the body in producing a greater amounts of the anabolic(without oxygen) hormones, testosterone, which is a hormone that will induce hair to grow, progesterone, a hormone that is normally produced by the ovaries in the female and cortisone.

Sarsaparilla's power is concentrated in the nerve fibers and tissue of the entire nervous system.   Plant alkaloids and the saponins in this herb are considered to be responsible for the softening of hardened dense tissue masses such as in Multiple Sclerosis.

• The alkaloid molecules of Sarsaparilla join themselves to microbes and weaken these disease producing organisms.

• Sarsaparilla is a blood purifying herb for nitrogen-based waste products such as uric acid.

• Sarsaparilla is used as a treatment for, liver problems, rheumatism, hormone excesses and skin disorders.

• Sarsaparilla is used to treat infants infected with venereal disease.

• Sarsaparilla is used as a natural steroid for the production of testosterone, this is particularly useful for body building as a source of the muscle building hormone.

• It is beneficial for the treatment of psoriasis and eruptive skin disorders.

• Sarsaparilla is an excellent antidote for poison.

• It is beneficial in relieving inflammation and gas and will increases the flow of urine. Also used to promote perspiration.

• Sarsaparilla is used in glandular balance formulas. It is known for increasing the metabolism rate and stimulates breathing in problems of congestion.

- By increasing circulation to rheumatic joints, Sarsaparilla is a remedy for gout.

Age spots	Impotence
Blood cleanser	JOINT ACHES
BLOOD PURIFIER	Liver problems
Boils	MALE HORMONES
Catarrh	Menopause
Colds	Mucus build-up
Dropsy	Perspiration
Eczema	Poison antidote
Edema	Prostatitis
Epilepsy	Psoriasis
Eyewash	Rheumatism (chronic)
FEMALE HORMONES	Ringworm
Fevers	SEXUAL PROBLEMS
Flu	SKIN DISEASES (ERUPTIONS)
Gas	Stress
Gonorrhea	Syphilis
GOUT	Urinary problems
Hair growth	Venereal diseases
Heartburn	Weakness (physical)
HORMONE REGULATION	Worms
HOT FLASHES	

SASSAFRAS (Sassafras officinalis, S. albidium)
A.K.A.,: Ague Tree, Smelling-stick, Cinnamonwood.

BODILY INFLUENCE: Alterative, Anti-rheumatic, Aromatic, Blood Purifier, Carminative, Diaphoretic, Diuretic, Emmenagogue, Parasiticide, Stimulant.
PART USED: Root, Bark.

As an item of interest, a mix-up of names in regard to the Sassafras Tree was when the Spanish first saw the tree in Florida in the 16th century they thought it was a Cinnamon Tree, thus the error continues in regard to one of the common names still in use for the Sassafras tree.

Sassafras has been used for hundreds of years as a tonic for the blood. The Nature is versatile and intuitive. It has been found that when the Sassafras plants mature in the spring, they contain mineral salts that can thin the blood to help man survive the hot summer months, and then when these same plants matures in the fall they develop mineral salts that thicken the blood, for those cold winter months. Sassafras is used to treat many kinds of skin diseases. It has been used to treat such venereal diseases as

Syphilis. It has been used to help with addictions to alcohol and tobacco.
• The Indians and early settlers used Sassafras for the treatment of Syphilis.
• The Sassafras roots, along with Sarsaparilla, are the original sources of natural root beer.
• The Sassafras root bark contains antiseptic properties making it a workable remedy for skin wounds and sores.
• Sassafras has been helpful for relief from the itching of poison ivy and poison oak.
• The gummy core of the branches of Sassafras has been used to soothe tired eyes.
• Sassafras stimulates liver action which clears toxins from the body making it excellent treatment for all internally caused skin disorders such as acne, eczema and psoriasis.
• After childbirth, Sassafras makes a good tonic.
• Sassafras by it blood cleansing abilities helps relieve pain brought on by inflammatory skin diseases and arthritic conditions, rheumatism and gout.
• An infusion of Sassafras roots is used by the Indians to bring down fevers.
• When used to purify the blood, Sassafras is usually combined with other alterative herbs.
• In helping to adjust the hormone balance in the body, the ingredients of Sassafras aids the pituitary gland in releasing an ample supply of protein.

NOTE: The oil is toxic and should never be taken internally for any reason.

ACNE
After-birth pains
BLOOD PURIFIER
Boils
Bronchitis
Colic
Cramps (stomach)
Diarrhea
Gas
Hair Growth
Kidney problems
Menstruation (painful)
OBESITY
Perspiration (increases)
Poison ivy/oak
PSORIASIS
Rheumatism
SKIN DISEASES
Spasms
Toothache
Varicose ulcers
WATER RETENTION

SAW PALMETTO   (Serenoa repens)
A.K.A.,: Windmill Palm, Sawtooth Palm.

BODILY INFLUENCE Anti-catarrhal, Anti-galactagogue, Anti-inflammatory, Antiseptic, Anti-spasmodic, Aphrodisiac(mild), Astringent, Diuretic, Expectorant, Hormonal, Nervine, Nutritive, Parasiticide, Sedative, Stimulant, Tonic.
PART USED: Berries.

Saw Palmetto is an old American tonic, dating to the Maya Indians or even further. John Lloyd, a famous early American medicinal botanist, observed that animals fed on these berries grew sleek and fat.

The Saw Palmetto berry when eaten has a noticeable effects on body weight, general health and disposition, tranquilization, appetite stimulation and reproductive organ health.

Saw Palmetto berries historically have been used to treat several related disorders of the genito-urinary system, including inflammation, rupture and blockage. These historical uses prompted European researchers to investigate the clinical use of Saw Palmetto berry extracts in BPH (benign prostatic hyperplasia). The educated guesses based on clinical findings concerning the cause of BPH is that testosterone levels build up in the prostate. Within the prostate, testosterone is converted to an even more potent compound (dihydrotestosterone). This compound causes cells to multiply excessively, which leads to prostate enlargement. Studies have shown that the fat-soluble Saw Palmetto berry extract prevents the conversion of testosterone to dihydrotestosterone.

In herbal combinations, Saw Palmetto's inclusion with other herbs, is to provide necessary nutritive that diabetes and other diseases of the glands and organs require. In combination with other herbs, Saw Palmetto helps stimulate the appetite, improve digestion and increase assimilation. As a nutritive tonic, Saw Palmetto functions to increase the size and secreting ability of the mammary glands, decreasing ovarian and uterine irritability.

Saw Palmetto berries act specifically on the enlarged prostate, reducing inflammation and pain. It increases the bladder.s ability to contract and expel its contents. Saw Palmetto is a specific in all formulas for male impotence, sterility and reproductive problems and to reduce inflammation and swelling of the prostate. Saw Palmetto is a urethra toning herb that increases blood flow to the sexual organs.

Saw Palmetto berries assist the thyroid to regulate sexual development, normalizing the activity of those glands and organs.
• Saw Palmetto is recommended in all wasting diseases because it has an effect upon all the glandular tissues.)
• Saw Palmetto is quieting to the nerves and acts as an

antiseptic.
- Saw Palmetto is claimed to increase the size of the breasts of women of childbearing age.
- Excessive mucus in the head and nose are relieved by Saw Palmetto, as well as the membranes of the throat, air passages and in cases of chronic bronchitis and lung asthma.
- Diseases of both male and female reproductive organs have been helped by Saw Palmetto.

Alcoholism
Asthma
Bladder
BREAST ENLARGEMENT
Bright's disease
Bronchitis
Catarrhal problems
Colds
Diabetes
DIGESTIVE AID
GLANDS
Frigidity
HORMONE REGULATION
Mucus discharge (head area)
IMPOTENCY

Infertility
Kidney diseases
Lung congestion
Nerves
Neuralgia
Obesity
PROSTATE GLAND
  (ENLARGEMENT)
REPRODUCTIVE ORGANS
SEXUAL STIMULANT
Sore throat
Urinary tract infections
WEIGHT GAIN (PROMOTES)
Whooping cough

SCHIZANDRA (Schisandra chinensis)
A.K.A.: Chinese (Wu Wei Zi).

BODILY INFLUENCE: Adaptogen, Antiseptic, Aphrodisiac, Astringent, Bitter, Expectorant, Sedative, Tonic (urogenital & hepatic).
PART USED: The berries.

As an astringent tonic, Schizandra strengthens the tissues and retains body energy. It is known as a calmer to the body and helpful in treating forgetfulness. It contains mild adaptogens, which regulate bodily functions and enables the body to handle stress. It is helpful with coughing, lung weakness, asthma, night sweats and prolonged diarrhea.

Schizandra is a cherished item among the Chinese women as a sexual enhancer and youth invigorator.

Schizandra is synergistic with Eleutherococus senticosus (Siberian ginseng) for anti-stress, weight loss and sports endurance formulas and aids in supporting sugar levels and liver function.

Schizandra improves digestion of fatty foods through its ability to cleanse the liver and increase the production of bile which then functions, when delivered to the G.I. tract, as digestant for splitting the fat in the food to fatty acids and glycerin. An improved utilization of the digested foods provides much improved blood and thus aids in setting up the atmosphere for healthy skin, problem free.

Schizandra allows the body to more quickly respond to stress, increases the body's capacity for work and decreases fatigue, increases blood circulation and bile production while lowering blood pressure. It increases the contraction of the heart muscle and the uterus. All the improved functions described above indicate one thing and that is improved digestion, which spells out better blood and thus better function.

• Schizandra as adaptogen herb increases the energy supply of cells in the brain, muscles, liver, kidney, glands, nerves and in the entire body.

• It is an adaptogen herb in that it promotes long life of the cell.

• Schizandra is capable of building the body's immune system and supporting the body against damage due to stress.

• It contains the capability to increase energy, strengthen the veins and relax the muscles of the eye, thereby, improving vision.

• Schizandra protects against free radical damage.

• It aids in balancing body functions, normalizes body systems and is effective in post surgery well being and recovery.

• Schizandra can protect against radiation, counteracts the effects of sugar, boosts stamina and also protects against infections.

AGING (ANTI)
Anxiety
Arteriosclerosis
Asthma
Blood pressure (normalizes)
Coughs
DIABETES
Diarrhea (chronic)
Digestive problems
Dropsy
Edema
ENERGY (INCREASES)
Exhaustion (nervous)
FATIGUE
Gastritis (chronic)
Heart palpitation
Hepatitis

IMPOTENCY
Insomnia
Infections
Kidney problems
Lung problems
MENTAL ALERTNESS
Motion sickness
NERVOUS DISORDERS
Night sweats
Radiation
Seminal emission
Skin conditions (allergic)
STRESS TONIC
Urination (frequent)
Uterine problems
Vision (improves)

SCULLCAP (Scutellaria lateriflora)
A.K.A., Mad Dogweed, Helmet Flower, Madweed.

BODILY INFLUENCE: An-aphrodisiac, Anti-bacterial, Anti-convulsive, Anti-pyretic, Anti-spasmodic, Aromatic, Astringent(slight), Diuretic(somewhat), Nervine, Sedative, Tonic.
PART USED: The whole plant.

The popular and generic name is derived from the Latin, "scutella' meaning a small dish in reference to the shape of the appendage to the flower, which resembles a cap in appearance, thus the name Scullcap. Scullcap was given the common name of mad Dogweed, as it was considered in olden times to be a remedy for hydrophobia (rabies).

Scullcap calms the nervous system without narcotic properties, quiets the person and often brings about, natural sleep. Dr. Shook said, "Scullcap is a slow-working, but sure remedy for practically all nervous affections, but it must be taken regularly over a long period of time to be a permanent benefit."

Scullcap's sphere of influence is on the central and sympathetic nervous systems. Many herbalist's will tell you that Scullcap is the best nervine. It acts through the cerebrospinal centers and sympathetic nervous system to control most nervous irritations. Scullcap has been used for nervousness and neuralgia and is known to have been used as an excellent nerve tonic. It gives the feeling of well being and inner calm allowing relaxed sleep.

It is an effective herb to ease the problems associated with drug and alcohol withdrawal and drug use. It has detoxification properties that tends to lessen the severity of such withdrawal symptoms as delirium tremers.

Scullcap is well noted for its abilities in spasmodic afflictions as with St. Vitus's Dance (involuntary jerking motion), epilepsy; etc., acting to quiet the nerves. Scullcap can be used in neurasthenia, a disease following depression in which the individual suffers from chronic exhaustion.

• Scullcap acts on the nervous system, calming nervous excitement.

• Scullcap relieves spasms and increases the flow of urine.

• Scullcap helps rebuild nerve endings in the brain.

• Scullcap has been used traditionally to help with infertility.

• Scullcap is used for upper respiratory infections, helps with extreme fatigue caused by blood poisons, soothes inflamed tissue and absorbs toxins from the bowel.

• Scullcap has been known to help with digestion problems.

• It is also beneficial to use for headaches arising from excessive coughing due to a nervous condition.

Alcoholism	Lock-jaw
ANXIETY	Menstruation (promotes)
BLOOD PRESSURE (HIGH)	Mental illness
Child diseases	Migraine headaches
Circulation	Mumps
CONVULSIONS	MUSCLE TWITCHING
Coughing (incessant)	NERVOUS CONDITIONS
Delirium tremens	NEURALGIA
Diuretic	Neuritis
Drug withdrawal	PALSY
EPILEPSY	Paralysis
Excitability	Poisonous bites
EXHAUSTION (NERVOUS)	Rabies
FEVERS	RESTLESSNESS
Fits	RHEUMATISM
Gout	Rickets
Hangovers	SLEEPLESSNESS
Headaches	Smoking
Hypertension	Snake bites
Hysteria	Spasms
Hypoglycemia	St. Vitus' dance
Indigestion	Tremors
INFERTILITY	Urinary problems
INSOMNIA	

SENECA   (Polygala senega)
A.K.A.,: Senega Snake Root, Mountain Flax, Milkwort.

BODILY INFLUENCE: Diaphoretic, Diuretic(mild), Emmenagogue(mild), Expectorant, Stimulant, in large doses, Cathartic and Emetic.
PART USED: Root.

Herbalist's have used preparations made from Senega roots to bring up phlegm in cases of asthma and bronchitis. Senega root contains mucilaginous compounds that thins mucous fluid and increases its production. The result is to loosen mucous so as to better enable the system to eliminate it from the system, thus making Senega root effective for colds, flu and asthma and other respiratory system problems.
• Senega aids in the second stage of acute bronchial catarrh or pneumonia.
• Senega root is an expectorant useful in respiratory problems.
• Senega root is used for upper respiratory infections, it helps with extreme fatigue caused by blood toxin, soothes inflamed tissue and absorbs toxins from the bowel.
• Senega root is a good antidote for many systemic poisons.

Asthma
Blood poisoning
BLOOD PRESSURE (HIGH)
BRONCHITIS (CHRONIC)
CATARRH (CHRONIC)
CONVULSIONS
CROUP
Dropsy
Drugs(side effects)
Epilepsy
FEVERS

INFERTILITY
INSOMNIA
LUNG CONGESTION
MUCUS
NERVES
Pleurisy
PNEUMONIA
Rheumatism
Small pox
SNAKEBITES
Whooping Cough

SENNA   (Cassia acutifolia)
A.K.A.,: Alexandrian Senna, Ringworm Bush.

BODILY INFLUENCE: Cathartic, Laxative, Purgative, Vermifuge.
PART USED: Leaves, bark and seed.

Senna is used as a cathartic.   Its griping effect necessitates a carminative such as ginger to be taken with it. It is to be combined with other herbs when it is used for bowel elimination's so as to reduce it from a cathartic to an effective laxative. It is suggested to use Senna by itself only in acute constipation.
• Senna has been used externally by the Arabians for skin afflictions.
• Senna is habit-forming as a cathartics and should only be used briefly, as in a cleansing.
• Due to its cathartic and vermifuge qualities, Senna can well be used in parasite cleansing programs.
• Senna can work well in cleansing the system during fasting, and with large quantities of water is can be effective in treating fevers.   Senna has an astringent toning effect on the digestive system and also effectively cleans the elimination system.

CAUTION: NOT TO BE TAKEN DURING PREGNANCY UNLESS TAKEN IN A LAXATIVE COMBINATION.

Biliousness
Breath (bad)
Colic
CONSTIPATION
Gallstones
Gout
JAUNDICE

Menstruation
Mouth sores
Obesity
Pimples
Rheumatism
Skin diseases
WORMS

SHEPHERD'S PURSE (Capsella bursa-pastoris)

A.K.A.,: Caseweed, Mother's-heart, Shepherd's Sprout, Shovelweed.

BODILY INFLUENCE; Anti-hemorrhagic, Anti-pyretic, Astringent, Diuretic, Hemostatic, Laxative, Stimulant, Styptic, Urinary antiseptic.

PART USED: The whole Plant.

Another name for Shepherds Purse comes from the plant's heart-shaped seedpods, which resemble pointed shovels and thus the name Shovelweed.

However the pods were more often compared to the leather pouches in which the shepherds carried their food, thus the name Shepherd's Purse

Most of the drugs that controlled bleeding were manufactured in Germany prior to World War II, and with the onset of the war these were no longer available to the Allies to include Great British. The British doctors knowing of the ancient use of the extracts of Shepherd's Purse were able to make good use of it as a suitable substitute.

Though Shepherds purse is a valuable herb for healing, most of what is necessary to say can be said briefly and to the point. Shepherd's Purse has astringent qualities and as such is an effective blood coagulant used to control bleeding. It can be used to control excessive menstrual flow. Externally it can be applied to bleeding sores, cuts, wounds, nosebleeds and bruises.

The American Indians used the plant for its nutritional properties.

- Shepherd's Purse is very valuable remedy for diarrhea.
- Shepherd's Purse is used for hemorrhages after childbirth, excessive menstruation, internal bleeding of the lungs, colon and hemorrhoids.
- Shepherd's Purse aids in constricting the blood vessels, therefore it is used to regulate blood pressure and the action of the heart in cases where there is either low and high pressure.
- Shepherd's Purse works to help remove catarrh of the urinary tract which is indicated by mucus in the urine.
- Shepherd's Purse works to control difficult urination, bedwetting.

NOTE: Be careful in the use of Shepherds Purse. It is an astringent, but may be used with care for after-birth bleeding control.

Arteriosclerosis
BLEEDING
BLOOD PRESSURE (RAISES & NORMALIZES)

BLOODY URINE
Constipation
Cystitis
Diarrhea

Dropsy
Dysentery
EAR AILMENTS
Heart
HEMORRHAGE
Kidney
Lumbago

MENSTRUATION (PAINFUL)
POSTPARTUM BLEEDING
Spleen
Urinary problems
Uterus (stimulates labor)
Vagina
Water retention

SHEEP SORREL (Rumex acetosella, R. acetosa)
A.K.A.,: Field Sorrel, Red Top Sorrel, Garden Sorrel, Greensauce.

BODILY INFLUENCE: Anti-pyretic, Anti-scorbutic, Antiseptic(mild), Astringent, Diuretic, Laxative, Nutritive.
PART USED: Leaves, Flowers, Roots.

Sheep Sorrel has green arrow shaped leaves and was commonly grown in European vegetable garden from the middle ages until the 1700's. It first came to America as a salad green. Sorrel leaves were eaten mixed with a vinegar and sugar dressing as a salad and this mixture mashed as a greensauce was used on cold meat, thus the plants name of Greensauce. The herb has a sharp taste from its oxalic acid and vitamin C content. It was used to prevent scurvy as the story goes in folk medicine. Oxalic acid can be reduced by parboiling before cooking.

Today Sheep Sorrel can be found in damp meadows and on shorelines in Europe and Asia. It is less abundant in North America. Sorrel has astringent qualities useful in treatment of hemorrhages for the stomach and with excessive menstrual bleeding.

Medicinally Sheep Sorrel is being used in Canada for cancer and other degenerative diseases. It makes an excellent poultice for a variety of uses.

• Sheep Sorrel works as a remedy for kidney trouble. It loosens, helps dissolve and aids in the expelling of gravel from the kidneys, aiding the body to function properly, thus helping the entire body feel better. This aids the skin to look much clearer.

Boils
DEGENERATIVE DISEASES
FEVERS
Gravel (kidneys)
Jaundice
Kidney problems

Menstruation (excessive)
Scurvy
Skin diseases
Stomach hemorrhaging
Tumors

SHIITAKE   (See Mushrooms)

SIBERIAN GINSENG   (See Ginseng)

SLIPPERY ELM   (Ulmus fulva)
A.K.A.,: Indian Elm, Red Elm, Rock Elm, Moose Elm.

BODILY INFLUENCE: Astringent(mild), Demulcent, Digestive, Emollient, Expectorant, Mucilant, Nutritive tonic, Pectoral, Vulnerary.
PART USED: Inner Bark.

The healing powers of the native Slippery Elm were first used by the American Indians. When Slippery Elm's inner bark gets wet the gummy mucilaginous substance surrounding its fibers swell, producing a soothing softening ointment. They used the salve externally to treat skin problems ranging from chapped lips to burns and wounds. The Indians used Slippery Elm as natures chapstick. Slippery Elm's principle ingredient is a mucilage, a polysaccharide similar to that in flax seed.

Slippery Elm is a demulcent and emollient and can be applied as a poultice to all wounds or ulcers to good effect. Internally it is used for stomach and intestinal ulcers. Slippery Elm is also used internally for lung problems. For external uses it is used for all inflamed surfaces, skin diseases, abscesses, warts, ulcers, etc. The poultice quickly disperses inflammation and draws out impurities. Slippery Elm makes an excellent bolus to be used rectally to soothe any lower bowel irritation

The main focus of the use of Slippery Elm is the GI Tract where it can provide nutrition, a soothing coat over stomach and intestinal ulcers, soothing the colon, either taken orally or as a bolus used as a suppository or added to enemas.

Slippery Elm is often encapsulated and can be purchased. An interesting side note concerning the Historical use of Slippery Elm. George Washington's Army during the bitter winter at Valley Forge was kept alive by eating the inner back of the Slippery Elm Tree. During the days of our forefathers who moved west, they often found themselves without food and were able to survive eating the innerbark of the Slippery Elm Tree, where present.

Slippery Elm can be mixed into a thin and perfectly smooth paste with cold water. It then may be mixed in a number of ways to create a tonic. The drink can be flavored with cinnamon, nutmeg, lemon rind or other flavorings. This mixture is known as Slippery Elm Gruel. It is important to make the cold water paste first and to stir steadily while adding a hot tonic as the mucilage in Slippery Elm will not dissolve in liquid. It will, however, swell as the mucilage soaks up the hot liquid tonic causing the drink to become thick.

• Slippery Elm is soothing to any inflamed or irritated area such as ulcers, or any ulcerated condition.

• Slippery Elm can neutralize stomach acidity and absorb foul gases.

• Slippery Elm helps in the digestion of dairy products. It protects against irritation and inflammations of the mucous membranes.

• When there is difficulty in holding and digesting food, Slippery Elm may be used as a food.

• Slippery Elm protects the body from impurities allowing the body to heal itself by coating the irritated areas with its mucilaginous properties.

• Slippery Elm is a good remedy for irritated kidneys and inflamed lungs.

• Slippery Elm helps to feed the adrenal glands and produces the cortin hormone which stimulates the entire body.

• Slippery Elm helps to lubricate the bowel, thus allowing for smooth and softer elimination's.

ABSCESSES	Hayfever
Appendicitis	Hemorrhage
ASTHMA	Herpes
Bladder problems	Hoarseness
Boils	INFECTION (CATARRHAL)
BRONCHITIS	Hemorrhoids
BURNS	Inflammation (internal)
Cancer	Jaundice
COLITIS	Kidney disorders
COLON	LUNGS
CONSTIPATION	Nutrition (weak & debilitated)
COUGHS	Pain
Cramps	Perspiration (strong)
Cystitis	Phlegm
Diabetes	Pneumonia
DIAPER RASH	Skin diseases
DIARRHEA	Sore throat
DIGESTIVE DISORDERS	Stomach problems
Diverticulitis	Syphilis
Dysentery	Tonsillitis
Eczema	Tuberculosis
Eyes	ULCERS
Female problems	Urinary tract infections
Fevers	Vaginal discharge
Flu	Venereal disease
Fractures	Warts
Gangrenous wounds	Worms (expels)
Gas	Wounds

SPEARMINT (Mentha spicata)

A.K.A.,: Garden mint.

BODILY INFLUENCE: Alterative(mild), Anti-emetic, Anti-spasmodic, Aromatic, Calmative, Carminative, Diaphoretic, Diuretic(mild), Nervine, Y Stimulant, Stomachic.

PART USED: Leaves or the entire herb.

Spearmint has similar qualities as Peppermint but it milder in its actions. It is better used on children's complaints due to this milder action. However it does have a stronger diaphoretic and diuretic than does Peppermint. This spicy herb is very similar to Peppermint in medicinal properties. Unlike peppermint, it should never be boiled to make a tea. When infusing Spearmint it should be done in a closed container so as not to loose its volatile oil.

Spearmint is used for stomach problems. It helps settle the stomach in the case of vomiting and nausea and is helpful for morning sickness during pregnancy.

• It's calming and soothing to the stomach and intestine. It increases the circulation in the stomach.

• There is no toxicity in Spearmint so it is an excellent herb for even the sickest person to tolerate.

• Spearmint is excellent in treating morning sickness or vomiting in pregnancy.

• Spearmint relieves smooth muscle spasms, increases blood circulation, promotes sweating, which helps to relieve pain.

• Spearmint is gentle and effective for colic in babies.

• Spearmint will relieve suppressed, painful or burning urine.

• Spearmint is also helpful for gas in the stomach.

Appetite	Hysteria
Bladder	INDIGESTION
COLDS	Insomnia
COLIC	Kidneys (inflammation)
Cramps	Menstrual cramps
Diarrhea	MORNING SICKNESS
Digestion	Muscle aches
Dizziness	NAUSEA
Dropsy	Nervousness
Fevers	Spasms
FLU	Stones
GAS	Urination (burning)
Headache	VOMITING
Hemorrhoids	

SPIRULINA   (Algae pratensis)
A.K.A.,: Blue-Green-Algae.

BODILY INFLUENCE: Nutritive, Polarity(corrects), Tonic.
PART USED: The whole plant.

When first introduced on the open market as a food supplement Spirulina was touted a the Greatest food supplement on the Market. Now several years later and after several new and wonderful supplement have arrived on the scene Spirulina is still high on the list, if not the highest of miracle foods.

Spirulina is a one-celled form of algae that multiplies in warm, alkaline fresh-water bodies. The name .Spirulina. is derived from the Latin word for .helix. or .spiral,. referring to the physical configuration of the organism when it forms swirling, microscopic strands.

Germs and scum, are associated with microorganisms of disease. Spirulina grows in this type of surroundings but it is in fact one of the cleanest, most naturally sterile foods found in nature. The ability of Spirulina to grow in hot and alkaline environments ensures its hygienic status, as no other organisms can survive to pollute the waters in which this algae grows.

Spirulina is the highest source in the world of Beta carotene, vitamin B12 and gamma linolenic acid (GLA). Spirulina contains most of the known amino acids. It contains all nine essential amino acids that the body must derive from food.

Spirulina has many times more the Beta-carotene than carrots. It contains 250% more vitamin B-12 than liver. It contains four times the protein of beef. Spirulina is 65-71% protein as compared to beef, which is about 18%. Proteins of Spirulina are 80-85% assimilated as compared to 20% for beef protein.

Spirulina is an algae which contains 26 times the calcium of milk, lots of phosphorus and niacin.   Spirulina can be stored for many years with any preservatives and still contain a high percentage of its nutrients.

Spirulina is a complete food with one acceptation, it is lacking in carbohydrates. It is beneficial for any and all ailments that exist, due to a deficient diet, hair can grow, eyes can see, ears can hear, taste buds are improved, strength is gained, all life is better as a result of ingesting Spirulina.

Spirulina remains among the most efficient blood, cell and tissue builders, as well as being an extremely potent and health energy booster. Spirulina helps to satisfy hunger naturally and balance blood sugar levels.

Spirulina provides good nutrition for the brain giving greater mental clarity and alertness.

Spirulina has only one deficiency and that is in its carbohydrate content. The body could convert its high protein content to energy supplying carbohydrates, but harm would result and could not be recommended. While it is a complete food, in that it contains all the life sustaining nutrients it needs an added ingredient to make it a complete beneficial food, carbohydrates.

• Spirulina is considered one of Nature's whole foods.
• Spirulina is a RNA/DNA balancer, it is a complete protein, and the entire B complex of vitamins, trace minerals, and essential fatty acids.
• Spirulina boosts the immune system, it is a cholesterol reducer and aids mineral absorption.
• It curbs the appetite and is very high in chlorophyll and iron.
• It has been recommended to keep one alert both physically and mentally.
• Spirulina aids the body in cleansing itself by helping it to remove toxic poisons in the body.

Allergies	Goiter
Anemia	Gout
Appetite suppressant	Hypoglycemia
Arthritis	Liver disease
BLOOD BUILDER	Pancreatitis
BLOOD CLEANSER	Poisoning (heavy metal)
Blood pressure (regulates)	Rejuvenation
Diabetes	Senility
Diets	Skin problems
DISEASES (CHRONIC)	TONIC
Energy	Ulcers
Eye complaints	Weight reduction
FOOD SUPPLEMENT	

SQUAW VINE   (Mitchella repens)
A.K.A.; Checkerberry, Partridgeberry.

BODILY INFLUENCE: Astringent, Diuretic, Emmenagogue, Parturient(childbirth), Uterine Tonic.
PART USED: The entire Herb.

The plant Partridgeberry, often called Squaw Vine, by this name alone is identified with the American Indians and especially with the Indian women. It was used especially for any function associated with child bearing.

Here is a list of uses and reason for the uses that the Indian women made of Squaw Vine.

• During the final weeks of pregnancy, women drank a tea made from the leaves of Squaw Vine to ease childbirth and nursing mothers applied a lotion made from the leaves to their breasts to relieve soreness.

- Squaw Vine was used to strengthen the uterus for safe and effective childbirth.
- Squaw Vine stimulates and regulates the amount of contraction which is necessary for safe and easy delivery.
- The herb is also recognized for encouraging the kidneys to eliminate urine and for correcting diarrhea in the bowels.
- The plant was also used extensively to treat several uterine difficulties, including painful menstruation and threat of miscarriage.
- Mixed in equal parts with Red Raspberry leaves and in an infusion form, Squaw vine will assist to ensure a safe and easy delivery in birthing
- Squaw Vine was used two to four weeks before the expected delivery date.
- Noted for its ability to ease childbirth, it was a popular Indian remedy, thus the name, Squaw Vine.

Those who are knowledgeable in the use of herb among the non- Indian population also use Squaw Vine for any and all female uses.
- For any urinary disease, Squaw vine is a valuable diuretic, tonic and alterative.
- Combinations that include Squaw Vine are used in several female corrective tonics.
- Squaw Vine is a uterine tonic and will relieve congestion of the uterus and ovaries.
- Squaw vine's is known to work on the uterine muscle during delivery, to speed up delivery and regulate contractions.
- Squaw vine has been used mostly for ailments of the female organs. It was also used for dropsy, suppression of urine and diarrhea.
- It is a healing herb that promotes urination as well as tones body tissue.
- Squaw Vine is extremely useful for the treatment of water retention.
- When used as a wash, Squaw Vine gives wonderful relief to sore eyes.

Anxiety	Hemorrhoids
Bladder	Inflammation
Bleeding (stops)	Insomnia
CHILDBIRTH (EASIER)	LACTATION
EYES (SORE)	MENSTRUAL IRREGULARITIES
Edema	MENSTRUATION (PAINFUL)
Gravel	Muscle spasms (erratic)

Nerves
Pain
Post-partum depression
SKIN PROBLEMS

Urinary problems
UTERINE DISORDERS
Varicose veins
Wounds

STEVIA (Stevia rebaudiana)
A.K.A.,: Sweet Herb.

BODILY INFLUENCE: Sugar substitute. Affects the pancreas and adrenals.
PART USED: Leaves.

Stevia is a natural herbal sweetener, claimed to be 50 to 60 times sweeter than sugar. It is said to be safe for diabetics, hypoglycemics and Candida sufferers. It is non-caloric so when used for baking it hold down the extra calories that sugar would have provided. Stevia being green in color changes the color of a white cake. Stevia adds a slightly anise taste to whatever you are cooking.
* Stevia can be made into an infusion by putting a spoonful in a cup of warm water and then adding it by the teaspoon to whatever you want to sweeten.
* Stevia is sold in a liquid concentrate that is used by the drops.
* Clinical studies indicate that Stevia is safe to use even in cases of severe sugar imbalance.
* Stevia is found to be non-toxic and safe to use as a harmless sweetner.

Addictions
DIABETES
FOOD CRAVINGS
Hypertension

HYPOGLYCEMIA
SUGAR SUBSTITUTE
TOBACCO CRAVINGS
WEIGHT REDUCTION

STILLINGIA (Stillingia sylvatica)
A.K.A.,: Queen's Delight, Queen's Root, Silver Leaf, Yaw Root.

BODILY INFLUENCE: Alterative, Expectorant, in large doses: Emetic, Cathartic, Cholagogue.
PART USED: Root.

Stillingia is a North American plant that is an herb in the throws of discovery. It has been found to be one of the best treatments for syphilis according to many doctors. It has become the alterative of choice in the last 100 years. Stillingia has been used to treat tuberculosis and also cancer and other conditions are being researched where an alterative is needed. Stillingia as a pronounced glandular stimulant is of great use in Cystic Fibrosis.

Stillingia is a great aid to protein digestion. The herb is a blood purifier and combines well with Prickly Ash.
• Stillingia is useful for long lasting skin problems, (especially acne, eczema and psoriasis.)
• Stillingia is an effective glandular stimulant.
• Stillingia is used to rid the system of the toxic drugs used in the chemotherapy treatment for cancer.
• Stillingia should be used with caution and is best when used in combination with other herbs.
• Stillingia is very effective as a stimulant for the liver.

ACNE
BLOOD PURIFIER
Bronchitis
Constipation
ECZEMA
LIVER PROBLEMS

RESPIRATORY PROBLEMS
SKIN PROBLEMS
Sore throat
SYPHILIS
Urinary problems

SUMA   (Pfaffia paniculata)
A.K.A.,: Brazilian Ginseng.

BODILY INFLUENCE: Adaptogen, Demulcent, Energy Tonic, Immuno-stimulant, Nutrient.
PART USED: Bark and Root.

Suma is an ancient herb dubbed as "para todo" by the Brazilian Indians meaning for everything. Suma is like the Siberian ginseng; but should not be confused with the oriental Ginseng of the Panax family.

Suma increases energy, strengthens the immune system, fortifies hormones (especially estrogen), reduces tumors and cancers and regulates blood sugar.

Suma has successfully been used with outstanding results on many varieties of cancer, (especially leukemia, Hodgkin's disease and diabetes.)

Suma enhances energy and vitality and shows great promise as a healing agent in chronic disorders believed to result from a lowered immune system.

(Both Chronic Fatigue Syndrome and Epstein-Barr virus may benefit from the use of Suma.)

Suma has been just recently discovered here in the United States and has had great results in overcoming problems in a modern society, such as fatigue and hormonal imbalance. It is a great booster for the immune system and has been used to rebuild the system from the ravages of cancer and diabetes.

Since it is an adaptogen herb, it has been credited with long life and longevity.

In Brazil, Suma was reported to be more powerful than Ginseng and it is referred to as Brazilian ginseng.

The two hormones found in Suma, sitosterol and stipmasterol, have been found beneficial to the heart and aids in lowering high cholesterol levels in the blood. It is antioxidant in nature as it contains germanium so it fights free radicals.

- Suma is an adaptogen herb, normalizes functions in the body heals and prevents disease.
- Suma relieves stress and helps the body to adapt to many and varied environment and psychological stresses.
- Suma helps to restore sexual function in both men and women.
- It protects against viral infections and benefits in cancer by its blood and system purification.
- The Japanese discovered a chemical in Suma that is unique and tends to inhibit tumor cell growth.
- It helps protect the immune system by providing a balanced environment.
- Suma helps in hormonal levels by balancing estrogen levels.

Anemia	Hypoglycemia
Arthritis	IMMUNE SYSTEM
Bronchitis	Joint diseases
CANCER	Menopause symptoms
CHOLESTEROL	Osteomyelitis
CIRCULATION PROBLEMS	Osteoporosis
Colds	Premenstrual problems
DEGENERATIVE DISEASES	Skin problems
Diabetes	STRESS
Emotional swings	Strokes
Energy booster	TONIC
Fatigue	Tumors
Heart disease	VITALITY
HORMONE REGULATOR	Wounds
Hot flashes	

TAHEEBO   (SEE PAU D'ARCO)

THYME   (Thymus vulgaris)
A.K.A.,: Garden Thyme.

BODILY INFLUENCE: Antiseptic, Anti-spasmodic, Aromatic, Carminative, Diaphoretic, Disinfectant, Emmenagogue, Expectorant, Nervine, Parasiticide, Sedative, Stimulant, Tonic, Vulnerary.
PART USED: The whole plant.

In ancient Greece, if a person was told that they smelled of Thyme it was considered a great compliment. To the Greeks, Thyme was a symbol of bravery. The generic title, thymus, was from the Greek word, thymos, which meant "strength" and referred to its "invigorating" odor.

The early Greeks learned to use Thyme for nervous conditions. They found it to be a good tissue cleanser and a help to heal wounds. (In addition, the anti-spasmodic use was discover which was found to help in cases of an asthma attack and other respiratory problems.) It was found to be helpful in quieting stomach cramps and gastrointestinal complaints and it even helped with whooping cough.

Thymol, the oil of Thyme, is a powerful germicide with a pleasant odor. It is used as a pharmaceutical product in gargles, mouthwashes and in toothpaste. Its best known use is in Listerine, the world famous antiseptic compound.

Additional uses of Thyme are for uterine and bowel problems, it being helpful in gastro-intestinal disorders as it relaxes spasms and inhibits flatulence, it has a soothing sedative effect on nerves, thyme.s disinfectant and germicidal effects are greatest in diseases of the upper respiratory passages.   Externally, use with a hot fomentation pad on abscesses, boils and other swellings.

• Thyme reportedly helps to dissolve and remove tumors, while relieving spasms and encouraging menstruation.

• Thyme is also said to be a general tonic with antiseptic qualities that promote healing. Thyme is also used to fight infection. The oil is occasionally used as a deodorant in the sick room or to control the odor of foul discharges.

• Thyme reportedly controls fungal infections such as athlete's foot as well as skin parasites such as scabies, crabs and lice.

• Some research has given that Thyme may be effective in the elimination of free radicals.

• Thyme has been reported to remove mucus from the head, lungs and respiratory passages.

• Thyme tea has been used as a remedy for shortness of breath.

Abscesses (external)
Alcoholism
Appetite stimulant
Asthma
Boils (external)
Bowel problems
BRONCHITIS (ACUTE)
Bruises
Catarrh
Cholesterol (lowers)
Colds
Colic
Cramps
Diarrhea
DIGESTIVE DISORDERS
Dyspepsia
Epilepsy
Fainting
Fever
Flu
GAS
Gastritis
GOUT
Hangover
HEADACHE
Heartburn
Hysteria
Indigestion (acid)
Infection

LARYNGITIS
Leprosy
LUNG CONGESTION
Mastitis
Menstruation (suppressed)
Migraine headaches
Mucus
Nervous conditions
Nightmares
Paralysis
Parasites
Perspiration
Phlegm
Respiratory problems
Rheumatism
SCIATICA
Shingles
Sinuses
Sore throat
Spasms
Sprains
Stomach (weak)
Stomach cramps
Swellings (external)
THROAT PROBLEMS
Tumors
Warts
WHOOPING COUGH
WORMS

USNEA (Usnea barbata)
A.K.A.,: Beard lichen, Old Man.s Beard.

BODILY INFLUENCE: Anti-bacterial, Antibiotic, Anti-fungal, Anti-viral, Astringent, Diuretic, Parasiticide, Tonic, Tuberculostatic.
PARTS USED: The whole plant, which is a lichen growing on branches of trees.

The name "Usnea' may have originated at the time of the Arabian school of medicine and pharmacy.
Paracelsus, a Swiss physician has been recognized as the popularizer of the famous "Doctrine of Signatures". This doctrine is a man-centered view of nature teaching that not only were plants created for man's use, but also each plant demonstrated a clear sign - a signature - to show the purpose for which the plant was intended. Usnea, or "Old Man's Beard," hangs in gray-green

strands from pines, oaks, Douglas fir, apple trees and other fruit trees in orchards and forests throughout the northern hemisphere and was, due to its appearance, a specific for the hair and scalp.

Usnea is used both internally and externally for fungus infections and for viral and bacterial infections. It is excellent in combinations with Echinacea used as a general herbal antibiotic and anti-fungal. These medicinal qualities are due to lichen acid, particularly usinic Acid. These present a wide range of medical applications. Usnea is good for the treatment of pneumonia, tuberculosis, lupus, internal infections, strep, staph, Trichomonas and other infected wounds.

By definition, a lichen is not really a single plant, but two or more organisms living as one in a symbiotic partnership. A lichen has a fungus base which provides a platform that a chlorophyll-bearing algae can gather and provide food sugars for all. It has been described a nature's solar collector. Usnea is effective against Trichomonas, a parasite which can cause, among other things, a serious infection of the uterine cervix.

"Usnea may also be superior to the drug Flagyl (metronidazole). Flagyl is widely prescribed for Trichomonas infection, but it can also cause cancer. After oral administration, it can be found in the bloodstream, cerebrospinal fluid and breast milk. Nursing mothers should strictly avoid this drug. (Physician's Desk Reference, 1983, P. 1874.)

Usnic acid is toxic, but happily it is poorly and slowly absorbed when in a tea or alcoholic solution, reducing the cause for concern. Usnic acid is barely water soluble. Thus, usnic acid at times is rendered unavailable to the site of the infection, offering the advantages of slow absorption or slow, steady and longer lasting release into a site of infection. This is one reason why so many of the European anti-bacterial, anti-fungal creams and balms are made from Usnea. Due to its strong selective anti-bacterial activity, Usnea has the great advantage in offering support to the natural defenses of the body.

Very few lichens are poisonous. The exceptions are two bright yellow or orange alpine species, Letharia vulpina and Cetraria penastri. It would be best to avoid the use of any bright-colored lichens growing in the high mountains. Large quantities of a strong tea of some lichens could cause gastro-intestinal upset, because of the irritating nature of the lichen compounds.

As with all herbal medicines, it is best to start with a low dose and slowly work up to a full therapeutic or nutritional dose. This allows the body to adjust to the energy of the particular herb or combinaton, and if one pays attention, is a way to determine whether it is the right remedy, or one that might prove to irritate or in some way be unsuitable.

Athlete's foot	Pleurisy
Bronchitis	Pneumonia
Burns	Respiratory tract infections
Catarrh	Ringworm
Colds	Scalp
Dropsy	Sinus infection
Epilepsy	Strep throat
Flu	Trichomonas
Fungal infections	Tuberculosis
Hair	Urinary tract infections
Impetigo	Whooping cough
Lupus	Wounds

UVA URSI   (Arctostaphylos uva-ursi)
A.K.A.,: Bearberry, Kinnikinnick(American Indian name), Bear's Grape, Coralillo(Mexico).

BODILY INFLUENCE: Anti-lithic, Aromatic, Astringent, Disinfectant, Diuretic, Lithontriptic, Sedative(renal), Stimulant(mild), Tonic, Urinary Antiseptic.
PART USED: Leaves.

Historically, the Chinese, Europeans, and American Indians considered Uva ursi a kidney herb. They used the leaves and fresh berries for treating bladder infections, kidney stones, incontinence, and like ailments. One tribe of North American Indians used an infusion of Uva ursi for sore gums, canker sores and as a mouth wash.

Marco Polo, in the 13th century, reported that the Chinese physicians were using this herb as a diuretic, to treat kidney and urinary problems. Kubla Khan learned of Uva ursi during his invasions of China. The early colonists found that the American Indians used Uva ursi and mixed its leaves with tobacco to create the smoking mixture they called "kinnikinnick," one of Uva ursi's common names.

The chief constituent of the leaves is a glycoside called arbutin. Medical herbalists explain that the diuretic action of Uva ursi comes from arbutin, which is largely absorbed and unchanged and is excreted by the kidneys. During its excretion, arbutin produces an antiseptic effect of the urinary mucous membrane. Tannic acid is also contained in the leaves and berries of Uva ursi. In addition, this herb helps balance the pH of urine that is high in acid.

Uva ursi strengthens the urinary passages and is good for inflammation in any part of the urinary system. Uva ursi stimulates kidney activity and can be used as a urinary antiseptic for kidney and bladder infections being very effective for acid urine and to treat blood in the urine. It has a direct sedative and tonic effect to the bladder walls, imparting tone and decreasing excessive discharges.

Uva ursi is an astringent herb with strong affinity for the urinary system. It has been used to help correct bedwetting, bladder diseases, cystitis, kidney congestion and infections of the kidneys and urinary tract. It is also said to have the ability to dissolve kidney stones. Due to the proximity of the prostate to the urinary tract in males, it has also been used in prostate remedies. Uva ursi produces potent antiseptic action in the kidney tubules.

Uva ursi has been shown to work in various types of bladder and kidney diseases. These include pyelitis, nephritis, urolithiasis, and urinary catarrh. Uva ursi has also been used in cystitis and urethritis, for urogenital inflammations and as a urinary antiseptic. Uva ursi also increases the flow of urine and cleanses the spleen.

Uva ursi is used for womb problems and is very good as a post-partum remedy to prevent infections. Uva ursi added to a hot tub of water makes a good bath for after childbirth, inflammations, hemorrhoids and skin infections. It can be used as a douche (infusion), for vaginal infections and other problems in the pelvic region.

• Uva ursi is a remedy for excessive sugar in the blood and as such is a help in controlling diabetes.

• This herb contains allantoin, which spurs the healing of wounds.

• This herb is useful for arthritis and inflammation throughout the body.

• Uva ursi has been shown to be strongly antibiotic against many organisms including Staph and E. Coli.

• Today, Uva ursi is used as a tonic and is specific in cases involving weakened liver, kidneys and other glands.

• Uva ursi's influence is most prominent in the urogenital system and for this reason, has been used traditionally for inflammation of the kidney or bladder and prostate problems.

• It is especially good in cases of gravel or ulceration of the membrane of the urinary tract. Uva ursi has achieved a reputation as a solvent for calculi deposits in the urinary tract. In chronic inflammation of the bladder and kidneys, it has no equal.

• The leaves are powerfully astringent.

• Uva ursi is effective in the treatment of incontinence. Incontinence is defined as the involuntary loss of bladder control.

• Uva ursi seems to be a tonic for the sphincter muscle of the bladder so as to prevent loss of bladder control.

• Uva ursi also works as a urinary disinfectant.

• Uva ursi effectively cures urinary infections and is unresponsive to pharmaceutical antibiotics.

- Uva ursi has been useful for arthritis.
- Uva ursi reportedly has invigorating and body strengthening qualities.
- (The herb has a large amount of tannins, which could cause stomach upset in large quantities and should not be given to children under the age of two. Begin with smaller amounts of Uva ursi at first and increase if necessary. You may notice that the herb often turns urine a dark green. Do not become alarmed, this is normal.)
- Uva ursi is reported to aid in treating the sexually transmitted disease gonorrhea.
- Uva ursi is considered a digestive stimulant.
- Uva ursi stimulates the uterus to contract, pregnant women should not take it.

Arthritis
Back pain (lower)
Bedwetting
BLADDER INFECTIONS
BRIGHT'S DISEASE
Bronchitis
CYSTITIS
DIABETES
Diarrhea
Digestive disorders
Dysentery
Female problems
Fevers
Gallstones
GONORRHEA
Gravel
Heart muscle (strengthens)
Hemorrhoids
KIDNEY INFECTIONS
Kidney stones
Liver
Lung congestion
Menstruation (excessive)
Mucous membranes
NEPHRITIS
Obesity
Pancreas
Prostate gland weakness
Rheumatism
SPLEEN
URETHRITIS (CHRONIC)
Uric acid
Urinary disorders
UTERINE ULCERATION
Vaginal discharge
Venereal diseases
Water retention

VALERIAN   (Valeriana officinalis)
A.K.A.,: Capon's Tail, All-heal, Garden Heliotrope, English Valerian.

BODILY INFLUENCE: Anodyne(mild), Anti-diuretic, Anti-spasmodic, Aromatic, Carminative, Cathartic, Diuretic, Hypnotic, Nervine, Parasiticide, Sedative, Stimulant, Tonic.
PART USED: Root.

Valerian root has been used for many centuries to calm all kinds of nervous disorders. It slows the action of the heart, while increasing its general force. In centuries past, it was supposedly taken as often as coffee by ladies in Germany, resulting in lack of nervousness irritability.

The volatile oil of Valerian contains esters (compounds created from the union of an alcohol and an acid with loss of water) similar to those in Rosemary. The development of the "dirty socks or 'rotten cheese" odor of Valerian comes during the drying process, when these esters undergo a chemical decomposition or change to produce iso-valerianic acid.

Valerian root is a primary sedative and is used when sleep disorders are the result of anxiety, nervousness, exhaustion, headache or hysteria. Valerian root has been used for these purposes since pre-Christian times and is cited in virtually every pharmacopoeia in the world.

Valerian has an influence on the cerebrospinal system and is employed as a sedative of the primary nerve centers for afflictions such as St. Vitus Dance, nervous unrest, neuralgia pain, epileptic fits, hysteria, restlessness and wakefulness.

Valerian root is playing an important role in the somewhat ardous process of rehabilitaion for many an addict. Often it serves as a substitute for Valium to help the addict sleep easily, relax and mellow out. The best results have been obtained in cases of hysteria and hypochondria, where the primary causes of difficulty are emotional or mental.

• Nature's tranquilizer, Valerian, calms the nerves without the side effects of comparable orthodox drugs.

• Besides acting upon the circulatory system, it stimulates secretion and peristalsis of the stomach and intestines.

• The herb is a proven sedative, but it also improves coordination and antagonizes the hypnotic effects of alcohol.

• Valerian is suggested for cases of heart palpitation, because it slows down the heart rate while increasing the strength of the beats.

• It is also used for circulatory problems and to stimulate the stomach and intestinal motility.

• Valerian is often used for hypochondria.

• It can be said that this herb is anti-spasmodic and equalizing, therefore, can be said to act as a sedative in states of agitation and a stimulant in fatigue.

• Today, the best known use of Valerian is as a natural tranquilizer.

• Valerian has long been used as a stomachic, anti-spasmodic, carminative, and antidote to the plague. It has also been used since ancient times in the treatment of epilepsy.

• Valerian may work by affecting the central nervous system, thus it is more a psychological drug than a physiological one.

• Valerian root works to calm the nerves and also relieves pain and spasms.

• Valerian root has a sedative effect, acting to decrease anxiety

and aggression and aiding in insomnia. It is one of the best herbal sources of calcium and magnesium.
- Valerian is used to relieve stomach cramps and stress.

AFTER-BIRTH PAINS
Alcoholism
Arthritis (pain)
Bladder
Bladder (gravel)
BLOOD PRESSURE (HIGH)
BRONCHIAL SPASMS
Colds
Colic
Constipation
Contagious diseases
CONVULSIONS
Coughs
Cramps
Digestive disorders
Drug addiction
Fever
Despondency
Epilepsy
Fatigue
Gas
Headaches
HEART PALPITATIONS
Hypoglycemia
HYSTERIA

HYPOCHONDRIA
Insomnia
Measles
Menstrual cramps
Menstruation (promotes)
Migraine headaches
MUSCLE SPASMS
NERVOUS BREAKDOWN
NERVOUS CONDITIONS
PAIN RELIEF
Palsy
Paralysis
Restlessness
Scarlet fever
Shock
Skin eruptions
SLEEPLESSNESS
Spasms
Stomach problems
Stomach (ulcerated)
Stress
Twitching spasms
Ulcers
Worms (expels)

VERVAIN   (Verbena officinalis)
A.K.A.,: Herb-of-the-Cross, Pigeon.s Grass, Wild Hyssop.

BODILY INFLUENCE: Alterative, Anti-spasmodic, Astringent, Cholagogue, Diaphoretic, Emmenagogue, Galactogogue, Nervine, Parasiticide, Sedative, Stimulant, Tonic.
PART USED: Tops.

Vervain is common in form and plentiful, but is highly regarded in its usage. It was used by the Romans to purify their temples and homes as well as using it medicinally. Vervain is said to worked into Catholic beliefs as the plant that stanched the bleeding of Christ on Calvary which gained the name, "Herb of the Cross".

Vervain gained a reputation as for being something for all things. Colds, fevers, nervous complaints, gout and skin infections were among the disorders it could cure.

What of Today, Vervain is still used usefully for liver congestion and related disorders. Vervain is helpful for painful or irregular menses. Vervain can also be used as an infusion for severe symptoms of colds, flu's and fevers.

Vervain is an effective nerve builder, liver stimulant, urinary cleanser and fever remedy, Vervain's flowering tops help mothers milk production and is used during labor to encourage contractions. Vervain has many topical uses including sores, wounds and gum disorders.

Vervain is one of the 12 original flower remedies which Dr. Bach's used to treat mental stress and overexertion, with insomnia and constant tension.

A hot infusion of Vervain is excellent for insomnia, nervous tension and to stimulate sweating and to speed up the immune system in feverish conditions.

Vervain has a relaxing nervine effect on the liver, it is said to be good for all ills of man, especially valuable for fevers, nervous disorders, including paralysis and mental stress; excellent for averting convulsions, for liver complaints, gallstones, weak heart, pulmonary ailments including asthma, pneumonia, tuberculosis; externally for weak, sore and inflamed eyes, sore mouth and throat ulcers of the mouth and gums or for any external sores; will expel worms when everything else fails; good for sleeplessness, nervous headache; will remove obstructions in the bowels, colon, Bladder; good in stomach troubles, when breathing is short and there is wheezing).

• Vervain is a great cleanser and will rapidly reduce fevers.

• Vervain is good for colds and for expelling phlegm from the throat and chest. It helps clear congestion where there is wheezing.

• Vervain helps to increase the flow of mother's milk.

• Vervain can be used in a poultice for insect bites, sprains and bruises. An ointment may be helpful on eczema, wounds and weeping sores and also painful neuralgia. A mouthwash in the form of a infusion has been found to be beneficial for mouth ulcers and soft, spongy gums.

Ague (malaria)	Digestion (sluggish)
Asthma	Eczema
Bladder	Eyes (sore)
Bowels	FEVERS
Catarrh	Flu
Circulation (poor)	Gallstones
Cirrhosis	Gout
COLDS	GUM DISORDERS
CONGESTION (GENERAL)	Headache (nervous)
CONVULSIONS	Heart (weak)
COUGHS	Hemorrhage

Hepatitis
Insect bites
Insomnia
Jaundice
Lactation
LIVER CONGESTION
Mastitis
Menstruation (painful & irregular)
Mental stress
Mouth ulcers
Mouthwash
Nervousness
Neuralgia

Paralysis
PHLEGM
Skin infections
Sleeplessness
Sores
Sprains
Stomach problems
Throat
Tuberculosis
Urinary problems
Wheezing
Worms
Wounds

VIOLET (Viola odorata)
A.K.A.,: Sweet Violet.

BODILY INFLUENCE: Alterative, Anti-neoplastic, Anti-pyretic, Antiseptic, Anti-spasmodic, Demulcent, Expectorant, Vulnerary. Larges doses: Emetic.
PART USED: Flowers and Leaves.

The Violet was a favorite of both the Romans and Greeks and was the national flower of Athens. The ancient writer Pliny wrote of the medicinal virtues of Violet, prescribing it for gout and spleen disorders and added that a garland of Violets worn about the head would banish headaches and dizziness.

Since about 500 B.C., the fresh Violet leaves have been used as a poultice to treat skin cancer. In the 1930's, Violet was widely used for breast and lung cancer and may today be a feature in alternative cancer therapies, especially after surgery to prevent the development of secondary tumors.
• The leaves and flowers have antiseptic and expectorant properties.
• Violet is used to soften hard lumps such as tumors and cancerous neoplasms(tumor).
• Violet has been used to treat respiratory disorders, as a gargle, in cough mixtures and as a diuretic.
• Violet is used as a syrup for sore throats, dryness of the upper respiratory tract, chronic coughs and asthma with associated dryness.
• Violet can be used for healing internal ulcers. It is also helpful for tumors, boils, abscesses, pimples, swollen glands and malignant growths.
• Violet will give relief to severe headaches, by relieving pressure in the head.

ASTHMA	Migraine headaches
Breathing difficulties	Mouth infections
BRONCHITIS	PHLEGM
CANCER (BREAST & LUNG)	Scrofula
COLDS	SINUS CATARRH
COUGHS (DRY)	Sores
Gout	Sore Throat
Headaches	Syphilis
Head congestion	TUMORS
Hoarseness	ULCERS
Lungs	Whooping cough

WATERCRESS (Nasturtium officinale)
A.K.A.,: Scurvy Grass.

BODILY INFLUENCE: Anti-scorbutic, Bitter, Blood purifier, Depurative, Diuretic, Emmenagogue, Expectorant, Laxative, Nutritive, Stimulant, Stomachic, Tonic.
PART USED: The Whole Plant.

Early settlers brought Watercress to America because of its anti-scurvy properties. Watercress was later identified as being rich in vitamin C.

As the Latin words nasus tortus, or "twisted nose," imply, Watercress gives off a pungent odor that makes the nose wrinkle. The leaves and edible seedpods have a sharp, peppery taste, which accounts for Watercress's longtime popularity as a salad green. Watercress is a succulent, aquatic perenial.

This evergreen thrives in clear cold water, where it forms dense masses along the edges of slow-moving streams. When collecting Watercress, be sure to gather only the Watercress, since the poisonous water hemlocks, which somewhat resemble the carrot plant, often grow nearby. The Watercress usually sways and floats on top of the water and is distinguishable from any nearby plants.

On the American continent, Coronado during his explorations, found it growing in abundance near the Gila River in Arizona. The native Indians reportedly used Watercress for liver and kidney troubles and to dissolve gallstones.

Watercress is strongly alkaline due to its high potassium content. It is useful in treating acidity and purifying the blood. Watercress juice and a raw fruit and vegetable diet aids arthritis and rheumatism and clears up acne spots. Watercress is high in vitamin C content and therefore, was extensively used to prevent scurvy in the last century. Watercress is literally a storehouse of natural vitamins, minerals and trace elements.

• Watercress is used to treat water retention, mucus in the lungs

and indigestion. It also stimulates metabolism and promotes bile metabolism.
* Known simply as Cress in Great Britian, it is rich in ascorbic acid.
* Watercress eaten fresh daily is a very useful blood purifier and tonic to help supply needed vitamins and minerals.
* Watercress increases blood circulation and increases energy.
* Watercress is used for urinary (bladder) problems, promotes kidney function, helps heart disease by relieving fluid retention, relieves indigestion and stops gas formation, by stimulating the rate of metabolism.
* Watercress is mainly used as a tonic for regulating the metabolism and flow of bile. It increases physical endurance and stamina.
* Watercress is a powerful intestinal cleanser, blood cleanser and builder.

Acne
ANEMIA
Appetite stimulant
Bladder
CRAMPS
Cysts
Eczema
Heart (strengthens)
Joints (stiff)
KIDNEY PROBLEMS
Kidney stones
Lactation
LIVER PROBLEMS
Lungs
Mental disorders
Mucus in lungs
NERVOUS PROBLEMS
RHEUMATISM
TONIC
Tuberculosis
Tumors
Uterine cysts
WATER RETENTION

WHEATGRASS   (Poaceae spp.)   (SEE CHLOROPHYLL)
A.K.A.,: Bluebunch (spicatum), Western (smithii), Crested (cristatum), Desert (desertorum), Slender (trachycaulum).

BODILY INFLUENCE: Blood Cleanser, Blood Builder, Blood Purifier. Nutritive tonic.
PART USED: The tender blade (the first 5-7 inches before the first joint appears) as soil-grown wheat.

The Wheatgrass chlorophyll, when taken in conjunction with a cleansing program will do much as a tonic aid toward relieving pain and suffering of all so-called "incurable" diseases and will promote general healing to the body.
Wheat Grass juice is considered to be one of the "Chlorophyll super foods" used for treating cancerous growths and other degenerative diseases. Research has shown that about one hundred pounds of fresh Wheat Grass has the nutritional value of

about one and a half tons of vegetables. There have been reported success with Wheat Grass juice inserted into the colon for cancer cases.

"Dr. Chiu-Nan Lai, a biologist at M.D. Anderson Hospital and Tumor Institute, has discovered that eating green vegetables will stop the progress of cancer in the colon. Dr. Lai found that extracts of sprouts, particularly from wheat, counteract carcinogens. It was further demonstrated that chlorophyll accounted for most of the extract's anti-cancer effect." (Vegetarian Times, July/August 1979).

The Chlorophyll in Wheat Grass juice is one of the best breath freshners available.

• Wheat Grass juice, due to its high Chlorophyll content will stop the development of unfriendly bacteria.

• Red blood cell counts are known to return to normal after using Wheat Grass juice because of its high Chlorophyll content.

• Wheat Grass juice is good for body building and for increasing energy.

• Wheat Grass Juice is best for expelling metals in the body.

• Wheat Grass juice can be used in douches and for sore throats.

• Wheat Grass juice is good for the colon when taken orally or taken directly into the colon as a cleansing agent. It may be used for high enemas or colonics.

• Wheat Grass juice is beneficial for lungs.

Arthritis
Bruises
Burns
Cancer
Constipation
Emphysema

Gangrene
Leukemia
Poison oak
Rheumatism
Skin abrasions
Wounds

WHITE OAK BARK   (Quercus alba)
A.K.A.,: Tanner's-oak.

BODILY INFLUENCE: Antiseptic, Astringent, Hemostatic, Parasiticide, Tonic.
PART USED: Inner Bark, Leaves, Acorns.

White Oak was for centuries, vital in wooden ship construction, from the English ships made from the English Oaks that brought our forefathers to this continent to the gun deck of the famous frigate Constitution and to the keels of World War II minesweepers and patrol boats.

The North American colonists also used the American Oak for barrel making because the wood when wet, swells up, seals the barrel enabling it to hold liquids, including the all-important rum. Rum at that time, represented our foreign trade and unfortunately the slave trade was tied to Rum.

Medicinally, White Oak Bark is the classic example of an astringent. Due to its high calcium and tannins content, it acts by precipitating the tissue protein to tighten them. For externally use, boil or steam the bark and/or the leaves and apply them over the area needing treatment to relieve bruises, injuries, varicosities, swollen tissues and bleeding. This also helps strengthen capillaries.

- The White Oak has been used to treat diarrhea, dysentery and bleeding.
- Use the fomentation as the means of transportation of the medicinal ingredients into injured and ailing body tissues, apply overnight to swollen glands, tumors, mumps, goiter and lymphatic swellings.
- In cases of a loose tooth, it will help to strengthen the tissues and helps the tooth to set well in place.
- It is taken to reduce the deleterious effects of poisonous medicines, especially if ulceration of the bladder and bloody urine occurs.
- White Oak Bark is a strong astringent, and is used for both external and internal hemorrhage. It has an cleansing effect on inflamed surfaces of the skin or mucous membranes.
- The bark can be used for chronic diarrhea, chronic mucous discharges and passive hemorrhage.
- White Oak bark is used as a goiter remedy.
- White Oak bark has been used to expel pinworms and in the cleansing of the entire gastrointestinal tract.
- Its highly astringent qualities have made it very popular for use on varicose veins and hemorrhoids.
- White Oak bark stops bleeding in the stomach, liver, lungs and bowels.
- It increases the flow of urine and acts as a good antiseptic and astringent.
- It will stop spitting up of blood.
- White Oak Bark supports the bladder and is used in douches and enemas.
- White Oak Bark can be used for external and internal bleeding.
- White Oak Bark aid in the healing of damaged tissues in the stomach and intestines.
- White Oak Bark has been used for excess mucus with common complaints such as sinus congestion and post-nasal drip.
- White Oak Bark is known to increase the flow of urine.
- White Oak Bark Removes kidney stones and gallstones.
- White Oak Bark in fevers, brings down temperature.

- White Oak Bark relieves the stomach by toning it for better internal absorption and secretion, improving metabolism.

Bladder infections
Bladder (ulcerated)
BLEEDING (EXTERNAL &
    INTERNAL)
BLEEDING (STOMACH, LIVER,
    BOWELS)
Bruises
Cancer
Canker sores
Dental problems
Diarrhea
Enemas
Fevers
Fever blisters
Gallstones
Gangrene
Gingivitis
Glandular swellings
Goiter
Gums (bleeding)
Gums (sore)
Hemorrhage
HEMORRHOIDS
Indigestion
Insect bites
Jaundice
Kidney problems
Kidney stones
Leucorrhea

Liver problems
MENSTRUAL PROBLEMS
Mouth gargle
MOUTH SORES
Nausea
Prostate problems
Pyorrhea
Skin diseases
SKIN IRRITATIONS
Snake bites
Sores
Spleen problems
TEETH (LOOSE)
THRUSH
Tonsillitis
Toothaches
THROAT (STREP)
Tumors
ULCERS
Urinary problems
URINE (BLOODY)
Uterus (prolapsed)
Vaginal discharge
Vaginitis
VARICOSE VEINS
Venereal diseases
Vomiting
WORMS (PIN THREAD)
Wounds (external)

WHITE PINE BARK   (Pinus strobus)
A.K.A.,: Pumpkin Pine, Soft Pine.

BODILY INFLUENCE: Aromatic, Astringent, Expectorant, Circulatory Stimulant.
PART USED: Inner bark.

The native white pine forests in northeastern America were so vast, as the story goes, that a squirrel could travel all its life without coming down from the trees.   So common was the tree that it was the emblem on the first flag of the Revolutionary forces during the War for Freedom from England.

White Pine possess a powerful medicinal resin in its bark. In India, the resin from a similar species of tree is successfully used to treat the most severe forms of venereal disease, including gonorrhea.

White Pine is a warming, circulation stimulant, used traditionally in herbal combinations to overcome or prevent the onset of colds and flu by raising circulatory action.

White Pine Bark was used by the Indians to treat colds, coughs, kidney troubles, scurvy and chest congestion. A poultice of White Pine Bark was used to treat sores and wounds. White Pine Bark is also used as an expectorant in cough syrups.

The best records for the use of White Pine Bark come from the Iroquois and Micmac Indians. The Indians used the White Pine bark as a panacea using it in most of their remedial herbal healing combinations.

• White Pine Bark is an excellent expectorant to reduce mucus secretions in colds and helps in its elimination.

• The Indians soaked the bark in water until it became soft and then applied it to wounds. They also boiled the inner bark of saplings and drank the liquid for dysentery.

BRONCHITIS	LUNG CONGESTION
CATARRH	MUCUS
COLDS	Rheumatism
Croup	Scurvy
DYSENTERY	Strep throat
FLU	Tonsillitis
Kidney problems	WHOOPING COUGH
LARYNGITIS	

WHITE WILLOW BARK   (SEE WILLOW)

WILD CHERRY BARK   (Prunus virginiana, P. serotina)
A.K.A.,: Chokecherry.

BODILY INFLUENCE: Anti-tussive, Aromatic, Astringent, Bitter, Carminative, Expectorant, Nervine, Parasiticide, Pectoral, Sedative, Stomachic, Stimulant, Tonic.
PART USED: Bark.

The Indians, used Wild Cherry Bark tea for treating diarrhea and ailments of the lungs. Early colonists learned of Wild Cherry Bark's medicinal value from the American Indians. The colonists used the bark from this plant for cough syrup. The bark was also used as an ingredient in tonics and as a decoction or extract to expel worms. Extracts of this tonic were used as a poultice to treat ulcers and abscesses.

The Wild Cherry makes an outstanding tonic for convalescence. It also is a valuable remedy for all catarrhal affections. Wild Cherry's tonic action is mild, soothing and slightly astringent to the mucous membranes, especially those of the respiratory organs. Wild Cherry has a volatile oil that acts as a local stimulant in the alimentary canal and increases the appetite, aiding with digestion.

Wild Cherry calms the respiratory nerves and allays cough and asthma. It also is an outstanding remedy for weakness of the stomach with irritations, such as ulcers, gastritis, colitis, diarrhea and dysentery. It is a remedy for heart palpitations when it is caused by a stomach disorder. It is a tonic for the stomach and improves digestion by stimulating the gastric glands. It soothes nerve irritations of both the stomach and lungs and loosens mucus in the throat and chest.

- Wild Cherry is a very useful expectorant.
- Wild Cherry is commonly used as a remedy for all catarrhal conditions.
- A volatile oil of Wild Cherry acts as a local stimulant in the alimentary canal and aids in digestion.
- Wild Cherry is best used for bronchial disorders that are caused by hardened accumulation of mucus.
- Wild Cherry loosens phlegm in the throat and chest. Asthma can be improved by use of this herb.
- Cherry has been a source of food and drink since time immemorial.
- Wild Cherry wood has been used in furniture making.

ASTHMA
BLOOD PRESSURE (HIGH)
BRONCHITIS
CATARRH (LOOSENS)
COUGHS (LOOSENS)
Diarrhea
Dyspepsia
Eyesight
FEVER (ERRATIC)

Heart palpitations
MUCUS (HARDENED)
PHLEGM (LOOSENS)
Scrofula
Spasms
Stomach (irritated-G.I. tract)
TUBERCULOSIS
Worms (intestinal)

WILD LETTUCE   (Lactuca spp.,)
A.K.A.,: Opium Lettuce, Prickly Lettuce, Horse Thistle, Compass Plant.

BODILY INFLUENCE: Anodyne, Bitter, Diuretic, Hypnotic, Narcotic, Nervine, Sedative(mild).
PART USED: Milky latex.

History has it that the Roman emperor Augustus built a statue of the physician who had prescribed Lettuce for him, as he believed that the plant had cured him of a serious disease. No doubt it was Prickly Lettuce. This ancestor of all lettuce plants was valued as a sedative and pain reliever. It was considered an opium substitute into the 19th century. Once known as ,poor man,s opium,. Also called compass plant because its leaves turn to follow the sun during the day. Prickly Lettuce is bitter to people but horses delight in it.

When dried, Wild Lettuce leaves, the milky substance of which is called lactucarium is often used to induce sleep and treat severe nervous disorders, it is known to calm restlessness, anxiety, and to subdue irritating coughs.

It is effectively against whooping cough bringing relief to those suffering from bronchitis. Sometimes Wild Lettuce is called "little opium" due to its use as a sedative and a hypnotic. Milder than opium, less reliable, but was preferred because it causes no addiction or digestive problems that are associated with opium.

Wild Lettuce increases urine flow and soothes sore inflamed mucus membrane and chapped skin. The leaves contain sedative properties that act like morphine, only milder. It is the dried leaves which are used to induce sleep and treat severe nervous disorders.

• Wild Lettuce exhibits a mild sedative effect, which relieves pain, insomnia, cramps, urinary tract infections, bronchitis.
• Wild Lettuce relieves pain caused by arthritis.
• Wild Lettuce also reduces cough irritability experienced in whooping cough.

Asthma
BRONCHITIS
Colic
Coughs
CRAMPS
Diarrhea
Dropsy
Heart palpitations

Insomnia
Lactation
NERVOUS DISORDERS
PAIN (CHRONIC)
Skin irritations
SPASMS
Urinary tract infections
WHOOPING COUGH

WILD YAM   (Dioscorea villosa)

A.K.A.,: Colic Root, Devil.s Bones, Mexican Wild Yam, Rheumatism Root.

BODILY INFLUENCE: Anti-bilious, Anti-catarrhal, Anti-emetic, Anti-inflammatory, Anti-rheumatic, Anti-spasmodic, Bitter, Blood Purifier, Carminative, Cholagogue, Diaphoretic, Diuretic, Expectorant, Hepatic, Laxative, Nervine, Relaxant, Stimulant, Stomachic, Tonic.

PART USED: Root.

There is no record telling us how Wild Yam came to be called devil's bones, but the name makes sense. They consist of long, thin, twisted roots that meander along below the surface of the soil and have a skeletal look.

Wild Yam roots were employed for bilious colic and abdominal cramps by physicians in the Army of Confederate States during the Civil War.

Wild Yam is used for biliary colic, pains of gallstones, menstrual cramps, arthritic and rheumatic pains, abdominal and intestinal cramps. It is also good for chronic problems associated with gas or flatulence.

Wild Yam's steroid-like substances are used in the making birth control pills. Wild Yam is used in gland balancing formulas. Wild Yam is a valuable anti-spasmodic and is used for abdominal cramps, bowel spasms and menstrual cramps.

It is combined with other blood cleaners and will aid in removing wastes from the system, relieving stiff and sore joints.

Wild Yam is one of the best herbal anti-catarrhal agents. It is very valuable in pulmonary and catarrhal conditions. Wild Yam is beneficial in all cases of nervous excitability as a stimulant, relaxant and anti-spasmodic.

Wild Yam has an overall effect on liver health due to its ability to lower blood cholesterol levels and lower blood pressure. These properties indirectly help the liver by increasing its efficiency and reducing stress.

Wild Yam root yields an important alkaloid substance which relaxes the muscles of the stomach walls and the entire abdomen region. This alkaloid also acts as a sedative on the nerves governing these areas.

Wild Yam has a potent tonic effect on the uterus when taken throughout the period of pregnancy. The Indians of North America for hundreds of years used the Mexican Wild Yam for birth control very effectively. Wild Yam is used as an anti-spasmodic that prevents cramping.

Mexican Wild Yam was the original contraceptive pill before the pharmeceuticals started making their synthetics. It contains a progesterone precursor. It has been used historically for those with exhausted adrenals. It certainly is in competition with Licorice Root which has become famous for problems with the adrenals and low blood sugar.

There are clinics in California who have used the Mexican Wild Yam in balancing out the male hormonal side of the female. It certainly helps with hot flashes and discharge problems.

Today, quantities of Dioscorea species are collected in the wild or cultivated in Mexico to supply diosgenin, the basic substance from which birth control pills and several other steroid drugs are made with an estimate of more than 200 million prescriptions a year sold with derivatives of this herb in them.

• Wild Yam is very relaxing and soothing to the nerves, for people who get excited easily. It is useful for pain with gallstones.

• Wild Yam will also help expel gas from the stomach and bowels.

• Wild Yam is known for its ability to soothe nerves, treat liver related problems, and help with general pains during pregnancy.

• Wild Yam is a useful glandular balancing formula for treating nausea in pregnant women.

• It has been found to be an excellent preventative of miscarriage. It relieves cramps in the region of the uterus during the last trimester of pregnancy.

NOTE: This herb is beneficial during pregnancy for pregnancy pain, nausea, cramping and will lessen the threat of miscarriage.

Abdominal pain	Intestinal irritation
Addison's disease	Jaundice
After-birth pain	LIVER PROBLEMS
ARTHRITIS	Lung congestion
ASTHMA (SPASMODIC)	MENSTRUAL CRAMPS
Blood purifier	Miscarriage
Birth control	MORNING SICKNESS
Boils	MUSCLE PAIN
BOWEL SPASMS	Nausea
Bronchitis	Nerves
Catarrh (stomach)	Neuralgia
Cholera	Pain (ovarian & uterine)
COLIC (BILIOUS)	Pregnancy
Cramps	Restlessness
Digestive disorders	Rheumatism
Diverticulitis	Scabies
Dysmenorrhea	SPASMS
Exhaustion	Stomach
Female problems	Sweating (promotes)
Gallbladder	Ulcers
GAS	Urinary problems
Hiccough (spasmodic)	Whooping cough
Inflammation (reduces)	

WILLOW (Salix alba)
A.K.A.,: White Willow, Red Willow.

BODILY INFLUENCE: Alterative, Analgesic, Anodyne, Anti-inflammatory, Anti-periodic, Anti-pyretic, Antiseptic, Antispasmodic, Astringent, Bitter, Diaphoretic, Diuretic, Febrifuge, Tonic, Vermifuge.
PART USED: Bark.

The Willow tree has often cited as one of nature's greatest gifts to man because its bark contains the glucoside salicin, an effective pain killer.

A infusion is made of the Willow Bark which contains the glucoside, salicin.

The Salicin is excreted in the urine as salicylic acid and related compounds. This ability renders this tea useful for kidney, urethra and bladder irritability's and acts as an analgesic to those tissues. Willow has an ageless reputation for reducing inflammation, and working as an astringent.

The bark of Willow contains salicin which is related to aspirin from which acetylsalicylic acid (Aspirin) was first derived.

White Willow Bark was the first aspirin like substance. When the synthetic aspirin is taken internally, it can cause the stomach to hemorrhage. It is estimated that a person will loose one to two teaspoons of blood. You may have the same benefits of aspirin, by taking White Willow Bark, but without the hemorrhaging.

White Willow Bark extract is good for the symptomatic relief of fevers, headaches and sciatic, arthritic, rheumatic and neuralgic aches and pains.

Aspirin is a synthetic copy of this extraction from White Willow Bark. Today aspirin contains no willow derivatives but is entirely synthetic. When the synthetic aspirin is taken internally, it can cause the stomach to hemorrhage. It is estimated that a person will loose one to two teaspoons of blood.

• Dioscorides prescribed in the first century A.D., Willow preparations for pain and inflammation.

• One of Willow's active principles is salicin. For 30 years, European chemists fiddled with salicin: An Italian produced salicylic acid from it, and a German took that and synthesized acetylsalicylic acid. (Aspirin)

• Willow is a valuable nerve sedative. It is the forerunner of aspirin, except that it does not cause the loss of blood through the stomach walls each time it is taken and perhaps other bad side effects.

• Willow is used as a first aid plant for the wood man, as it has strong benign antiseptic abilities for infected wounds.

• Willow is used to reduce fever, works on inflammation, is an

excellent herbal source of magnesium, helps to calm nerve, may be used for first-aid (wounds and abrasions).
• Willow is useful in all stomach problems, especially sour stomach and heartburn.
• Willow is mostly used for minor aches and pains of the body.

Arthritis
Bleeding
Chills
Colds
Corns
Dandruff
Diarrhea
Dysentery
Earache
ECZEMA
FEVERS
Flu
Gout
Hayfever
HEADACHES
Heartburn

Impotence
Infection
INFLAMMATION (JOINTS)
Muscles (sore)
NERVOUSNESS
Neuralgia
Night sweats
Ovarian pain
PAIN
RHEUMATISM
SEX DEPRESSANT
Tonsillitis
ULCERATIONS
Worms
WOUNDS

WINTERGREEN (Gaultheria procumbens)
A.K.A.,: Teaberry, Boxberry, Mountain Tea.

BODILY INFLUENCE: Analgesic, Anodyne, Anti-pyretic, Anti-rheumatic, Antiseptic, Anti-spasmodic, Aromatic, Astringent, Diuretic, Expectorant, Rubefacient(counter-irritant).
PART USED: The whole plant.

As far back as the 1800's, chemists discovered that there was an oil from the wintergreen leaves that has properties similar to aspirin. Wintergreen oil has been applied externally to treat inflammation of the joints and muscles and to reduce swelling.

Wintergreen is applied externally or taken internally or both, to relieve pain and allay rheumatic complaints. The leaves contain methyl salicylate which has anti-inflammatory properties similar to aspirin, making it useful for a wide variety of painful syndromes from headaches to arthritis.

Wintergreen is a cooling, fragrant analgesic. Crushed into a poultice, the leaves were an important Indian remedy to relieve aching, arthritic pain, or overtaxed exhausted muscles and joints. Poultices also relieved swellings, wounds, rashes, inflammations-even toothaches. Internally, wintergreen tea was taken to relieve fever, gonorrhea symptoms, sore throats, upset stomachs, and ulcers.

- Wintergreen's leaves and berries contain methyl salicylate, closely related to aspirin.
- Wintergreen is also effective taken in small frequent doses, to stimulate the heart and improve respiration. It is helpful in obstructions in the bowels. Valuable in colic and gas in the bowels.
- Wintergreen can be used as a tea for headaches, rheumatic pains, sciatica or joint or muscles pains.

ACHES
BACK PAIN (LOWER)
Cystitis
Diabetes
Digestive disorders
Diphtheria
Gas
GOUT
HEADACHES (MIGRAINE)

Inflammation
Leucorrhea
PAIN
Rheumatic fever
Rheumatism
Sciatica
Throat gargle
Urinary problems
Yeast infection

WITCH HAZEL   (Hamamelis virginiana) LT OK
A.K.A.,: Snapping Hazelnut, Winterbloom.

BODILY INFLUENCE: Anti-inflammatory, Antiseptic, Astringent, Hemostatic, Sedative, Styptic, Tonic.
PART USED: Bark, Leaves, Twigs.

Dossiers have been using for hundreds of years a forked twig from Witch Hazel trees as divining rods to locate water and minerals. The "witch" in the name Witch Hazel comes from the Anglo-Saxon word meaning "to bend".

The name Witch Hazel derives from the Old English word for "pliant", and in fact the limber branches were used to make archery bows.

The Indians drank Witch Hazel tea as a general tonic and used it as a gargle for mouth and throat irritations. Witch Hazel steam baths were very beneficial in helping to loosening heavy phlegm and coughing it up.

Witch Hazel has been one of the commonest home remedies in America. Consisting of a distillation of Witch hazel bark, twigs and leaves mixed with alcohol and water, it has been used mainly as an astringent. Witch Hazel can be applied fomentation to strained and bruised muscles, or as a cold compress over a fevered brow.

Witch Hazel has a strong astringent action and is effective in stopping bleeding both internally and externally. It reduces swelling and inflammation from bruises, hemorrhoids and helps relieve varicose veins.

The treatment of the various physical problems that exist in mankind is benefited by the variety of herb that have been placed here to be uses. However there are mainly two distinct categories to place these herbs in. There are the herbs that help alleviate pain and discomfort and some how allow man to continue living as he chooses without knowledge of a better way, these are the sedatives and stimulants and astringents. Then there are the herbs that contain the very necessary vital elements of life that for some reason man has not acquired in his daily intake of nutrients. These herbs supply in right and proper amounts these nutrients and in many case also contain those other ingredients that help sustain him over the interim, after he has begun to suffer the results of his past indiscretions.

Witch Hazel possesses a unique kind of astringency whose main focus of action is on the venous system, acting to restore tone, health and vigor throughout that system. As a first aid herbal it is excellent, it has hemostatic properties benefitting hemorrhoids, varicose veins, any minor bleeding, stops nose bleeding, scratches, etc., can be quickly mended with the application of Witch Hazel tincture or poultice. But the basic usefulness of Witch Hazel leaves is for treating female congestive conditions of the uterus, cervix and vagina, including vaginitis and prolapsus.

Witch Hazel is safe non-toxic herbal substance that can be used in the cleansing and toning of the skin and to help prevent an oily build-up on the tissues of the skin.

The tea or fluid extract is one of nature's best remedies for stopping excessive menstruation, hemorrhages from the lungs, stomach, nose, uterus, kidneys and rectum.

Witch Hazel used as a fomentation or poultice, is good for wounds or sores, sore and inflamed eyes, bed sores any oozing skin disease. One can not think of an inflamed condition internally or externally that will not benefit by this remedy.

• Witch Hazel has a slight sedative property when taken internally. It is very useful for treating inflamed or irritated sensitive tissues, like mucous membranes.

• Witch Hazel compresses are used to treat headaches, inflamed eyes, skin irritations, insect bites, burns and infections. An extract helps when applied to strained muscles and arthritic joints.

• Witch Hazel is used in great quantities for external use, as an astringent skin cleanser, body lotion, aftershave, massage liquid for body and scalp, and an aid in setting hair. The extract is also used for insect bites and sunburn.

Abrasions	Bleeding gums
Backaches	Bruises
BLEEDING (INTERNAL STOPS)	Burns

Cancer	Nervousness
Circulation	Nose bleeds
Colds	Phlegm
Coughs	Poison ivy
Cuts	Scalds
Diarrhea	Sinus
Eyes (inflammation)	Skin diseases (oozing)
Fevers	SORES (BED)
Gargle	Sore throat
GUMS	Stings
HEMORRHAGES	SUNBURN
HEMORRHOIDS	SWELLINGS
INFLAMMATIONS (EXTERNAL)	Tuberculosis
INSECT BITES	Ulcers
Menstruation (excess)	Vaginitis
Mouthwash	VARICOSE VEINS
MUCOUS MEMBRANES	Venereal disease
Muscles (sore)	WOUNDS (WASHING)

WOOD BETONY   (Betonica officinalis, Stachys officinalis)
A.K.A.,: Bishopwort, Lousewort, Beefsteak Plant.

BODILY INFLUENCE: Alterative, Anti-scorbutic, Aperient, Aromatic, Astringent, Carminative, Hepatic, Nervine, Parasiticide, Sedative, Stomachic, Bitter Tonic,
PART USED: The whole plant.

Wood Betony was used in medieval England to cure 'monstrous nocturnal visions, devils, despair and lunacy.' Betonic is the Celtic name of the plant and comes from ben (the head) and ton (good) in reference to the herb's abilities as a remedy for head complaints.

Wood Betony is an excellent remedy for head problems as with pain in the head, headaches and face twitching. Wood Betony is used in combination with other herbs for treating rheumatism and other diseases which stem from impurities of the blood. It will open obstructions of the liver and spleen, mildly stimulate the heart and expel worms from the system. It is also a tonic for general digestive disorders.

The glycosides of Wood Betony have recognizable hypotensive activity. This explains most of the understandable properties, since a substance that is hypotensive relaxes nervous tension as well as opens up constrictive blood vessels that are the basis for the headaches.

• Wood Betony is good for head and facial pains and nervous disorders.

• Snuff combined with Wood Betony was once used as a headache remedy.

- Wood Betony is calming to the nerves.
- Wood Betony acts as a gentle laxative and also tones the stomach. It can prevent or cure scurvy indicating its vitamin C content.
- It is a vascular dilator and excellent for headaches. Wood Betony is of great value when there is pain in the face and head.
- Wood Betony loosens congested areas of the liver and spleen. It cleans impurities from the blood and can be used for indigestion, heartburn, and cramps in the stomach.

Anemia
Anxiety
Arthritis
Asthma (bronchial)
Bedwetting
Bladder
Bleeding (internal)
Blood vessels (dilates)
Bronchitis
Colds
Colic
Convulsions
Consumption
Coughs
DELIRIUM
Diarrhea
Digestive disorders
Dropsy
Epilepsy
FEVERS
Gout
HEADACHES (MIGRAINE)
Headaches (nervous)
Heartburn
Heart stimulant
HYSTERIA
Indigestion
Inflammation

Insanity
Insomnia
JAUNDICE
Kidneys
LIVER PROBLEMS
Lung congestion
Menstruation
Mental illness
Muscle spasms
NERVOUS CONDITIONS
Neuralgia
Night sweats
Pain reliever
Palsy
Parasites
PARKINSON'S DISEASE
Perspiration
Rheumatism
Scurvy
Sores
Spleen obstructions
Stomach cramps
Ulcers
Urination (increases)
Varicose veins
WORMS
Wounds

WORMWOOD   (Artemisia absinthium)
A.K.A.,: Pasture Sagewort.

BODILY INFLUENCE: Anti-bilious, Anti-inflammatory, Antiseptic, Anti-venomous, Aromatic, Bitter, Carminative, Cholagogue, Diaphoretic, Emmenagogue, Febrifuge, Hemostatic, Hepatic, Narcotic, Parasiticide, Stimulant, Stomachic, Styptic, Tonic, Vermifuge.
PART USED: Root, Leaves, Flowering tops.

Wormwood has been used for centuries as anthelmintics (parasiticides) internally and as a hemostatic, externally. It was used medicinally for colds, sore eyes, as a hair tonic, to control menstrual flow and swelling wounds. Wormwood can counteract fevers, regulate the liver and treat anemia and arthritis. It is taken as a bitter tonic and given to eliminate intestinal worms.

This herb is helpful for stopping internal bleeding and and useful as an antidote for many poisonous mushrooms. Fomentations and compresses soaked in Wormwood tea are excellent in applications for rheumatism, swellings, sprains, bruises and local inflammation. The oil of Wormwood acts as a local anesthetic and is a good liniment when applied to relieve pains of rheumatism, neuralgia, arthritis, sprains, bruises, lower back pain and local inflammation.

• Wormwood is an invigorating, aromatic herb that has antiseptic qualities and is capable of expelling worms.

• Wormwood has been useful for all complaints of the digestive system such as constipation and indigestion. It stimulates sweating when experiencing dry fevers and for an acid stomach.

• Wormwood promotes menstruation, stimulates uterine circulation and will also help relieve menstrual cramps.

• Wormwood should be used in small quantities and for only short periods of time.

• Giving Wormwood to children is considered as not being safe.

• Wormwood can be used externally and internally to reduce hair loss.

• The bitter herb has long been used as an insect repellent.

CAUTION: This herb stimulates uterine contractions and can be toxic in large doses and therefore should be avoided during pregnancy.

Appetite stimulant	Breath (bad)
Arthritis	Bruises
Back pain (lower)	Childbirth pains
Blood circulation	Circulation
Boils	Colds

CONSTIPATION
DEBILITY
Diarrhea
DIGESTIVE AID
Dropsy
Earaches
Eczema
Female disorders
FEVERS
Gallbladder
Gas
Gastritis
Gout
Heart
Hepatitis
Indigestion
INFLAMMATION CONDITIONS
(G.I. TRACT)

Insect repellent
JAUNDICE
Kidney problems
LIVER PROBLEMS
MENSTRUAL CRAMPS
MENSTRUATION (PROMOTES)
Morning sickness
Nausea
Neuralgia
Obesity
Perspiration
Poisons (expels)
Rheumatism
Spasms
Sprains
STOMACH PROBLEMS
Swellings
WORMS (EXPELS)

YARROW (Achillea millefolium)

A.K.A.,: Bloodwort, Thousand-leaf, Milfoil(French), Milefolia(Spanish).

BODILY INFLUENCE: Alterative, Anti-bacterial, Anti-inflammatory, Anti-pyretic, Antiseptic, Anti-spasmodic, Aromatic, Astringent, Carminative,Y Diaphoretic, Digestant, Diuretic, Emmmenagogue, Hemostatic, Stimulant, Stomachic, Styptic, Tonic,Vulnerary.
PART USED: Leaves, Flowering tops.

"Achillea," Yarrow's generic name dates back in folklore to Achilles in his battle for the Conquest of Troy, is said to have used Yarrow to bind the wounds of his soldiers, that's one story, the other is that he used Yarrow to bind his Achilles heal. Either way, we have the generic name of "Achillea".

Yarrow is a strong, soothing diaphoretic. Taken as a hot tea, it will naturally increase body temperature, open skin pores, stimulate free perspiration, increase elimination and equalize the circulation, thus making it an important herb for cold and fevers. Yarrow purifies the blood of morbid waste material which must be eliminated in sickness. Yarrow balances the function of the liver and has an influence on secretion production throughout the alimentary canal. Yarrow's tonic action is most invigorating and will greatly assist nature's actions to remove congestion and disease. Yarrow has the ability to stop bleeding relatively quickly which assists in the healing process.

The following appears contradictory in its opposite interesting result.

Yarrow in the treatment of nosebleeds works in a peculiar way, you insert a roll of Yarrow into the nostril, the bleeding stops shortly. Now! For a severe sinus headache, insert a roll of Yarrow into the nostril. A nosebleed will result, relieving pressure on the head and thus the headache is relieved. If you have a bleeding nose and want to stop it, use Yarrow. If you don't have a bleeding nose, but need one, use Yarrow. It is a very accommodating plant.

Yarrow is also a good blood cleanser, helping to clean the blood of uric acid, thereby removing the cause of gout. This herb contains aromatic compounds that aid in shrinking inflamed tissue and promote sweating. Therefore, Yarrow is useful in treating inflammatory skin conditions.

The English had the reputation of colonizing a large part of the globe at one time and were often in the tropics and subject to exposure to all the varied diseases with their accompanying fevers. Over many years Quinine was the drug of choice for fevers. Yarrow apparently was one of the herbs that they took for their somewhat minor problems, thus the name Englishman's Quinine.

• In China, it is said that Yarrow grows around the grave of Confucius.

• Yarrow is considered very effective where there are symptoms of chills, constant nasal drip, catarrh and sensations of alternate cold and heat.

• For centuries, Yarrow has been used on wounds and in the 1950's, an alkaloid from the plant was found to have some ability to make blood clot faster.

• Nicholas Culpepper, the seventeenth-century British herbalist, recommended Yarrow for wounds.

• The Shakers knew Yarrow and included it in treatments for a variety of complaints from hemorrhages to flatulence.

• The Piute Indians called Yarrow "Wound Medicine."

• The Navajo Indians consider Yarrow to be a "life medicine" and chewed the leaves to stop toothache pain. These Indians make an infusion of the plant tops and pour it into the ears for earaches.

• Yarrow opens the pores of the skin permitting a greater discharge of internal poisons through the essentials of perspiration. The flowers contain an oil which saturates the bloodstream and chemically helps uric acid impurities.

• Yarrow effects two major actions on the system: (a) it works on the liver to produce bile, and (b) builds up the blood and stops internal hemorrhaging. Yarrow is effective against yeast infections in the female reproductive system.

• Yarrow has tannin and choline in its arsonal of active ingredients. The tannin or tannic acid in the flowers is a powerful

virus inhibitor.
- Yarrow usually breaks up a cold within 24 hours.
- Yarrow supports and regulates liver and pancreas function.
- Yarrow has a very soothing and healing effect on the mucous membranes.
- Yarrow aids with nausea and helps to control fungus.
- Yarrow stimulates sweating in dry fevers and is a quinine substitute.
- Yarrow is a tonic for run-down conditions and is used in skin and hair conditioners.
- Yarrow is sometimes used in childhood conditions involving skin eruptions.
- Yarrow tea is excellent for shrinking hemorrhoids, hemorrhages and bleeding of the lungs. It is sometimes used for diarrhea in infants.
- Yarrow can be used to control bleeding from the lungs and bowels.
- Yarrow regulates many urination problems. It soothes and heals mucous membranes and is effective against fevers and the flu.
- Yarrow grows nearly everywhere as a weed.

NOTE: This herb is a strong astringent and mild abortifacient and should not be taken during pregnancy except in combinations with other herbs.

Abrasions	Epilepsy
Appetite stimulant	Female problems
Arthritis	FEVERS
Bladder problems	FLU
Bleeding (lungs & bowels)	Gas
Bleeding (stops)	Hair loss
BLOOD CLEANSER	Headaches
Blood coagulant	Hemorrhoids
Blood pressure (reduces)	Hysteria
BOWELS (HEMORRHAGE)	Jaundice
Bright's disease	Kidney problems
Bronchitis	Liver problems
Bruises	LUNGS (HEMORRHAGE)
Bursitis	Malaria
Cancer	MEASLES
CATARRH	Menstrual bleeding
Chicken pox	Mucous membranes
COLDS	Night sweats
Cramps	Nipples (sore)
Cuts	NOSE BLEEDS
Diarrhea	Pleurisy
Diarrhea (infants)	Pneumonia

Rheumatism	Typhoid fever
Skin problems	Ulcers
Smallpox	Urinary problems
Sore throat	Urine retention
Spleen	Uterus
Stomach problems	Vaginal discharge
SWEATING (PROMOTES)	Yeast infections

YELLOW DOCK (Rumex crispus)

A.K.A.,: Curled Dock, Sour Dock, Garden patience, Narrow Dock.

BODILY INFLUENCE: Alterative, Anti-scorbutic, Anti-scrofulous, Anti-syphilitic, Astringent, Bitter, Cathartic, Cholagogue, Depurative, Hepatic, Laxative, Nutritive(leaves), Tonic.

PART USED: Root.

The generic name for Yellow Dock, rumex, is derived from the Latin "rumex" meaning a lance in reference to the shape of its leaves. Its species name, crispus, is from the Latin "crisped" in reference to its leaves being crisped at the edges.

Yellow Dock is an excellent blood cleanser, tonic and builder, working through increasing the ability of the liver and related organs to strain and purify the blood and lymph system, it achieves its tonic properties through the astringent purification of the blood supply to the glands. Yellow Dock roots has one of the highest iron contents in nature and is an effective tonic treatment for anemia during pregnancy and anemia in general. It is used to treat skin diseases, liver disorders and iron deficiency. It will also nourish the spleen.

It will tone up the entire system and is good for diseases such as skin infections, tumors, liver and gallbladder problems, ulcers and skin itch. It makes an excellent salve for itchy skin diseases and swellings of glands or otherwise. It acts as a laxative because it stimulates the flow of bile.

- Externally, Yellow Dock is applied to bleeding hemorrhoids and wounds.
- Yellow Dock tightens varicose veins.
- Yellow Dock is an excellent cleansing herb for the lymphatic system.
- Yellow Dock is a great endurance builder.
- Yellow Dock balances body chemistry with its high mineral content.
- Yellow Dock nourishes the glands.
- Yellow Dock builds the immune system.
- Yellow Dock tones the entire system, especially the pineal

gland.
- Yellow Dock is sometimes used in arsenic poisoning.
- Yellow Dock strengthens and tones the entire system. It is very valuable for cleansing the blood, boils, ulcers, and wounds. It is high in iron.

NOTE: This herb is beneficial during pregnancy as it aids iron assimilation and will help to prevent infant jaundice.

Acne
ANEMIA
Arsenic poisoning
Arthritis
Bladder
Bleeding
BLOOD CLEANSER
BLOOD DISORDERS
BLOOD PURIFIER
BOILS
Bowels (regulator & normalizer)
Bronchitis (chronic)
CANCER
CHICKEN POX (TOPICAL FOR ITCH)
Constipation
COUGHS
Dysentery
Ear infections
Eczema
Energy
EYELIDS (ULCERATED)
Fatigue
Fevers
Gallbladder
Glandular tumors
Hayfever
Hemorrhoids (external)
Hepatitis
HIVES
IRON DEFICIENCY

ITCHING
Jaundice
Leprosy
Leukemia
LIVER CONGESTION
Lymphatic system
Mucus
Paralysis
Pituitary gland
Poison ivy/oak
PREGNANCY (IRON SUPPLEMENT)
Psoriasis
RHEUMATISM
Scarlet fever
SCURVY
SKIN ERUPTIONS
SKIN DISEASES
SORES
Spleen
Stamina
Swellings
Syphilis
Thyroid glands
Tumors (glandular)
Ulcers
Varicose veins
Venereal disease
Vitality (lack of)
Worms
Wounds

YERBA SANTA   (Eriodictyon spp.,)

A.K.A.,: Sacred Herb, Mountain Balm, Bear's Weed, Consumptive Weed.

BODILY INFLUENCE: Alterative, Aromatic, Astringent, Bitter, Carminative, Expectorant, Sialagogue, Stimulant, Stomachic.
PART USED: Leaves.

The Spanish learned of this plant from the Indians who boiled the fresh or dried leaves and used the preparation for such problems as coughs, colds, sore throats, mucus, stomachaches, vomiting and diarrhea. Yerba Santa is used for upper-respiratory congestion as an infusion or syrup. It will also promote salivation and thus aid thirst, dryness and digestion.

Yerba Santa has a strong stimulant action which is most pronounced on the lungs. Yerba Santa acts as an expectorant, meaning it stimulates the lungs and respiratory tract to expel mucus. In conditions such as bronchitis, coughs, chest colds and other conditions where there is excessive mucus to be expelled from the body, Yerba Santa is an excellent choice.

Externally, Yerba Santa has been used as a poultice for wounds, bruises, sprains and insect bites.

Yerba Santa is a South American stimulanting and rejuvenating herb and naturally relieves fatigue. It protects against the effects of stress and is helpful in opening respiratory passages to overcome allergy symptoms. In addition to its inherent benefits, Yerba Santa is a catalyst substance that increases the healing effectiveness of other herbs.

• Yerba Santa is an old remedy for tuberculosis.

• Yerba Santa means "Sacred herb" in Spanish.

• Yerba Santa is excellent for bronchial congestion, as well as all chest conditions, acute or chronic and is effective when there is much discharge from the nose.

• Yerba Santa cleanses the blood, tones the nervous system, retards aging, stimulates the mind, controls the appetite, stimulates production of cortisone and is believed to enhance the healing powers of other herbs.

• Yerba Santa allieviates pain in rheumatism, helps enervate tired limbs, reduces swellings and heals sores.

ALLERGIES
Arthritis
ASTHMA
Bladder catarrh
Blood cleanser
BRONCHIAL CONGESTION
CATARRH
COLDS

Constipation
Coughs (dry)
Diarrhea
Digestion (improves)
Dysentery
Fatigue
Fevers
Flu

HAYFEVER
Headache
Hemorrhoids
Kidney problems
Laryngitis (chronic)
Lungs
Nose discharge
Obesity

Pulmonary conditions
Rheumatism
Sore throat
Stomachaches
Stress
Vomiting
Water retention

YOHIMBE   (Pausinystalia johimbe)
A.K.A.,: NONE.

BODILY INFLUENCE: Aphrodisiac.
PART USED: Bark.

The Yohimbe tree is native to Africa. It has become popular due to the reputation it is gaining as a strong aphrodisiac affecting both male and female impotency. A testosterone precursor, Yohimbe is an effective body builder. It is a hormone stimulant and is a strong athletic formula herb where increased testosterone is needed.

The bark of this tropical tree, Yohimbe, has been smoked, rubbed on the body, ingested and sniffed, for its effect on sexual interest and performance. The bark has long been valued as an aphrodisiac. The plant yields yohimbine, which in the form of an alkaloid salt, yohimbine hydrochloride, has been used in prescription formulas to improve sexual performance.

• The drug yohimbine dilates the blood vessels of the skin and mucous membranes, thus bringing the blood closer to the surface of the sex organs and simultaneously lowering blood pressure.

• The problem with Yohimbe as an aphrodisiac is that if the blood pressure is normally low, fatigue may produce temporary impotence instead of vigorous performance.

• Yohimbe should never be taken at the same time as foods or substances containing tyramine which is an amino acid. Foods high in tyramine include liver, cheese, and red wine as should certain diet aids and decongestants.

NOTE: This herb should be avoided if there is high blood pressure or heart arrhythmia.

YUCCA   (Yucca baccata, Y. glauca)
A.K.A.,: Spanish Dagger, Soapweed, respectively.

BODILY INFLUENCE: Alterative, Anti-bacterial, Anti-inflammatory, Anti-rheumatic, Astringent, Bitter, Blood Purifier, Laxative.
PART USED: Root.

The plant has a rich history in the South Western areas, primarily amongst the many American Indian Tribes in that area. The plant was used for almost everything, from making clothing to medical applications.

The most important variety of Yucca is a desert plant sometimes known as Spanish bayonet. Its root has a high content of natural saponins. When it is chopped up in water, it makes a natural lather and is an effective soap substitute. The most common folk name applied to this plant is soap rope. Early settlers learned from the Indians that processed Yucca root made a sudsy shampoo or general purpose soap, particularly for clothing.

Yucca's root has a high content of natural saponins. Extracts from Yucca roots make excellent shampoo and soap, When it is chopped up in water, it makes a natural lather and is an effective soap substitute. A soap-like material, Yucca will actually lather like soap, because it holds water agaisnt the skin. This is why Yucca is used as a soap.

Testing further reveals it to be a hormonal material, a steroid. The adrenal hormone, cortisone is a steroid. Yucca has a definte action upon the intestinal bacteria, or intestinal flora, living within the human intestines, which actually helps with the digestion of food and prevents certain types of harmful bacteria from flourishing which could cause sickness if too many accumulate.

It is now known that Yucca's roots high content of natural saponins does not enter the bloodstream, but acts only on the intestinal flora to regulate the balance of the bacterial colonies in the colon. By stimulating friendly flora and inhibiting others, Yucca saponins may indirectly stimulate the absorption of other nutritional factors and decrease the amount of toxins available for absorption from the digestive system. The eliminative systems of the body (kidneys, liver, lymph, and blood) are thus less taxed to remove poisons from the body. This lowers the build-up of toxins in the joints and elsewhere which seem to be related to degenerative diseases like arthritis. The saponins provide a healthy alkalinity to an otherwise acid-ridden system full of toxic impurities. It has been found by its action, that the saponins somehow improves digestion and reduces the tendency to develop accumulations of undigested toxic waste which decompose in the colon, producing foul-smelling gases.

In some clinics in the Sonoran desert region of Arizona, Yucca is the remedy routinely prescribed against arthritis, with impressive results. Yucca can occasionally be purgative and cause some intestinal cramping. For this reason, it is good to combine it with other complimentary anti-rheumatic herbs.

Yucca is most often included in formulas designed to "break up obstructions" especially to reduce the inflammation in joints, which include the chronic degenerative diseases, arthritis and rheumatism. Yucca has the ability to break up inorganic mineral obstructions and deposits.

- Yucca is high in fiber an can be beneficial for intestinal problems.
- Scientists have discovered that Yucca roots contain a high concentration of saponins, natural substances which are similar to steroids such as cortisone.
- Yucca reduces inflammation of the joints and so is primarily used for arthritic and rheumatoid conditions.
- Yucca has been used as a natural cortisone.
- Extracts from Yucca roots make an excellent shampoo and soap.
- It is known to aid digestion and help conditions such as urethritis and prostatitis.

Addison's disease	Gonorrhea
Allergies	Gout
ARTHRITIS	Inflammation (joint)
BLOOD PURIFIER	Liver problems
BURSITIS	Osteo-arthritis
Cancer	Prostatitis
Cataracts	RHEUMATISM
CHOLESTEROL (REDUCES)	Scalp problems
Colitis	Skin problems
Dandruff	Skin inflammations
DETOXIFIER	Urethritis
Gallbladder	Venereal disease

HERB COMBINATIONS

Herbalists who have devoted their lives to understanding the medicinal properties of nature's healers, believe that many herbs work best when used in combination with other herbs. This is because some act as catalysts, encouraging other herbs to work more effectively.

Seldom can we isolate one single deficiency or excess as the cause of a medical problem. Illness is generally the result of an accumulation of ailments, thus herbal combinations are often the most effective treatment. "The Little Herb Encyclopedia" takes the guesswork out of herb combinations by suggesting some of the most beneficial herbal formulas. As with single herbs, time and experimentation will determine which work best for your body. Depending upon where we live and the foods our bodies are accustomed to, some herbs and herb combinations will have a rapid and dramatic effect. Others will work more slowly. Realize that some contagious diseases must run their course, and although herbal formulas may be helpful in treating the symptoms, the body must cure itself. The herb combinations listed here and their uses are only suggested for your benefit. "The Little Herb Encyclopedia" does not attempt to diagnose or prescribe.

Stories continue to abound telling of the tremendous benefits people have received from using herbs.

ALLERGIES

Horseradish, Mullein, Fenugreek seeds, Fennel fruit, Boneset.

BODILY INFLUENCE: Antispasmodic, Decongestant, Expectorant, Mucilant.
SPECIFIC CONDITIONS: Allergies-respiratory, Asthma, Bronchial congestion, Bronchitis, Congestion-respiratory, Cough-expectorant, Diarrhea, Dyspepsia, Earache, Emphysema, Hayfever-decongestant, Indigestion, Inflammation, Lymphatic congestion, Sinus congestion, Pneumonia, Swollen glands.

This combination was designed by Master Herbalist, Jeanne Burgess to give maximum relief for allergy sufferers. This product has a long and proven tract record.

ALLERGIES

Concentrated Ephedra, White Willow bark, Valerian, Lobelia, Golden Seal, Bee Pollen, Capsicum.

BODILY INFLUENCE: Analgesic, Anti-inflammatory, Calmative, Expectorant, Stimulant.
SPECIFIC CONDITIONS: Hayfever, Allergies, Sinus congestion, Bronchial spasms, Head congestion, Asthma, Bronchitis, Mucus, Colds, Lung problems.
This combination was designed to be a natural decongestant by helping to reduce swollen membranes allowing nasal and sinus passages to drain.

ANTI-GAS

Papaya fruit, Ginger, Peppermint, Wild Yam, Fennel, Dong Quai, Spearmint, Catnip.

BODILY INFLUENCE: Antacid, Aromatic, Carminative, Stomachic.
SPECIFIC CONDITIONS: Bloating, Foul belching, Gas-expel or prevent, Heartburn, Hiatal hernia, Indigestion, Sour stomach.
A healthy digestive system will efficiently digest food and eliminate undesirable materials. This product is helpful when there is bloating and gas due to improper digestion. This may be the result of a hiatal hernia or improper food combining.

ANTI-GAS

Papaya fruit, Peppermint.

BODILY INFLUENCE: Antacid, Carminative, Stomachic.
SPECIFIC CONDITIONS: Gas-expel or prevent, Heartburn, Sour stomach, Indigestion.

Papaya mint chewable tablets nutritionally support the digestive system, but they can also be used as a tasty breath mint. Papaya fruit contains proteolytic enzymes that function in the digestion of protein, while peppermint leaves contain aromatic compounds capable of triggering the production of digestive fluids. Together they work to support the digestive system. It.s great for children.

ARTHRITIS/RHEUMATISM

Bromelain, Hydrangea, Yucca, Horsetail, Celery seed, Alfalfa, Black Cohosh, Catnip, Yarrow, Capsicum, Valerian, White Willow, Burdock, Slippery Elm, Sarsaparilla.

BODILY INFLUENCE: Alterative, Analgesic, Bitter, Diuretic, Lithotriptic.
SPECIFIC CONDITIONS: Arthritis, Bursitis, Calcium deposits, Gout, Lupus, Neuritis, Rheumatism, Stiffness-general, Fibrositis.

This combination helps to aid arthritis sufferers from joint stiffness. It is rich in easily-absorbed calcium, it detoxifies and neutralizes uric acid and is a solvent for calcium deposits.

ARTHRITIS/RHEUMATISM

Yucca, Willow, Hydrangea, Alfalfa, Burdock, Black Cohosh, Sarsaparilla, Parsley, Slippery Elm, Redmond clay, Capsicum, Pan Pien Lien.
(SEE ARTHRITIS ABOVE)

ASTHMA

Blessed Thistle, Pleurisy, Scullcap, Yerba Santa.

BODILY INFLUENCE: Anti-spasmodic, Expectorant, Decongestant, Nervine.
SPECIFIC CONDITIONS: Allergies, Pollen, Asthma attacks, Bronchitis, Congestion-general, Cough-dry and hard, Hayfever, Mucus, Pleurisy, Pneumonia, Headache, Lung problems, Respiratory distress-upper, Lymph congestion.

This herbal combination stimulates natural antihistamines. It is a nutritional aid for the nervous, respiratory and muscle systems.

ASTHMA

Mullein and Pan Pien Lien.

BODILY INFLUENCE: Anti-spasmodic, Astringent, Expectorant, Nervine.
SPECIFIC CONDITIONS: Asthma, Pleurisy, Bronchitis, Mumps, Lymph congestion, Tuberculosis, Glandular swelling.
Mullein is astringent in nature increasing the production of mucus by decreasing the thickness of the mucus so the body can eliminate the waste.

Pan Pien Lien is similar in action to Lobelia which is a great nervine that relaxes bronchial passages so that breathing is improved.
(SEE ASTHMA ABOVE)

BLOOD PRESSURE EQUALIZING
Garlic bulb, Capsicum fruit, Parsley, Ginger, Siberian Ginseng, Golden Seal.

BODILY INFLUENCE: Hypertensive, Hypotensive.
SPECIFIC CONDITIONS: Arteriosclerosis, Blood Pressure-high or low, Heart palpitations, Plaque-helps dissolve.
This provides nutrients necessary for proper function of the circulatory systems. Garlic has been credited as one of nature's most all-around nutritive herbs. Siberian ginseng, one of the most extensively studied of all herbs, is used by Soviet athletes and many others as a regular dietary supplement. Parsley is rich in chlorophyll and potassium, a natural deodorizer.

BLOOD PRESSURE EQUALIZING
Fumitory(Fumaria officinalis), Knollensonnenblume (Helianthus tuberosus), Persian Garlic, Onion, Strawberry leaves, Raspberry leaves, Garlic, Citruce (lime and orange peel), Cichoriumintybus, Pear, Calcome, Rueprechtskraut(Geranium purpureum Vill), Vite(Vitis vinifera L.), Licorice root.

This herbal combination nourishes the circulatory system.
(SEE BLOOD PRESSURE EQUALIZING ABOVE)

BLOOD PRESSURE REDUCER
Capsicum, Garlic, Parsley.

BODILY INFLUENCE: Antiseptic, Aromatic, Hypotensive, Stomachic.
SPECIFIC CONDITIONS: Arteriosclerosis, Blood pressure-low /high, Bronchitis, Chills, Circulation-poor, Colds-general formula for, Cough, Earache, Emphysema, Fatigue-stimulant, Fever, Flu, Hemorrhoids, Infection, Kidney infection, Lymphatic congestion, Mucus-expels, Pneumonia, Tonsillitis, Cholesterol-lowers, Herbal penicillin, Hypertension, Heart-strengthens.

This herbal formula is useful in enhancing overall circulation, and in toning and strengthening the heart. It is believed to be useful in stabilizing the blood pressure.

BLOOD PRESSURE REDUCER
Capsicum, Garlic.
(SEE BLOOD PRESSURE REDUCER ABOVE)

BLOOD PRESSURE REDUCER
Garlic, Parsley.
(SEE 1ST BLOOD PRESSURE REDUCER ABOVE)

BLOOD PRESSURE REDUCER
Garlic, Capsicum, Golden Seal Root, Parsley, Ginger, Eleurherococcus senticosus.

BODILY INFLUENCE: Antibiotic, Diuretic, Hormonal, Stimulant.
SPECIFIC CONDITIONS: Blood pressure-low or high, Bronchitis, Chills, Circulation, Colds, Coughs, Congestion, Infection, Kidney and Bladder infection, Flu.

When you have high blood pressure, the first place you should look is to the kidneys. This formula is used to reduce down swelling also.
(SEE 1ST BLOOD PRESSURE REDUCER ABOVE)

BLOOD PURIFIER
Freeze-dried Shark cartilage, dehydrated Reishi mushroom, Pau D'Arco herb, Burdock root, Sorrel, Turkish Rhubarb, Cress.

This is a combination of herbs put together to boost the immune system and especially designed with anti-cancer and anti-tumor qualities.

BLOOD PURIFIER/DETOXIFIER/CANCER
Burdock, Pau d' Arco, Red Clover tops, Yellow Dock, Sarsaparilla, Dandelion, Cascara Sagrada, Buckthorn, Peach Bark, Barberry, Stillinga, Prickly Ash, Yarrow.

BODILY INFLUENCE: Alterative, Bitter, Blood Purifier, Cholagogue, Diuretic.
SPECIFIC CONDITIONS: Acne-blood cleansing, Anemia-builds liver, Boils, Cancer, Chronic weakness, Contagious diseases, Eczema, Gangrene, Jaundice, Poison ivy/oak, Ringworm, Skin-inflammation of, Toxemia, Toxic blood, Tumors, Abscesses, Addictions, AIDS.

This combination of herbs traditionally is used to nutritionally support the quality of the blood and the functions of the kidneys and the liver. The original formula was put together by Dr. John Christopher, N.D.

BLOOD PURIFIER/DETOXIFIER
Red Clover tops, Burdock root, Pau d' Arco bark, Spice.

BODILY INFLUENCE: Alterative, Blood Purifier.
SPECIFIC CONDITIONS: Cancer-immune booster, Toxic blood, Tumors, Leukemia.

Red Clover is one of the major herbs in the Hoxsey formula. This combination when used in tea form has historically been used to dissolve down tumors and eliminate cancer. It is good support for the liver and other immune system organs. This original formula was developed by Sir Jason Winters and what was supposed to be his death bed. He has since been knighted by the queen and travels the world preaching about health.

BLOOD PURIFIER /DETOXIFIER
Burdock root, Sheep Sorrel herb, Slippery Elm bark, Turkish Rhubarb root.

This herbal combination was originally developed in Canada by Rene Caisse. She acquired this combination from the Obijy Indians. This combination has been used for cancer and a mulitude of degenerative diseases for at least 60 years. This product comes both in tea form and in concentrated capsules. In tea form, generally two ounces of the prepared liquid to six ounces of water. Two capsules are equivalent to one cup of tea.
(SEE BLOOD PURIFIER/DETOXIFIER/CANCER ABOVE)

BLOOD PURIFIER/DETOXIFIER
Gentian root, Irish Moss plant, Cascara Sagrada, Golden Seal, Slippery Elm, Fenugreek, Safflower, Myrrh gum, Yellow

Dock, Parthenium, Black Walnut, Barberry, Dandelion, Uva Ursi, Chickweed, Catnip, Cyani flowers.

BODILY INFLUENCE: Alterative, Laxative-mild, Parasiticide. Works best when used with Psyllium hulls, an herbal laxative and plenty of water.
SPECIFIC CONDITIONS: Arthritis, Body odor, Breast lumps, Cancer-cleansing, Constipation-mild, Cysts, Parasites, Toxemia, Tumors, Fibroid cysts, Lou Gerig's disease, Polyps, Tumors-fatty, Headache, Pain reliever, Cleanser-general.

This special formula was put originally put together by an Indian Medicine Man by the name of Chief Sundance. He was arrested 17 times for curing cancer in the state of Utah and Idaho and was never convicted once. It is one of the best blood cleansers available today.

BLOOD PURIFIER/DETOXIFIER
Gentian, Catnip, Bayberry, Golden Seal, Myrrh gum, Irish Moss, Fenugreek, Chickweed, Yellow Dock, Prickly Ash, St. John's Wort, Blue Vervain, Evening Primrose, Cyani flowers.

This product was designed by a very famous naturopathic physician from Utah and has a long proven tract record.
(SEE BLOOD PURIFIER/DETOXIFIER/CANCER ABOVE)

BOWEL BUILDER
Psyllium hulls, Algin, Cascara Sagrada bark, Bentonite clay, Apple pectin, Marshmallow root, Parthenium root, Charcoal, Ginger root, Sodium copper chlorophyllin, Vitamin C, E, Beta-carotene, Betaine HCL, Bile salts, Pancreatin, Pepsin, Selenium, Zinc.

BODILY INFLUENCE: Absorbent, Laxative, Mucilant.
SPECIFIC CONDITIONS: Diverticulitis, Toxic bowel, Bloating, Crohn's disease, Colitis, Diarrhea, Irritable Bowel Syndrome, Prolapsed colon.

This combination contains products that are necessary for cleansing and detoxifying of the bowel. It contains both bulking and fibrous agents. It also contains agents for digestion such as Betaine HCL, pepsin, pancreatin and bile salts. Because of the bulking fibrous agents in this product that are moisture absorbent, adequate amounts of water must be consumed.

This product was designed for long term use where there has

been long term bowel problems. UCLA has said when doing autopsies, that they have found impactions in colons that they have estimated have been there for as long as twenty five years.

CALCIUM RICH
Alfalfa, Marshmallow, Plantain, Horsetail, Oatstraw, Wheat Grass, Hops.

BODILY INFLUENCE: Bitter, Mucilant, Nutritive.
SPECIFIC CONDITIONS: Arthritis, Bedwetting, Breast milk-enrich, Cartilage damage, Cramps, Eczema, Gout, Menstrual disorders, Muscle spasms, Tooth decay, Multiple Sclerosis, Sciatica, Shingles-relieve pain, Teeth grinding, Backache, Insomnia, Pain, Nerve sheaths-rebuilding (calcium is catalyst), Leg cramps, Baldness, Mineral deficiency.

This is an herbal combination that the pure vegetarian can use for extra calcium. This combination has been called a 'knitter, healer' combination and has been used also for wounds and surgery that would not seem to heal.

It is designed to work on bones, muscle and cartilage and is helpful with bruises, sore joints and all structural parts of the body.

CALCIUM RICH
Oatstraw, Horsetail, Comfrey leaves, Pan Pien Lien.
(SEE CALCIUM RICH ABOVE)

CALCIUM RICH
Slippery Elm, Marshmallow, Golden Seal, Fenugreek seed.

BODILY INFLUENCE: Cell Proliferant, Soothing.
SPECIFIC CONDITIONS: Bites/Stings-apply externally, Blood poisoning, Cuts, Hiatal hernia, Inflammation, Sores-soothing poultice, Swelling, Ulcerations, Wounds, Sciatica, Pain, Bruises, Burns, Ulcers, Arthritis, Bone knitter, Aches.

This combination is specially formulated to be mixed and used as a poultice to be applied externally to aid healing and soothe painful sores and aches. Use internally as a knitter and healer.

CALCIUM RICH
Yarrow, Mullein, Plantain, Rehmannia.

BODILY INFLUENCE: Cell Proliferant, Diaphoretic, Expectorant, Mucilant, Nutritive.
SPECIFIC CONDITIONS: Asthma, Bronchitis, colds, Croup, Digestive disorders, Heals wounds, Painful joints, Rheumatism, Ulcers.

This combination is designed to give the body the capability of healing and rebuilding degenerative conditions for the tissues and joints. It helps to cleanse and support the mucous membranes of the respiratory and digestive tract. It has all the healing qualities that herbalists have come to expect in healing plants such as Comfrey. This combination can also be used internally as a knitter, healer.

CANCER PREVENTATIVE
Dietary Indoles, Multiple Cruciferous vegetables.

BODILY INFLUENCE: Nutritive.
SPECIFIC CONDITIONS: Anti-cancer, Bulking and fiber agent, Nutritive, Immune system.

This combination has been concentrated through a freeze-dried process where they vaccumed off the cellulose that held these plants together. The end result was up to 2 lbs. of broccoli, cauliflower, kale and other cruciferous vegetables in one capsule. Research was done in New York for three years under a grant by the National Institute of Health proving the value in cancer treatment and prevention.

CANDIDA/ANTIFUNGAL
Pau d'Arco bark, Garlic bulb, Golden Seal root, Yucca root, Lemon Grass herb, Rose Hips concentrate, Hesperidin complex, Citrus bioflavonoids, Caprylic acid, Vitamin A, E, C, Pantothenic acid, Biotin, Zinc, Selenium,

BODILY INFLUENCE: Anti-fungal, Immuno-stimulant.
SPECIFIC CONDITIONS: Candida Albicans, Yeast infections, Immune builder.

This is an extra strong anti-fungal combination for deep systemic candidias.

Caprylic acid from coconut has been proven to kill fungus on contact. In combination with the rest of these herbs is a good place to start to bring the body back into chemical balance and boost the immune system.

CANDIDA/ANTIFUNGAL
Caprylic acid, Black Walnut hulls, Red Raspberry leaves, Pau d'Arco bark.
(SEE CANDIDA/ANTIFUNGAL ABOVE)

CANDIDA/ANTIFUNGAL
Caprylic acid, Pau d. Arco, Echinacea, Vitamin E, odorless Garlic, Black Walnut hulls, Selenium with natural herbal essential oils as flavorings.
(SEE CANDIDA/ANTIFUNGAL ABOVE)

CIRCULATION/CHOLESTEROL
High profile chelated vitamin formula, EPA (fish lipid concentrate), High potency Garlic, Black Currant oil, Guggul lipid.

This is a combination of herbs and vitamins put together to help support the circulatory system and to aid the body in bringing the cholesterol in balance within the system.

COFFEE SUBSTITUTE
Roasted Barley, Malt, Chicory, Rye, flavorings.

BODILY INFLUENCE: General Nutrition.

Herbal Beverage is the perfect coffee substitute, with the taste and aroma of coffee, without the caffeine or acids found in coffee. Herbal Beverage is made with healthy roasted grains and herbal flavorings and can be enjoyed hot or cold, plain or sweetened with honey.

COLDS/FLU/FEVER
Ginger, Capsicum, Golden Seal, Licorice.

BODILY INFLUENCE: Antipyretic, Aromatic, Stomachic.
SPECIFIC CONDITIONS: Colds, Cramps-stomach, Diarrhea, Fever, Flu-general, Motion sickness, Nausea, Stomachache,

Vomiting, Chills, Abdominal pain, Water retention.

The original formula was put together by Dr. Daniel Mallory, Ph.D. Dr. Mallory says that he can knock the flu out of anyone in 24 hours. Suggested use from Dr. Mallory is to start with 8 for the first dose, then take 4 to 5 capsules until you have a strong ginger taste in the mouth. Then stop. Starting the next day with the same dosage, continuing this procedure until the flu is gone. This combination nutritionally supports the digestive, immune and lymph systems.

COLDS/FLU/FEVER
Fenugreek seed, Thyme.

Helps the body by dissolving mucus helping to move it out of the body. Also helps with fever and chills.
(SEE COLDS/FLU/FEVER ABOVE)

COLDS/FLU/FEVER
Extract of Ephedra, Horehound, White Willow, Licorice root, Pan Pien Lien, Chickweed, Mullein, Echinacea, Golden Seal root, Cayenne, Wild Cherry bark, Rose Hips.

BODILY INFLUENCE: Antibacterial, Antibiotic, Anti-inflammatory, Bitter, Calmative, Expectorant, Mucilant, Stimulant.
SPECIFIC CONDITIONS: Coughs, Colds, Congestion, Nasal decongestant, Relieves headaches due to colds.
(SEE COLDS/FLU/FEVER ABOVE)

COLD REMEDY
Rose Hips, Chamomile, Slippery Elm, Yarrow, Capsicum, Golden Seal, Myrrh gum, Peppermint, Sage, Lemon Grass.

BODILY INFLUENCE: Antibiotic, Astringent, Nutritive, Stimulant.
SPECIFIC CONDITIONS: Colds-general formula for, Flu, Tonsillitis, Sinus, Bronchitis, Ear and Viral infection.

This combination provides nutrients needed for the immune system. This original formula was designed by Dr. Airola, N.D. Many herbalists will put together multiple combinations to get a greater synergistic action for faster and more complete healing.

COLD REMEDY

Rose Hips, Chamomile, Slippery Elm, Yarrow, Capsicum, Golden Seal, Myrrh gum, Peppermint, Sage, Lemon Grass, Parthenium, Horseradish, Mullein, Fenugreek seeds, Fennel, Boneset.

This is a combination of herbs put together with special attention to the respiratory system during times of colds and lung congestion.
(SEE COLD REMEDY ABOVE)

COLD REMEDY

Bayberry, Ginger, Willow, White Pine, Cloves, Capsicum.

BODILY INFLUENCE: Analgesic, Aromatic, Astringent, Stimulant,
SPECIFIC CONDITIONS: Colds, Congestion, Sinuses, Headaches, Fevers, Bronchials, Neuralgia and pains in the muscles and joints, Flu, Nasal congestion, Eases congestion, Mucus.

This cold remedy has been around for a long time. The original remedy was called Herbal Composition Formula by Jethro Kloss, the author of 'Back to Eden.' It is especially great for moving out congestion and dissolving mucus.
It is designed to open sinus passages rapidly and to promote the healing of them.

COLDS/VIRUS

Dandelion, Purslane, Indigo, Thlaspi, Bupleurum, Scute, Pinellia, Cinnamon, Licorice.

BODILY INFLUENCE: Anti-viral.
SPECIFIC CONDITIONS: Herpes Simplex, Cold sores-to prevent, Viruses, Flu, Epstein-Barr virus, AIDS, Candida Albicans, Thrush, Canker sores-internal, Fever blisters, Mononucleosis.

The Chinese have been using this formula for years for viruses of all kinds. This herbal combination helps with chronic viral infections and will benefit those with chronic immune deficiencies and who have had many bouts with antibiotics. It helps to reduce glandular swelling and protects the liver while stimulating the immune system.

COLITIS

Slippery Elm, Marshmallow, Ginger, Wild Yam and Dong Quai.

BODILY INFLUENCE: Laxative bulk, Mucilant, Nutritive, Stomachic

SPECIFIC CONDITIONS: Colitis, Celiac disease, Constipation, Convalescence, Debility, Intestines-inflammation of, Ulcerations-internal, Diarrhea, Colon-irritable, Crohn.s disease, Irritable Bowel Syndrome.

Extra Slippery Elm should be added to this combination for effectiveness.

All citrus fruits should be eliminated while this condition exists. Also cold liquids should not be taken. Acidophilis supplements need to be taken on a regular basis before retiring at night.

COLON FIBER ENHANCER

Psyllium hulls, Oat bran, Apple fiber, natural flavors.

BODILY INFLUENCE: Mucilant, Soothing, Laxative bulk, Cholesterol-lowers, Absorbent. Drink plenty of water when taking this product.

SPECIFIC CONDITIONS: Constipation-bulk, Laxative, Cholesterol-high, Weight control, Diarrhea, Hemorrhoids, Irritable Bowel Syndrome, Multiple Sclerosis, Hyperlipidemia.

Psyllium provides bulk to any diet and has a high mucilaginous quality. It is the highest soluble fiber known in a plant. Lack of fiber has long been associated with helping to prevent heart disease. Apple pectin has long been credited with lowering cholesterol along with Oatbran. Products of this type have even helped with weight loss and maintaining weight. It certainly gives the body regular normal bowel eliminations and the fastest rising cancer in the U.S., is cancer of the colon. This type of product can be added to drinks, cereals, soups, cottage cheese, salads, casseroles and pancakes. The list is endless.

COLON FIBER ENHANCER
Psyllium hulls, Hibiscus flower, Licorice.

BODILY INFLUENCE: Laxative bulk, Mucilant, Absorbent, Cholesterol-lowers.
SPECIFIC CONDITIONS: Cholesterol-lowers, Constipation-bulk laxative, Diarrhea, Bowel-toxic, Hemorrhoids, Multiple sclerosis.

These types of products can be taken in bulk or if preferred in capsules.
Be sure to drink plenty of water.
(SEE COLON FIBER ENHANCER ABOVE)

COLON FIBER ENHANCER
Psyllium husk, Fructose, Apple fiber, Acacia gum, Guar gum, Oat bran, Cinnamon, SynerPro herbal food blend (Broccoli, Cabbage, Watercress, Chinese cabbage, Turmeric, Rosemary, Carrot, Tomato and bioflavonoids), natural apple flavor.

Psyllium in this product is also going to give us fiber and Psyllium is one of the highest soluble fibers known. This undigestible fiber helps us to have healthy bowel eliminations. Nutritionists have always said that the American public needs to increase their intake of fruits and vegetables in our diets. Studies have been done on vegetables like the cruciferous vegetables and found that they slow sugar assimilation and carry unwanted fats from the body. Diets of this type have been linked to reducing blood cholesterol levels, thus reducing the risk for heart disease. Research has also shown the Indole 3's found in cruciferous vegetables boost the immune system helping to prevent and cure cancer.
(SEE COLON FIBER ENHANCER ABOVE)

COLON FIBER ENHANCER
Psyllium husk, Guar gum, natural Orange flavor, Hibiscus flower, natural Banana flavor, Caa Inhem extract, Licorice root, Peppermint, Cinnamon, Papaya, Garlic, Rhubarb, Alfalfa, Fenugreek, Slippery Elm, Ginger, Aloe Vera, Burdock, Black Walnut hulls, Red Raspberry, Pumpkin seed, Yucca root, Marshmallow root, Uva Ursi, Buchu, Capsicum, Clove seed, Chickweed, Cornsilk, Dandelion, Echinacea, False Unicorn.

This product contains two kinds of fiber - insoluble and soluble. The insoluble fiber passes through the system without dissolving in water. Its bulk helps make digestion cleaner and faster. Soluble fiber dissolves in water and, may, with a low-fat diet, help lower blood cholesterol. The product is designed to be a good-tasting powdered drink that provides ample high quality dietary fiber and herbs that are beneficial to the gastro-intestinal tract. It can be used as a colon cleanse and for colon health maintenance. High fiber intake may also help with weight control by contributing to a feeling of fullness without added calories.

DIABETES
Golden Seal, Juniper Berries, Uva Ursi, Cedar Berries, Mullein, Yarrow, Garlic, Slippery Elm, Capsicum, Dandelion, Marshmallow, Nettle, White Oak, Licorice.

BODILY INFLUENCE: Aperitive, Bitter, Diuretic.
SPECIFIC CONDITIONS: Blood sugar problems, Diabetes, Pancreatic weakness.

This combination has 14 different herbs in it for rebuilding and repairing of the pancreas. Insulin save lives, but insulin also kills. It should be the goal of all diabetics to get off of insulin before they lose their fingers, toes, hands, arms, legs, kidneys or go blind. Diet and exercise are very important to a diabetic.

DIABETES
Cedar Berries, Licorice, Uva Ursi, Golden Seal, Mullein, Capsicum.

Cedar berries helps restore the function of the pancreas, Licorice puts a governor on the pancreas by helping it to get control of itself and Golden Seal has natural insulin and regulates sugar levels.
(SEE DIABETES ABOVE)

DIABETES
Cedar Berries, Burdock, Horseradish, Golden Seal, Siberian Ginseng.

BODILY INFLUENCE: Adaptogen, Antibiotic, Stimulant, Tonic.

SPECIFIC CONDITIONS: Blood sugar-high, Pancreatic weakness, Diabetes, Pancreas, Insulin-lack of, Blood sugar imbalances, Adrenals, Hypoglycemia.

Dr. Christopher found that Cedar Berries could replace insulin injections. Golden Seal has the ability to lower blood sugar levels and is food for feeding the pancreas.

DIABETES

Golden Seal, Juniper Berries, Uva Ursi, Cedar Berries, Mullein, Yarrow, Garlic bulb, Slippery Elm, Capsicum, Dandelion, Marshmallow, Nettle, White Oak bark, Licorice, Chromium, Zinc chelated to the amino acids Glutamine, Leucine and Lysine.

BODILY INFLUENCE: Bitter, Antibiotic, Astringent, Diuretic, Tonic.
SPECIFIC CONDITIONS: Diabetes-build pancreas, Hypoglycemia, Pancreatic weakness.

Research has shown that when vitamins and minerals are combined together, they are chelated. This chelation process allows many times, this product to be absorbed into the system. 95% of all diabetics have a deficiency in Chromium. Chromium is called the glucose tolerance factor (GTF).

DIABETES

Chromium in a base of Red Clover tops, Yarrow flower, Horsetail.

BODILY INFLUENCE: Nutritive.
SPECIFIC CONDITIONS: Arteriosclerosis, Blood pressure-high, Fatigue, Hypoglycemia, Addictions, Diabetes, Pancreas.

Chromium has also been used with weight lifters to build muscle tone. It also helps with the liver, because of the fats in the blood. 95% of all diabetics have a deficiency in Chromium. Chromium is lost so easily because of the processing of our foods.

DIABETES

Gymnena Sylvestre, Papaya, Chromium picolinate.

BODILY INFLUENCE: Appetite suppressant, Sugar blocker, Breaks down fats.

SPECFIC CONDITIONS: Diabetes, Pancreas, Weight loss, Appetite control, Fat metabolism, Blood sugar problems Sugar craving, Obesity.

Gymnema Sylvestre has the ability to block up to 50% of those sugar calories and also blocks the taste of sweets and sugars. (SEE DIABETES ABOVE)

ALL OF THE FOLLOWING FORMULAS FOR DIGESTION WILL AID THE BODY IN DIGESTING ITS FOOD OF WHICH SOME ARE CHEMICAL AND SOME ARE HERBAL.

DIGESTIVE AID/ENZYMES

Lactase, Protease, Lipase, Beet fiber, Caraway seed, Ginger root, Fennel seed, Gentian root, Dandelion.

Many people think that their bodies have more than enough enzymes and if they don't, the food has all the rest that they need. WRONG! Most people eat food where the enzymes have been destroyed by cooking the food or the food was grown in depleted soil so that the food never developed the quality nor the quantity that should have been there. The human body has within it, enzymes that do a specific job. There are protease enzymes whose job is to be a protein digesting enzyme. Amylase enzymes break down carbohydrates. Lipase enzymes are fat digesting enzymes. Each enzyme only acts on a specific group of molecules. It is often named for the food it acts upon. Another example is the enzyme sucrase which breaks down the sugar called sucrose and lactase breaks down the milk sugar lactose.

This enzyme formula's #1 enzyme is lactase. This is the enzyme that breaks down lactose (milk sugar) in milk and other dairy products. The second important enzymes are lipase and protease. These break down the fat in milk. As we go through our teenage years, we slowly stop producing those enzymes needed for breaking down milk. God does this, as He designed milk for infants and children. Man discovered years ago this difficulty in consuming dairy products as they got older, so he learned to culture the products, so they would develop their own enzymes and help to digest themselves in the human body. Most black people were born with a lactate deficiency. So this product is ideal for them and those people who want to continue using dairy products past puberty.

DIGESTIVE AID/ENZYMES

Amylase, Glucoamylase, Invertase, Protease, Lipase, Cellulase enzymes, Beet fiber, Caraway seed, Ginger root, Fennel seed, Gentian root, Dandelion root.

This is a carbohydrate enzyme combination especially designed to help digest those carbohydrates that are in legumes (grains/beans), cruciferous vegetables (broccoli, cauliflower, cabbage, onions, etc.) and also whole grains. One of the enzymes, cellulase is there to help break down cellulose in the legumes. cell wall.

DIGESTIVE AID/ENZYMES

Lipase, Protease, Amylase, Cellulase enzymes, Beet fiber, Caraway seed, Ginger root, Fennel seed, Gentian root, Dandelion root.

This combination is specifically designed for people who have trouble digesting fats and oils. It also contains protease which helps in the digestion of protein. People who have trouble digesting the fats which are in foods will have liver and gallbladder problems. These individuals will develop circulatory problems and heart disease. Weight also becomes a great problem.

DIGESTIVE AID/ENZYMES

Protease, Amylase, Glucoamylase, Lipase, Pectinase, Cellulase enzymes, Beet fiber, Caraway seed, Ginger root, Fennel seed, Gentian root, Dandelion root.

This combination is designed to be a "full spectrum" general purpose enzyme product. It is designed to help in the proper digestion of all food types 'except dairy'. It does not contain hydrochloric acid which seems to be the # 1 cause of digestion. Without hydrochloric acid, the food will lay in the stomach and literally rot before the stomach releases it. This fermentation causes gas, flatulence, and bloating. If this is a problem, we should add a hydrochloric acid supplement with each and every meal.

DIGESTIVE AID/HERBAL
Papaya, Peppermint.

Papaya contains papain which breaks down protein into a digestable state. It is considered to be the highest enzymatic fruit known to man today. It has been used as an aid in cancer cures and peppermint is a stimulant. It aids in the production of HCL and activates the salivary glands to produce enzymes. It also helps to expel gas from the body. It has been used for lightheadedness and dizziness and helps with bad breath.

DIGESTIVE AID/HERBAL
Pancreatin, Papain, Ox bile, Pepsin, Bromelain, Betaine hydrochloride. Peppermint, Comfrey and Slippery Elm.
(SEE DIGESTIVE AID/ ENZYMES ABOVE)

DIGESTIVE AID/HERBAL
Papain and Prolase(from Papaya), Bromelain(from Pineapple), Chamomile extract, Peppermint leaves, Diastase(from Barley malt), Amylase(from starch digesting enzyme), Anise, Slippery Elm, Golden Seal, Fennel, Papaya melon extract, Papaya leaves.

This combination contains herbs and foods that are super high in digestive enzymes.
(SEE DIGESTIVE AID/HERBAL ABOVE)

DIGESTIVE AID/HERBAL
Peppermint, Fennel, Ginger, Wild Yam, Catnip, Cramp Bark, Spearmint, Papaya.

BODILY INFLUENCE: Aromatic, Calmative, Carminative, Digestant, Hepatic.
SPECIFIC CONDITIONS: Indigestion, Acidity, Stomach, Intestinal gas, Heartburn, Aids digestion, Colic, Soothes stomach spasms.
This combination helps with indigestion, settles an acid stomach due to heartburn and provides digestive enzymes.
(SEE DIGESTIVE/HERBAL ABOVE)

DIGESTIVE AID/PROTEIN
Betaine HCL, Pepsin.

BODILY INFLUENCE: Carminative, Stomachic; helps digest protein, not needed for starchy meals.
SPECIFIC CONDITIONS: Allergies, Appetite-lack of, Bloating, Cancer, Gas-prevent, Heartburn, Protein indigestion, Fibrositis, Food poisoning-to prevent, osteoporosis,

Dr. Kurt Donsbach told me one time that 95% of all allergies could be taken care of with the addition of hydrochloric acid. I have found this to be true. We are told that we are what we eat, but we are definitely what we digest and then we are what we assimilate and then what we circulate and then last but not least, what we eliminate. Many people eat $20 meals and only get 20 cents worth of value. Some people have the richest toilets in town. The U.S. public health service says that as we age, we produce less HCL. In fact, they say at age 45, the average person has a deficiency of HCL. They say at 55, the majority of people have this deficiency. Yet, if you are reading this at 85 and don't have a deficiency of HCL, you are the exception. You can die of malnutrition with a full stomach with a deficiency of HCL. WARNING: Do not chew or dissolve these tablets in the mouth, as they are acid. Swallow them immediately and let them go down into your acid stomach. Your stomach has a special lining of organic sodium to protect it from the HCL. You may have to supplement your diet with every meal for the rest of your life to keep from having bloating, flatulence, gas and stomach distension. It also prevents you from dying of degenerative diseases from malnutrition (poor digestion). HCL also destroys bacteria and parasites.

DIGESTIVE AID/HCL/ENZYMES
Betaine HCL, Bile salt, Bromelain, Lipase, Mycozyme, Pancreatin, Papain, Pepsin.

BODILY INFLUENCE: Aperitive, Carminative, Stomachic.
SPECIFIC CONDITIONS: Bloating, Cancer, Debility, Fatigue-chronic, Food allergies, Gas-prevent, Headache, Heartburn, Indigestion, Indigestion of fats, Pancreatic weakness, Cystic Fibrosis, Ulcers-duodenal.

Enzymes are needed for digestion of protein, fats and carbohydrates. Cooking foods destroy enzymes. Many things that we ingest destroy enzymes such as chemicals, even from water and

drugs. Processed foods have their enzymes destroyed and then our bodies have to deplete our own enzymes to help digest them. This depletion goes on long enough and the body develops diseases such as liver failure, diabetes, arthritis and heart failure.
(FOR INFORMATION ON HCL - SEE DIGESTIVE PROTEIN ABOVE)

ENERGY

Siberian Ginseng, Kelp, Bee Pollen, Schizandra fruit, Yellow Dock, Barley grass, Licorice, Gotu Kola, Rose Hips, Capsicum.

BODILY INFLUENCE: Adaptogenic, Hormonal, Stimulant.
SPECIFIC CONDITIONS: Fatigue-general, Endurance-lack of, Energy-lack of.

This combination was put together after much research by Master Herbalist, Joan Vandergriff. The herbs in this combination are adaptogenic herbs which are known to extend life to the cell and then there are herbs that feed the adrenals and boost the immune system. This combination can be taken more frequently when extra energy is needed.

ENERGY

Siberian Ginseng, Ho-Shou-Wu, Black Walnut, Licorice, Gentian, Fennel, Slippery Elm, Bee Pollen, Bayberry, Myrrh gum, Peppermint, Safflower, Eucalyptus, Lemon grass, Capsicum.

BODILY INFLUENCE: Tonic-general.
SPECIFIC CONDITIONS: Adrenal exhaustion, Endurance, Fatigue, Weak muscles, Tendonitis, Aging.

This combination was designed specifically for exercise and endurance and the side effect is long life and longevity and enjoying it while you.re doing it. It has a proven track record with athletes already, but many people take it just for good lasting energy.

ENERGY/STIMULANT

Bee Pollen, Siberian Ginseng, Gotu Kola, Capsicum, Licorice, Glutamine, Choline bitartrate, B-6, B-12, Vitamin C, Calcium, Folic acid, Iodine, Niacinamide, Pantothenic acid, Potassium, Phosphorus, Zinc.

BODILY INFLUENCE: Nutritive, Stimulant.
SPECIFIC CONDITIONS: Athletic endurance, Caffeine withdrawal, Endurance-lack of, Fatigue, Increases stamina.

Modern day herbalism has found that when combining vitamins, minerals and amino acids to herbs, a greater synergistic action can be attained. Harvey Ashmead proved this years ago, by combining amino acids to the vitamins and minerals. The assimilation of those products increased enormously. Greater benefit was then achieved with even smaller amounts of nutrients. This is called synergistic efficiency. Research done in Poland in the 70.s found that you could increase the assimilation of vitamins and minerals 4 to 5 times by simply ingesting them in a base of herbs.

ENERGY/STIMULANT
Chinese herbal tea extract, Siberian Ginseng extract, Gotu Kola extract, Bee Pollen, Calcium carbonate, Ascorbic acid, Kelp, Zinc gluconate, Manganese gluconate, Ferrous fumerate, Vitamin A palmitate, Calcium pantothenate, Vitamin D-3, Rose Hips, Pyridoxine HCL, Riboflavin, Thiamine mononitrate, Folic acid, Octacosanol, biotin, Cyanocobalamin.

BODILY INFLUENCE: Adaptogen, Antispasmodic, Nervine, Stimulant, Tonic.
SPECIFIC CONDITIONS: Caffeine withdrawal, Energy, Alertness, Endurance, Combats fatigue.

This combination helps to build energy and endurance to meet the challenges of extra activity that may be placed on the body.

ENERGY/STIMULANT
L-Carnitine, Kelp, Yellow Dock Psyllium hulls, Alfalfa, Zinc, Vitamin C, Vitamin B2, Vitamin B, Niacin, Vitamin B6, Vitamin B12 in a Guar Gum base.

BODILY INFLUENCE: Nutritive, Hormonal, Rejuvenative.
SPECIFIC CONDITIONS: Muscle toning, Endurance, Colon.

L-Carnitine is a natural amino acid that converts fat to muscle. Research has shown that when children with what they call mushy hearts (weak heart muscle), grow older and larger, the more life becomes precarious for them, because their weak heart can not support a large body. Research has shown that when giving L-Carnitine to these children, most of them are out playing with other children in as little as 72 hours. When L-Carnitine is given in a weight loss program, it helps the skin from becoming flabby.

EYES

Golden Seal, Bayberry, Eyebright, Red Raspberry.

BODILY INFLUENCE: Astringent.
SPECIFIC CONDITIONS: Cataracts, Conjunctivitis, Diarrhea, Edema, Eye infections, Eye problems-general, Glaucoma, Respiratory infections, Eye-Blood shot, Pink eye, Stye.

This combination may be used internally for strengthening the eye. It also can be used as an eyewash. If used as an eyewash, mix 1 to 2 open capsules in 4 to 6 ounces of reverse osmosis water. Heat to a simmer, cover and allow to cool. Strain the liquid as Golden Seal is gritty. Use coffee strainer, cheese cloth or heavy paper towel. Use the liquid to bathe the eyes, using an eyecup or syringe 2-3 times daily or as desired. Keep liquid refrigerated and make a new batch every 2 to 3 days to avoid contamination. Use internally and externally. People have been able to wash trigieum (a fatty growth that comes across the eye and can cause blindness) off the surface of the eye.

FASTING

Licorice, Red beet, Hawthorn, Fennel.

BODILY INFLUENCE: Antacid, Hypertensive, Tonic-general.
SPECIFIC CONDITIONS: Fasting, Fatigue, Toxemia, Compulsive eaters, Hepatitis, Arthritis, Liver problems, Acne, Allergies, Cancer, Gout, Jaundice, Lupus, Poisoning, Skin eruptions.

This combination was designed to control hunger and helps keep blood sugar levels at normal while on a fast. It was also designed to help support the liver and the heart during this time of stress. As we lose poisons, we can lose potassium from the cells. Hawthorn is high in potassium. Fennel helps to control gas that may develop and also controls hunger pains. Licorice keeps blood sugar levels at normal and feeds the pancreas. Always consume copious amounts of liquid during a fast and keep the bowels wide open.

FEMALE PROBLEMS

Golden Seal, Red Raspberry, Black Cohosh, Queen of the meadow, Althea, Blessed Thistle, Dong Quai, Capsicum, Ginger.

BODILY INFLUENCE: Bitter, Hormonal-female, Oxytocic, Emmenagogue.
SPECIFIC CONDITIONS: Acne-female hormones, Anemia, Edema, Female problems, Hot flashes, Infertility-female, Menopause, Menstrual cramps, Nephritis, PMS, Postpartum weakness, Puberty-female hormones, Uterine problems, Birth control side effects, Breasts, Hormone balancer, Morning sickness, Menstrual irregularity, Mood swings-hormonal, Menstruation-heavy flow, Bladder problems, Endometriosis, Cysts, Tumors.

This combination, as you can see by the specific conditions listed above, has a lot of work to do. Thanks to Steven Horne for researching those conditions. Many women suffer needlessly today, because they do not know that natural remedies are available. They continue to use drugs which only cover up the problem and then we arrive at the doctor.s final solution - the hysterectomy or the mastectomy.

FEMALE PROBLEMS

Red Raspberry, Dong Quai, Ginger, Licorice, Queen of the meadow, Blessed Thistle, Marshmallow.

BODILY INFLUENCE: Hormonal-female, Hypertensive, Oxytocic, Emmenagogue.
SPECIFIC CONDITIONS: Acne-female hormones, Dysmenorrhea, Female problems, Hot flashes, Infertility-female, Menopause, Menstrual cramps, PMS, Breasts-sore, Endometriosis, Fibroid cysts, Morning sickness, Female reproductive-balances,

This combination is much higher in Dong Quai than other formulas. Dong Quai is probably one of the most famous of the Chineses herbs as a female corrective. It has been credited with being able to enlarge the breasts of women. It has also been credited with helping in conditions such as arthritis and poor bowel elimination.

FEMALE PROBLEMS

Blessed Thistle, Golden Seal, Red Raspberry, Squaw Vine, Ginger, Cramp Bark, Capsicum, Uva Ursi, Marshmallow, Pan Pien Lien, False Unicorn.

This combination is a balancer and a cleanser of the female system.
(SEE FEMALE CORRECTIVE ABOVE)

FEMALE PROBLEMS
Golden Seal, Capsicum, Ginger, Uva Ursi, Cramp Bark, Squaw Vine, Blessed Thistle, Red Raspberry, False Unicorn.

BODILY INFLUENCE: Antibiotic, Diuretic, Emmenagogue, Hormonal, Stimulant.
SPECIFIC CONDITIONS: Edema, Nephritis, Pospartum weakness, Hormone balancer-female, Menstrual problems, Vaginal problems, Hot flashes, Menopause.

This combination does not contain Black Cohosh which produces natural female hormones. Some women do not need more female hormones when they are out of balance and consequently cannot handle Black Cohosh. This combination could be the answer to their problems. This formula originated with Dr. Christopher, N.D.

GALL BLADDER/LIVER
Barberry bark, Ginger root, Cramp Bark, Fennel seeds, Peppermint leaves, Wild Yam root, Catnip.

BODILY INFLUENCE: Bitter, Cholagogue, Stomachic.
SPECIFIC CONDITIONS: Age spots, Gallbladder-sluggish, Liver-sluggish, Jaundice, Indigestion.

This combination helps to aid in digestion and help the liver and gallbladder function properly. This combination was put together by Dr. Christopher to help improve appetite and the body,s production of digestive fluids. It is both a liver and blood cleanser that stimulates circulation while soothing inflammation of smooth muscles.

GLANDULAR BALANCER
Kelp, Dandelion, Alfalfa.

BODILY INFLUENCE: Alterative.
SPECIFIC CONDITIONS: Acne-glandular imbalance, Anemia, Endurance, Fingernails-weak or brittle, Glandular imbalance, Hair-dullness of, Pregnancy, Dermatitis, Growth-problems with.

This is a glandular balancer of the thyroid, pituitary and liver. This combination, when it first came out, was called K-9 and was used for animals as an herbal vitamin supplement and also helped keep fleas and ticks off them. I personally give 3 per day to my Rottweilers, along with 3 capsules of garlic. Their coat is smooth and slick and they are super healthy and I have never had to deworm them. The combination became so popular for humans, they dropped the name K-9. This combination contains all the known vitamins and minerals that man needs and has been used as a multiple/vitamin supplement by the puritan vegetarian.

GLANDULAR BALANCER

Licorice, Lemon Bioflavonoids, Asparagus powder, Alfalfa, Parsley, Kelp, Black Walnut, Thyme, Parthenium, Schizandra, Siberian Ginseng, Dong Quai, Dandelion, Uva Ursi, Marshmallow, Beta Carotene, Vitamin C, E, Zinc, Pantothenic acid, Manganese, Potassium, Lecithin.

BODILY INFLUENCE: Hormonal, Immuno-stimulant.
SPECIFIC CONDITIONS: Age spots, Aging, Glands-general, Glandular imbalance, Hormone imbalance, Breasts-enlarged, Growth-problems with, Hot flashes, Myasthenia Gravis.

This is another combination put together to balance out the hormonal system with the best nutrition available. The combining of the herbs and the vitamins together, we many times increase the assimilation and utilization factor and get faster results.

GLANDULAR BALANCER

Magnesium, Iodine from Kelp, Glutamic acid, Proline, Histidine.

BODILY INFLUENCE: Hormonal, Immuno-stimulant, Nutritive.
SPECIFIC CONDITONS: Glandular imbalance, Growth problems, Aging.
(SEE GLANDULAR BALANCER ABOVE)

HAIR RESTORER

Dulse, Horsetail, Sage, Rosemary.

BODILY INFLUENCE: Nutritive, Tonic.

SPECIFIC CONDITIONS: Fingernails-weak or brittle, Hair-split ends, Nails-problems with, Nerve sheaths-frayed, Pregnancy, Skin disorders, Baldness, Dandruff, Hair loss, Fractures.

This combination has not only been used for the hair, but also for the skin and nails. One of the herbs is Horsetail, which is the richest source of organic silica known to man. Silica is very necessary for utilization and is considered to be one of the youth minerals. It helps us to utilize calcium and keep bones flexible.

HEART
Hawthorn, Capsicum, Garlic.

BODILY INFLUENCE: Cardiac, Hypertensive, Hypotensive, Tonic-cardiac.
SPECIFIC CONDITIONS: Angina, Arteriosclerosis, Blood pressure-low or high, Cholesterol, Circulation-poor, Dropsy, Edema, Fatigue, Flu, Heart disease, Hyperlipidemia, Thrombosis, Weakness-general, Heart, Arrthythmias.

This combination strengthens the heart by increasing blood flow and helping to dissolve cholesterol. Hawthorn is the oldest known herb in the world for rebuilding tired and worn out hearts. It has been known to stop angina pains very rapidly. It can be taken frequently with no toxic effects. Capsicum has been proven to stop heart seizures.

HEART
(ENRICH)
Hawthorn, Capsicum, Lecithin.

SPECIFIC CONDITIONS: Arteriosclerosis, Cholesterol, Cardiac.

It helps to improve circulation as well as restores the heart muscle. This herbal combination also helps brain function due to the Lecithin which is a brain food.
(SEE HEART ABOVE)

HEART
Ginkgo Biloba leaves, Hawthorn berries.

BODILY INFLUENCE: Cardiac, Immuno-stimulant.
SPECIFIC CONDITIONS: Circulation-poor, Heart problems,

Inability to concentrate, Cold limbs, Numbness, Age spots, Blood pressure-low, Mitral valve prolapse, Memory problems.

Ginkgo is the oldest known tree on earth. It has outlasted the dinosaur and the Ice Age. It has become very popular in landscaping and has the amazing ability to take on all the pollution you can give it and still survive. This herb has been taken for years for long life and longevity. It has been used to boost the immune system and for the brain and memory. Hawthorn is one of the most respected herbs in the world for the heart. In Europe, and I don.t like to use the word, but I will; they say, 'It is the drug of choice for the heart.'

HEART/VALVES

Capsicum, Hawthorn, Co-enzyme Q10, Copper, Iron, Magnesium, Zinc chelated to Leucine, Histidine, Glycine.

BODILY INFLUENCE: Hypotensive, Tonic-cardiac.
SPECIFIC CONDITIONS: Angina, Blood pressure-high, Cancer, Fatigue, Gum diseases, Heart disease, Immune deficiency, Incontinence, Muscle weakness, Swelling, Thymus-underactive, Tumors, Teeth-loose, Heart valves.

Co-enzymes are in reality a vitamin-like substance. Q10 was first found to cure peridontal diseases. Scientists then discovered gum tissue and heart tissue were exactly the same and identical. Using CoQ10 on people who had cardic failure found three years later that 85% were still alive and kicking. With cardiac failure, you generally have 2 weeks to two months to live, whichever comes first.

HORMONE BALANCER

Siberian Ginseng, Parthenium, Saw Palmetto, Gotu Kola, Damiana, Sarsaparilla, Horsetail, Garlic, Capsicum, Chickweed.

BODILY INFLUENCE: Aphrodisiac, Hormonal-male/female, Adaptogen.
SPECIFIC CONDITIONS: Aging, Anorexia, Aphrodisiac-general, Chronic weakness, Endurance-lack of, Fatigue, Frigidity, Hormone imbalance, Hot flashes, Impotency, Infertility-male/female, Menopause, Night sweats, Nocturnal emissions, Senility, Sex drive-increase, Urine-turbid, Sex rejuvenator and stimulant.

This formula was originally designed by Dr. Airola, N.D. for male problems. The way it is designed now, it can benefit both males and females, especially hot flashes in the female. It is for impotency, sterility and long life. First thing to go in aging is the reproductive system. Putting it back into good working order, and aging seems to go away.

HORMONE BALANCER

Suma, Eleutheroerococcus senticosus, Damiana, Sarsaparilla root, Gotu Kola, Saw Palmetto, Licorice root, Ho-Shou-Wu, Ginger root, Nettle, Zinc, Amino acid chelate, Vitamin E.

BODILY INFLUENCE: Adaptogen, Aphrodisiac, Hormonal male/female, Stimulant, Tonic.
SPECIFIC CONDITIONS: Aging, Weakness, Endurance, Fatigue, Frigidity, Hormone imbalance, Hot flashes, Impotency, Infertility-male/female, Nocturnal emisions, Senility, Sex drive-increase, Sex rejuvenator.

In this day and age, we have so much stress, both job and home related, less time to relax, that relations seem to be put on a back burner. This combination is designed to keep your energy levels up and to promote long life and longevity. The reproductive system is one of the first to go in aging and this is an anti-aging formula. This formula is used for both males and females.

HORMONE BALANCER

Siberian Ginseng, Sarsaparilla, Black Cohosh, Licorice, Golden Seal, Periwinkle, Damiana, Alfalfa, Kelp.

BODILY INFLUENCE: Adaptogen, Aphrodisiac, Glandular tonic, Hormonal, Stimulant.
SPECIFIC CONDITIONS: Aging, Endurance, Energy, Frigidity, Infertility-male or female, Senility, Menopause, Sex rejuvenator.

This combination was designed for both males and females to bring their hormones into balance. This combination extends the life of the cell and makes living worth living. It boosts the immune system to ward off disease. It is designed to keep your glands young.

HORMONAL BALANCER

Elk Antler, Canadian Ginseng, Bee Pollen, Echinacea, Ginger, Cinnamon, Capsicum.

BODILY INFLUENCE: Adaptogen, Antibiotic, Aphrodisiac, Stimulant, Tonic.

SPECIFIC CONDITIONS: Impotency, Infertility, Energy, Digestion, Longevity, Increases stamina, Increases circulation, Stress reduction.

The Chinese have used horns and antlers for thousands of years as an aphrodisiac. They have been known to pay hundreds of dollars for just a sliver of these products. They claim that it promotes extended sexual life.

Elk Antler is a precious renewable resource that promotes longevity and good health through nutritionally supporting the circulatory system. Other benefits that may be derived from Antler Velvet include, support of the healing process, improved sexual performance, an overall feeling of well-being, nourishment of the body's natural immune system, promoting natural body balance and a preventative supplement rather than a curative one. These naturally ocurring ingredients are designed by nature to work in harmony with one another to provide nutritional balance.

HYPOGLYCEMIA

Licorice, Safflowers, Dandelion, Horseradish.

BODILY INFLUENCE: Aperitive, Stimulant, Tonic.

SPECIFIC CONDITIONS: Blood sugar imbalance, Blood sugar problems, Dizziness, Hypoglycemia, Pancreatic weakness, Anemia, Sickle cell, Anorexia-balance blood sugar, Hypoglycemia, Energy, Mood swings, Diabetes

Hypoglycemia is low blood sugar and is a precursor to diabetes. This individual would need to eat 5 small meals a day to keep blood sugar levels normal. This herbal combination is designed to help replenish blood sugar imbalances by feeding the organs that regulate carbohydrate metabolism.

HYPOGLYCEMIA

Licorice, Juniper, Wild Yam, Dandelion, Horseradish.

(SEE HYPOGLYCEMIA ABOVE)

IMMUNE BUILDER
Blue-green algae in a base of Alfalfa; this algae contains high amounts of minerals, vitamins and Beta carotene.

Blue-green algae is a very powerful immune and a very high nutritional food. The populations of the world have used this for survival. It helps to cleanse and detoxify the body. In Romania, they have used this for curing cancer and AIDS. It is one of the righest sources of chlorophyll known to man and also is an energy builder.

IMMUNE SYSTEM
Pycnogenol in a base of Cruciferous vegetables (Broccoli, Cabbage, watercress, Chinese cabbage, Turmeric, Rosemary, Carrot, Tomato) and Bioflavonoids from citrus fruits.

Pycnogenol is an antioxidant which helps neutralize "free radicals," which are highly reactive molecules and able to damage or weaken body tissue. They may even reduce the oxygen supply needed by body cells. Studies have shown that proanthocyanidins (similar to compounds in Bilberry) are up to 50 times more effective than Vitamin E as an antioxidant. Unlike other known antioxidants, proanthocyanidins readily crosses the blood-brain barrier to help protect vital brain and nerve tissue from oxidation. Cruciferous vegetables which have been shown to contain antioxidant nutrients. Cruciferous vegetables have been winning acclaim for the strong protective factors they provide for the body. Antioxidants are bioflavonoids and they play an important role in the strength of blood capillaries, which deliver oxygen and nutrients to the body's tissues and remove poisonous wastes.

IMMUNE SYSTEM
Garlic, Zinc gluconate, Bee Propolis, Echinacea, Pau d' Arco, Rutin, Golden Seal Root, Selenomethionine, Peppermint, Cloves.

BODILY INFLUENCE: Anti-oxidant, Antibiotic.
SPECIFIC CONDITIONS: Candida Albicans, Immune deficiency, AIDS, Cancer, Epstein-Barr virus, Recurring infections.
This combination is classified as an OTC which means it is an over the counter product. The Food and Drug Administration

has approved the fact that this is a product that has nutritional support for the immune system.

IMMUNE SYSTEM
Siberian Ginseng, Korean Ginseng, White Willow, Echinacea Purpurea, Spices, Psyllium hulls, deodorized Garlic.

BODILY INFLUENCE: Adaptogen, Alterative, Anti-viral, Hormonal, Immuno-stimulant, Nutritive.
SPECIFIC CONDITIONS: Low immune system response, Infections, Viral infections, Energy, Bulking agent for the colon.

This combination was designed to boost the immune system when under stressed conditions. It increases stamina, energy and longevity.

IMMUNE SYSTEM/CANCER
Freeze-dried Shark cartilage, dehydrated Reishi mushroom.

BODILY INFLUENCE: Shark cartilage causes antoangigensis which stops the blood supply to the cancer/tumor robbing it of oxygen via the bloodstream causing it to die. Cartilage supplementation has been used for years to help in rebuilding the cartilage in our joints.

Experiments have been done around the world especially in Cuba, proving the benefits of this product. The major active ingredient in Shark cartilage is called mucopolysaccharides. This formula has added to it, the Reishi mushroom, sometimes known as Ganoderma. The Reishi mushroom has been used in China for a long time as an immune builder and for cancer. Bovine cartilage was used in original experiments for degenerative joints. Shark skeletons are 100% cartilage with a very low fat content. Shark cartilage has been proven to be many times more effective than bovine cartilage. Shark cartilage has also been found to be effective taken orally or administered as a retention enema.

IMMUNE SYSTEM/CANCER
Red Clover, Sheep Sorrel, Peach Bark, Barberry root, Enchinacea, Licorice root, Mahonia aquifolium root, Stillingia root, Cascara Sagrada root, Sarsaparilla root, Prickly Ash bark, Burdock root, Kelp, Rosemary.

BODILY INFLUENCE: Alterative, Antibiotic, Bitter, Blood Purifier, Cholagogue, Diuretic, Hormonal, Laxative, Tonic.
SPECIFIC CONDITIONS: Blood cleansing, Liver, Boils, Cancer, Contagious diseases, Eczema, Gangrene, Blood poisoning, Toxemia, Tumors, Abscesses, Addictions, AIDS, Anemia, Hormone balance , Infection fighter.

This combination was designed after the original Hoxsey formula. Dr. Hoxsey was the first natruopathic doctor to open up a cancer clinic in Mexico. He did so after being arrested for curing cancer under doctor.s supervision in a hospital. This formula is used for any type of degenerative condition known to man.

IMMUNE SYSTEM/MAINTENANCE

Barley Grass juice powder, Wheatgrass juice powder, Asparagus powder, Astralagus root, Broccoli powder, Cabbage powder, Ganoderma herb, Parthenium root, Schizandra fruit, Siberian Ginseng root, Myrrh gum, Pau d' Arco bark, Vitamins A, C, E, Zinc, Selenium.

BODILY INFLUENCE: Antioxidant, Free radical scavenger.
SPECIFIC CONDITIONS: Cancer-prevention, Candida Albicans, Immune deficiency, AIDS, Epstein-Barr virus, Myasthenia Gravis, Spinal meningitis, Infections-reoccurring, Low immune response.

This herbal/vitamin combination is designed for the person who wants to maintain a good working immune system at all times. It contains many antioxidants and cruciferous vegetables along with extra vitamins and minerals that have been proven to do so. This combination is for the person who is on the go all the time with a lot of physical and mental stress, which can break down the immune system. It is very popular also with the elderly who.s immune system is fragile at best. They add a Homeopathic remedy that helps to prevent immune breakdown in place of the sometimes very dangerous inoculations they receive at different times of the year. An example of this, is the swine flu shots that so many took and so many died or were paralyzed permanently.

IMMUNE SYSTEM/THYMUS

Rose Hips, Beta Carotene (2,000 IU), Broccoli powder, Cabbage powder, Siberian Ginseng, Parsley, Red Clover flowers, Wheat Grass powder, Horseradish.

BODILY INFLUENCE: Adaptogen, Alterative, Corrects polarity, Immuno-stimulant, Nutritive.
SPECIFIC CONDITIONS: Infection, Low immune response, Lyme's disease, Cancer-immune booster, Colds-build immune system, Flu, Addictions, AIDS, Candida Albicans, Epstein-Barr virus, Hepatitis, Myasthenia Gravis, Thymus-underactive, Self-esteem-low.

This combination was designed to specifically feed and support the thymus, a little BB size organ that sits in the chest. The thymus produces all the T- helper cells that fight off any and all viruses that invade the body (colds, flu, AIDS, etc.). The thymus also fights off fungus in the body. This is definitely an immune builder combination.

INDIGESTION (SEE DIGESTIVE AID)

INFECTION FIGHTING
Parthenium, Yarrow, Golden Seal, Capsicum.

BODILY INFLUENCE: Antibiotic, Antipyretic.
SPECIFIC CONDITIONS: Abscesses, Natural antibiotic, Bile-excess, Bites/Stings-use internally, Bronchitis, Colds-fights infection, Contagious diseases, Ear infection, Emphysema, Enteritis, Fever-infection, Flu, Gastritis, Infection, Jaundice, Lymphatic infection, Swollen glands, Tonsillitis, ulcerations;

This combination was designed to be used in all types of infections. This can be used for both children and adults. The only caution is that hypoglycemics should use infection fighters without Golden Seal. Golden Seal has a tendency to affect blood sugar levels and if the blood sugar is already low, it may lower it even more.

INFECTION FIGHTING
Parthenium, Echinacea, Golden Seal, Burdock, Dandelion, Capsicum.
(SEE INFECTION FIGHTING ABOVE)

INFECTION FIGHTING

Parthenium, Yarrow, Myrrh gum, Capsicum.

BODILY INFLUENCE: Antibiotic, Antipyretic.
SPECIFIC CONDITIONS: Antibiotic, Bites/Stings-use internally, Blood poisoning, Bronchitis, Colds-fights infection, Contagious diseases, Ear infection, Emphysema, Fever-infection, Flu-infection, Lymphatic infection, Swollen glands, Tonsillitis, Breasts-sore, Sinuses, Gangrene.

This is a combination to combat infection. This herbal combination works very similarly to the one mentioned above, except this combination is especially formulated for hypoglycemics since it does not contain the herb Golden Seal.

INFECTION FIGHTING

Echinacea, Parthenium, Myrrh gum, Capsicum.

This herb combination works very similarly to the one mentioned above, except this combination is especially formulated for hypoglycemics since it does not contain the herb Golden Seal. They have used Echinacea in Europe for curing cancer. It has antibiotic, antiviral and anti-inflammatory properties. It has been proven to increase the quantitiy and quality of white blood cells.
(SEE INFECTION FIGHTING ABOVE)

INFECTION FIGHTING

Golden Seal, Black Walnut, Althea, Parthenium, Plantain, Bugleweed.

BODILY INFLUENCE: Antibiotic, Antipyretic.
SPECIFIC CONDITIONS: Antibiotic, Bites/Stings-use internally, Bronchitis, Cold limbs, Ear infection, Emphysema, Fever-infection, Flu, Infection, Kidney infection, Lymphatic infection, Prostate-inflammation, Tonsillitis, Swollen glands, Breast infection, Rheumatism, Measles.

The credit for this original combination has to go to Dr. John Christopher, N.D. It is a very good antibiotic combination to be used for all types of infections.

INTESTINAL CLEANSER
Marshmallow, Pepsin.

BODILY INFLUENCE: Antacid, Stomachic.
SPECIFIC CONDITIONS: Cancer-prevention, Heartburn, Indigestion, Mucus-breakup for better food absorption, Tones large and small intestines, Soothes gastric and digestive systems, General digestive aid, Helps eliminate gas by helping to digest protein.

Marshmallow has a high mucilage content and is used as a substitute for Comfrey. Pepsin is needed to digest proteins. This combination is designed to dissolve down heavy mucus coating in the intestinal wall which prevents absorption of nutrients.

IRON HERBAL/ANEMIA
Red Beet, Yellow Dock, Red Raspberry, Chickweed, Burdock, Nettle, Mullein.
BODILY INFLUENCE: Alterative.
SPECIFIC CONDITIONS: Anemia-supplies iron, Fatigue-anemia, Pregnancy-iron, Sickle cell, Oxygen-deficiency in the blood, Cramps, kidneys, Herbal iron supplement, Blood builder, Glandular balancer.

This is an herbal combination designed to supply iron to the body without becoming constipated, nauseous and the stool turning black. Many ladies should be interested in this statement. Iron is called the frisky horse as we need it for energy and to carry oxygen to the cells.

IRON/ANEMIA
Rose Hips, Mullein, Chickweed, Thyme, Yellow Dock, Iron, Vitamin C, Calcium.

BODILY INFLUENCE: Nutritive.
SPECIFIC CONDTIONS: Ambition-loss of, Anemia, Appetite-lack of, Depression, Fatigue-anemia, Hair loss, Heart palpitations, Irritability, Itching, Muscle weakness, Skin-lack of tone, Slow growth.

In the 70's in Poland, they found if you put vitamins and minerals into a base of herbs, you would raise the assimilation of those vitamins and minerals 4 to 5 times from what it was originally. The iron found here is in a base of herbs.
(SEE IRON HERBAL/ANEMIA ABOVE)

IRON/ANEMIA

Iron fumerate, Copper gluconate, B-12(cobalamin conc.), Folic acid, Yellow Dock, Dandelion, Kelp.
(SEE IRON HERBAL/ANEMIA ABOVE)

KIDNEY/BLADDER

Juniper Berries, Parsley, Uva Ursi, Dandelion, Chamomile.

BODILY INFLUENCE: Diuretic, Lithotriptic.
SPECIFIC CONDITIONS: Backache, Bedwetting, Bladder problems-general, Bloody urine, Cysts, Edema, Gonorrhea, Kidney diseases, Kidney stones, Nephritis, Pregnancy, Urethritis, Urination-scant, Uterine bleeding, Incontinence, Prostate infections, Cleanses and strengthens.

Herbal kidney combinations are designed not only to help the kidneys, but used for the entire urinary system. They are designed to flush, clean and to aid in elimination. They are also designed not to rob the body of minerals, especially potassium. They help to prevent and dissolve kidney stones. They can also strengthen the bladder in problems of incontinence and bedwetting.

KIDNEY/BLADDER

Juniper Berries, Golden Seal, Parsley, Marshmallow, Watermelon seeds, Uva Ursi, Pan Pien Lien, Ginger.
(SEE KIDNEY/BLADDER ABOVE)

KIDNEY/BLADDER

Dong Quai, Golden Seal, Juniper Berries, Uva Ursi, Parsley, Ginger, Marshmallow.

BODILY INFLUENCE: Antiseptic, Diuretic, Lithotriptic.
SPECIFIC CONDITIONS: Backache, Bedwetting, Bladder infections and stones, Bloating, Edema, Kidney problems, Pregnancy, Urination-scant, Prostate infection, Strengthens and cleanses.

This formula originated with Dr. John Christopher. It has been reformulated and can been used as a female corrective. This combination is helpful for restoring weakened sexual function, especially in the male.
(SEE 1ST KIDNEY/BLADDER ABOVE)

KIDNEY/URINARY SYSTEM
Uva Ursi, Hydrangea, Parsley, Dandelion, Siberian Ginseng, Schizandra fruit, Dong Quai, Cornsilk, Horsetail, Hops, Lemon Bioflavonoids, Vitamin B-1, B-2, C, D, Folic acid, Magnesium, Niacinamide, Pantothenic acid, Potassium.

BODILY INFLUENCE: Diuretic.
SPECIFIC CONDITIONS: Edema, Kidney problems, Incontinence, Bladder infections.
Combining vitamins and herbs together synergistically raises the assimilation factor 4 to 5 times what it was before. This herbal/vitamin/mineral combination is designed to build, strengthen and support the urinary system, thereby giving tone and strengthen to the kidney and bladder. It repairs damaged tissues and improves circulation, while increasing urine flow to control body/blood fluid balances and pressures.
(SEE KIDNEY/BLADDER ABOVE)

KIDNEY/BLADDER
Parsley, Marshmallow, Gravel root, Ginger, Juniper Berries, Uva Ursi, Black Cohosh, Watermelon seed, Pan Pien Lien.

BODILY INFLUENCE: Diuretic, Lithotriptic, Stimulant.
SPECIFIC CONDITONS: Kidney problems, Edema, Water retention, Bladder problems, Incontinence, Bedwetting, Backache, Stones.
(SEE 1ST KIDNEY/BLADDER ABOVE)

KIDNEY/BLADDER
Uva Ursi, Juniper Berries, Shave Grass, Cornsilk, Parsley, Queen of the meadow, Buchu leaves, Goldenrod, Cubeb Berries, Cranberries, Watermelon seeds.

BODILY INFLUENCE: Diuretic.
SPECIFIC CONDITIONS: Kidney and bladder problems, Nephritis, Edema, Swelling, Bloating.
This combination is an OTC (over the counter) formula which means the FDA has approved it to eliminate excess water. It is formulated to relieve the body of temporary water weight gain.

LAXATIVE

Cascara Sagrada, Buckthorn, Licorice, Capsicum, Ginger, Barberry, Turkey Rhubarb, Couch Grass, Red Clover tops.

BODILY INFLUENCE: Bitter, Laxative-stimulant, Parasiticide, Tonic-colon.

SPECIFIC CONDITIONS: Colitis, Constipation-laxative, Diverticulitis, Jaundice, Obesity, Worms/parasites-expels, Stool softener.

This lower bowel cleanser was originally designed by Dr. Stan Malstrom, N.D. This combination is designed not only to cleanse, but to rebuild and restore the muscular action of the colon. Herbal laxative combinations are not habit-forming, but mainly restorative. Herbal laxatives can be taken with each and every meal if necessary, to feed the colon. The best results are when they are taken as far away from a meal as possible, preferrably just before going to bed.

LAXATIVE

Cascara Sagrada, Barberry, Raspberry, Fennel, Senna, Pan Pien Lien, Ginger, Golden Seal, Cayenne.

BODILY INFLUENCE: Laxative, Parasiticide, Stimulant, Tonic.

SPECIFIC CONDITIONS: Lower bowel cleanser, Bad breath, Gastrointestinal, Normalizing peristaltic activity, Relieving constipation.

Dr. Stan Malstrom originally put this combination together. (SEE LAXATIVE ABOVE)

LAXATIVE

Dong Quai, Cascara Sagrada, Turkey Rhubarb, Golden Seal, Capsicum, Ginger, Barberry, Fennel, Red Raspberry.

BODILY INFLUENCE: Bitter, Laxative stimulant, Parasiticide.

SPECIFIC CONDTIONS: Colitis, Constipation-laxative, Digestion-poor, diverticulitis, Liver imbalance, Worms/parasites-expels, Intestinal mucus, Strengthens the colon and increases peristalsis.

This original combination was designed by Dr. John Christopher. (SEE 1ST LAXATIVE ABOVE)

LAXATIVE

Cascara Sagrada and Aloe Vera in a base of other herbs.

BODILY INFLUENCE: Bitter, Laxative, Nutritive, Parasiticide, Tonic.
SPECIFIC CONDITONS: Constipation, Increases peristalsis.

This combination is considered to be an OTC (over the counter) product which the FDA has approved as being laxative in nature.

LAXATIVE

Senna leaves, Fennel seeds, Ginger, Catnip.

BODILY INFLUENCE: Bitter, Laxative.
SPECIFIC CONDITIONS: constipation-severe, jaundice,

Herbal laxatives are no more habit-forming than a bowl full of prunes. Some combinations are stronger and some are milder. This is a fairly strong combination for some people. Laxatives should only be taken when needed.

LAXATIVE

Buckthorn, Senna, Psyllium, and Fennel.

BODILY INFLUENCE: Bitter, Laxative, Parasiticide.
SPECIFIC CONDITIONS: Constipation, Colitis, Diverticulitis, Stool softener, Increases peristalsis.
(SEE LAXATIVE ABOVE)

LIVER

Red Beet, Dandelion, Parsley, Horsetail, Liverwort, Black Cohosh, Birch, Blessed Thistle, Angelica, Chamomile, Gentian, Goldenrod.

BODILY INFLUENCE: Alterative, Bitter, Cholagogue, Hepatic.
SPECIFIC CONDITIONS: Age spots-liver support, Appetite-lack of, Depression, Gallbladder-sluggish, Gall stones, Hangover, Hepatitis, Liver problems, Jaundice, Alcoholism, Mononucleosis, Morning sickness, spleen, Detoxifies poisons, Speeds up blood cleansing.

The liver's #1 job in the body is to detoxify the bloodstream.

It can become polluted itself and need to be cleaned and repaired. This formula contains an herb that is famous for correcting liver problems, the Dandelion root.

LIVER

Dandelion, Golden Seal, Red Beet root, Yellow Dock, Bayberry, Oregon Grape, Pan Pien Lien.
(SEE LIVER ABOVE)

LIVER

Milk Thistle extract, Silymarin, Dandelion, Choline bitartrate, Inositol, Vitamin A, C, Iron.

BODILY INFLUENCE: Alterative.
SPECIFIC CONDITIONS: Liver problems, Exposure to toxic chemicals.

The liver has hundreds of functions, we really don,t know how many, nor what they all do. This combination contains milk thistle which is probably the single best herb for feeding and cleansing the liver. Again, adding herbs and vitamins together, we will get 4 to 5 times the assimilation we had before.

LIVER CLEANSER

Rose Hips, Red Beet root, Barberry, Horseradish, Dandelion, Parsley, Fennel.

BODILY INFLUENCE: Blood Purifier, Digestant, Hepatic, Tonic-liver.
SPECIFIC CONDITIONS: Blood sugar problems, Indigestion, Fat metabolism, Allergies-food, Toxic blood, Sluggish liver, Age spots-liver support, Alcoholism, Psoriasis.

This formula was put together by Master Herbalist, Jeanne Burgess. This type of combination has been put together to clean, flush and rebuild liver and gallbladder problems. The liver,s #1 job in the body is to detoxify the bloodstream and then handling the metabolizing. Sometimes the liver is so toxic, that we cannot metabolize well, which creates more toxins than the body can handle. The gallbladder becomes the recipient of these toxins that it can not do its job of distributing bile for the digestion of fats and also the distribution of cholesterol.

LONGEVITY

Suma root, Astragalus, Siberian Ginseng, Ginkgo Biloba, Gotu Kola.

BODILY INFLUENCE: Adaptogenic, Hormonal, Immuno-stimulant.
SPECIFIC CONDITIONS: Low immune response, Fatigue-general, Energy-lack of, Endurance-lack of, Weakness-general, Aging-to prevent Glandular imbalance, Immune deficiency.

Suma is called ₊para todo₊ in South America which means 'for everything'. Suma is called Brazilian Ginseng and like Astragalus, also contains many of Ginseng₊s properties, but are not true Ginsengs. This is a combination for rejuvenation and long life. It has been used to reverse the effects and damage from strokes.

LONGEVITY

Gotu Kola concentrate, Ginkgo Biloba concentrate.

BODILY INFLUENCE: Adaptogen, Anti-aging, Tonic.
SPECIFIC CONDITIONS: Brain-poor circulation to, Senility, Memory-loss of, Inability to concentrate, Aging, A.D.D.

This is a combination of two major anti-aging and memory herbs. Both herbs have been used singly for energy. Ginkgo has been used as an immune performance enhancer and even for heart problems.

LONGEVITY

Ginkgo Biloba, Siberian Ginseng, Sage, Bee Pollen, Capsicum.

BODILY INFLUENCE: Adaptogen, Circulatory, Nutritive, Stimulant, Tonic.
SPECIFIC CONDITIONS: Aging, Longevity, Memory, Fatigue, Endurance, Senility, Energy.

Ginkgo, one of the oldest known plants on the earth, is an herb that is considered to be a free radical scavenger. Siberian Ginseng contains both male and female hormones, so it can be used by both sexes.

LUNGS

Marshmallow, Chinese Ephedra, Mullein, Passion flower, Catnip, Senega, Slippery Elm.

BODILY INFLUENCE: Anti-histamine, Decongestant, Expectorant.
SPECIFIC CONDITIONS: Allergies, Asthma, Bronchitis, Chest pain, Colds-decongestant, Quiets coughing spasms, Emphysema, Hayfever, Hoarseness, Mucus, Pleurisy, Pneumonia, Sneezing, Respiratory congestion, Sinus congestion, Sinus headache, Sinus infection, Lung problems, Rhinitis, Stiff shoulders, Lymphatic swelling, Nasal congestion.

This formula was originally designed by Master Herbalist, La Dean Griffin. This combination was designed for deep-seated and long-term lung problems. So many people have breathing problems today because of the environment that they have to live and work in. Herbal lung combinations were designed also to protect the lungs.

LUNGS

Comfrey root, Mullein, Chickweed, Marshmallow, Slippery Elm, Pan Pien Lien.

BODILY INFLUENCE: Decongestant, Expectorant, Mucilant.
SPECIFIC CONDITIONS: Respiratory problems, Heals, soothes and relaxes bronchial tubes, Lungs, Allergies, Asthma, Colds, Coughing, Hayfever, Pleurisy, Pneumonia, Sinus and nasal congestion.

This combination is designed to give relief to the most stubborn lung problems. Pan Pien Lien has the same similar action as Lobelia. Lobelia is a dilator and will move blockages when nothing else will. It is a very effective mucus dissolver.
(SEE LUNGS ABOVE)

LUNGS

Lily of the Valley, Periwinkle, Mullein, Juniper Berries, Pan Pien Lien.

BODILY INFLUENCE: Anti-spasmodic, Astringent, Cardiac, Diuretic, Expectorant, Stimulant.
SPECIFIC CONDITIONS: Heart, Bronchials, Lungs,

Respiratory Congestion, Chest, Colds, Blood sugar levels, Kidneys, Hypoglycemia.

This combination is designed to benefit in all aspects of the respiratory system. It also strengthens the heart and has a calming action on the lungs and bronchials.

LUNGS
Fenugreek seed, Marshmallow root, Slippery Elm.

BODILY INFLUENCE: Decongestant, Expectorant, Mucilant, Nervine.
SPECIFIC CONDITIONS: Asthma, Bronchitis, Chest pains, Cough, Emphysema, Hayfever, Hoarseness, Mucus-loosens, Pleurisy, Pneumonia.

Marshmallow and Fenugreek are mucus dissolving herbs and with the addition of Slippery Elm which is a coating herb can be used for irritated membranes. This combination can be used for throat and nose problems also.

LUNGS
Comfrey root, Fenugreek, Yerba Santa, Hyssop, Wild Cherry.

BODILY INFLUENCE: Decongestant, Expectorant, Mucilant,
SPECIFIC CONDITIONS: Asthma, Bronchitis, Cough, Emphysema, Hayfever, Hoarseness, Pleurisy, Mucus, Respiratory congestion, Lymphatic congestion, Mucus in lungs, Pneumonia.

Wild Cherry has been used in cough syrups for years to dissolve down mucus and for its soothing action. The Bible tells us how great Hyssop is for any degenerative disease.

LYMPHATICS
Bayberry, Alfalfa, Chamomile, Echinacea Purpurea, Parthenium integrifolium, Siberian Ginseng Yarrow, Lecithin, Garlic bulb, CoQ10, Sodium copper chlorophyllin, Vitamins A, C, B-6, D, Magnesium.

BODILY INFLUENCE: Adaptogen, Antibiotic, Stimulant, Tonic.
SPECIFIC CONDITIONS: Lymphatic system, Immune system, Spleen.

There are more miles of the lymphatic system in the circulatory than the blood itself. It has been called the garbage dump system and certainly the immune system. In Iridology, we might possibly have a lymphatic rosary indicating that the lymphatic system was backing up. We can find lumps and bumps in strange places in the body indicating lymphatic blockages. This combination was designed with vitamins, minerals and herbs to increase its assimilation and tests have shown 4 to 5 times the assimilation when these ingredients are blended together. Homeopathics for lymphatics when used with this formula gives greater success.

MEMORY/ENERGY
Siberian Ginseng, Gotu Kola, Capsicum.

BODILY INFLUENCE: Adaptogen, Stimulant, Tonic-general.
SPECIFIC CONDITIONS: Aging, Endurance-lack of, Epilepsy, Fatigue-build endurance, Learning problems, Memory problems, Mental dullness, Prolonged illness, Senility, Brain anemia, Parkinson's disease, Inability to concentrate, Jet lag, A.D.D.

Gotu Kola is not only considered a brain and memory herb, but it is also used in mental institutions in Europe as an anti-depressant and memory restorer. It is the mainstay of the diets of the elephants. Did you ever hear that an elephant ever forgot anything? It is also considered to be anti-aging along with Siberian Ginseng. Siberian Ginseng gives us protection against viruses and is an energy booster.

MEMORY/ENERGY
Siberian Ginseng, Gotu Kola, Bee Pollen, Capsicum.

BODILY INFLUENCE: Adaptogen, Stimulant, Tonic.
SPECIFIC CONDITIONS: Aging, Exhaustion/energy, Fatigue, Vitality, Endurance, Longevity, Endurance, Memory, Senility, Learning problems, A.D.D, Brain anemia.

The addition of Bee Pollen in this combination is good, because it is one of the most perfect foods that there is. It contains both the RNA and DNA factors of the cell. This is the blueprint of the cell that we need to build a new healthy cell.
(SEE MEMORY/ENERGY ABOVE)

MEMORY/ENERGY

Gotu Kola concentrate, Ginkgo Biloba concentrate.

BODILY INFLUENCE: Adaptogen, Anti-aging, Tonic.
SPECIFIC CONDITIONS: Brain-poor circulation to, Senility, Memory-loss of, Inability to concentrate, Aging, A.D.D.

This is a combination of two major anti-aging and memory herbs. Both herbs have been used singly for energy. Ginkgo has been used for immune performance and even for heart problems.

MENOPAUSE

Black Cohosh, Licorice, Siberian Ginseng, Sarsaparilla, Squawvine, Blessed Thistle, False Unicorn.

BODILY INFLUENCE: Adaptogen, Anti-spasmodic, Aphrodisiac, Stimulant, Tonic.
SPECIFIC CONDITIONS: Acne-female hormones, Aphrodisiac, Fatigue, Hot flashes, Impotency, Infertility-female, Menopause, Menstrual cramps, Mood swings, Estrogen-low, Osteoporosis.

This combination was originally designed by Dr. John Christopher, N.D. One of the most difficult times in a woman.s life is going through the changes in menopause. Black Cohosh becomes the natural female hormone of choice. This combination helps the woman to be able to survive the hot flashes, the dry tract problem and the depression that accompanies this problem. Adding vitamin E at this time certainly helps.

MENOPAUSE

False Unicorn, Black Cohosh, Blue Cohosh, Cramp Bark, Pennyroyal, Bayberry, Ginger, Squaw Vine, Uva Ursi, Raspberry, Valerian, Blessed Thistle.

BODILY INFLUENCE: Aphrodisiac, Stimulant, Tonic.
SPECIFIC CONDITIONS: Hot flashes, Female hormones, Infertility, Menopause, Menstrual cramps, Mood swings, Osteoporosis.

It brings the hormones back into balance for a better life.
(SEE MENOPAUSE ABOVE)

MIGRAINE HEADACHES
Fenugreek seeds, Thyme.

BODILY INFLUENCE: Antiseptic, Anti-spasmodic, Decongestant.
SPECIFIC CONDITIONS: Asthma, Congestion-respiratory, Emphysema, Migraine/sinus headache, Sinus congestion, Dissolves and cuts mucus, Fevers, Flu, Congestion.

One of the major benefits of this combination is to dissolve mucus in the digestive tract and sinus passages. Fenugreek acts like a antioxidant so the body can utilize oxygen. The brain has the ability to protest when it does not get enough oxygen, thus the headache. Stress can also bring on migraine headaches. Thyme also has anti-spasmodic attributes.

MUCUS DIGESTANT
Fenugreek, Thyme.

BODILY INFLUENCE: Antiseptic, Anti-spasmodic, Decongestant.
SPECIFIC CONDITIONS: Asthma, Congestion-respiratory, Emphysema, Migraine/sinus headache, Sinus congestion, Fevers, Dissolves and cuts Mucus, Flu, Congestion.

One of the major benefits of this combination is to dissolve mucus in the digestive tract and sinuses passages. Fenugreek soothes inflamed tissues, removes phlegm and helps to expel wastes. Thyme has anti-spasmodic qualities which helps in relaxing the bronchioles, as well as, stimulates ciliary movement in the lung.

MUCUS DIGESTANT   (SEE INTESTINAL CLEANSER)

NAILS   (SEE HAIR)

NAUSEA
Ginger root, Peppermint, Anise seed, Catnip.

BODILY INFLUENCE: Carminative, Digestive, Stomachic.
SPECIFIC CONDITIONS: Nausea, Vomiting, Motion sickness, Flatulence, Bloating, Morning sickness, Dizziness.

This combination is considered to be an OTC (over the counter) product which the FDA has given approval to say that these herbs do help with motion sickness.

NERVES

White Willow, Black Cohosh, Capsicum, Valerian, Ginger, Hops, Wood Betony, Devil's claw.

BODILY INFLUENCE: Analgesic, Anti-spasmodic, Aromatic, Calmative, Nervine, Sedative.

SPECIFIC CONDITIONS: Alcoholism, Anxiety, Arthritis pain, Asthma, Drug addiction-nerves, Headaches, Hysteria, Menstrual cramps, Nerve sheaths-frayed, Nervous disorders, Smoking-calms nerves, Stress, Compulsive eaters, Multiple Sclerosis, Herbal tranquilizer, Insomnia, Spasms.

The herbs in this combination provide us with calmatives & nervine herbs. Nervine herbs rebuild the nervous system of the body. Calmatives calm you down naturally to your natural levels. This type of combination is not like a tranquilizer which is a downer that you may have to take an upper to get going again. It brings you to your normal.

NERVES

Chamomile, Passion, Hops, Fennel seeds, Marshmallow, Feverfew.

BODILY INFLUENCE: Anodyne, Anti-spasmodic, Calmative, Nervine, Relaxant.

SPECIFIC CONDITIONS: Stress, Nervousness, Anxiety, Pain, Addictions, Anorexia, Crohn's disease, Depression, Hyperactivity, Chest pain, Nervous disorders.

Chamomile is the #1 herb in this combination and is used widely throughout the world. This herb is used widely for sleep disorders because of its calming effect.   Here in the U.S., it carries the nickname Sleepytime.   Chamomile relaxes nervous tension and calms shattered nerves.

NERVES

Black Cohosh, Scullcap, Valerian, Hops, Capsicum, Wood Betony, Passion flower.

BODILY INFLUENCE: Analgesic, Emmenagogue, Nervine, Relaxant.
SPECIFIC CONDITIONS: Alcoholism, Anxiety, Drug addiction, Headache, Insomnia, Nervous disorders, Smoking-calms nerves, Stress, Schizophrenia, Shingles-relieves pain, Hyperactivity, Nervous breakdown.

This herbal combination seems to work best on the person who is both quiet and hyper at the same time - a person who holds anxieties within.

NERVES

Schizandra fruit, Choline bitartrate, PABA, Wheat germ, Bee Pollen, Valerian, Scullcap, Inositol, Hops, Citrus bioflavonoids, Vitamins C, B-1, B-2, B-6, B-12, Folic acid, Biotin, Pantothenic acid, Niacinamide.

BODILY INFLUENCE: Adaptogen, Calmative, Nervine, Relaxant, Sedative.
SPECIFIC CONDITIONS: Emotional problems, Nervousness, Stress, Alcoholism, Anorexia-nerves, Crohn's disease, Depression, Dermatitis-to stop itching, Drug withdrawal, Hyperactivity, Parkinson's disease, Schizophrenia, Chest pain, Nervous disorders.

This combination is designed both with vitamins and herbs so that it can many times increase its effectiveness to support and even to rebuild the nervous system. Studies done in Poland showed that by combining vitamins and minerals into a base of herbs, synergistically they would increase the absorption of those vitamins and minerals 4 to 5 times what it was before. This combination is for those who live in a world of stress. Stress can kill you or make you wish you were dead.

NERVES

Valerian, Hops, Wood Betony, Scullcap, Black Cohosh, Mistletoe, Pan Pien Lien, Capsicum, Lady's Slipper.

BODILY INFLUENCE: Analgesic, Anti-spasmodic, Aromatic, Calmative, Nervine, Relaxant, Sedative.
SPECIFIC CONDITIONS: Nervousness, Strengthens nerves, Nervous disorders, Stress, Hyperactivity, Hysteria, Anxiety, Insomnia, Spasms.

The first herb in this combination is world famous as it is the original source of valium which the body develops a drug dependency on. Herbalists have for years used Valerian to help bring a person down off of valium. Scullcap is a nervine and has been used to rebuild nerve endings.

NERVES
Valerian, Blessed Thistle, Scullcap.

BODILY INFLUENCE: Anti-spasmodic, Astringent, Sedative.
SPECIFIC CONDITIONS: Nervousness, Circulation, Liver, Heart.

This combination has herbs in it that are natural calmatives and also herbs to help rebuild the nervous system. Blessed Thistle is one of the finest herbs for the liver. By combining these, you have a beautiful combination to promote calm nerves and restful sleep.

NERVES
Valerian root, Scullcap, Hops, Thiamine mononitrate, Riboflavin, Nicotinamide, Calcium pantothenate, Pyridoxine HCL, Ascorbic acid, Schizandra chinensis, Piper methysticum, Folic acid, Cyanocobalamin, Biotin.

BODILY INFLUENCE: Anti-spasmodic, Nervine, Sedative, Tonic.
SPECIFIC CONDITIONS: Stress, Anxiety, Sleeplessness, Nervousness, calming, Fatigue from overwork.

This combination helps to combat stress due to overwork or fatigue, infections, after a time being sick and after surgery. It helps to restore strength and rebuild strong nerves.

PAIN RELIEF
White Willow, Valerian, Wild Lettuce, Capsicum.

BODILY INFLUENCE: Analgesic, Anodyne, Anti-inflammatory, Anti-spasmodic, Aromatic, Nervine, Sedative, Circulatory Stimulant.
SPECIFIC CONDITIONS: Aches, Afterbirth pain, Arthritis pain, Backache, Childbirth, Colds-aches and pain, Cramps, Earache, Flu-with aches, Headache, Heart pain, Hysteria, Pain-general, Pain-acute, Smoking, Tension, Fibrositis, Herbal aspirin, Sore throat, Menstrual cramps, Muscle pain.

White willow bark is the original source of aspirin, but is not harmful to the body. It does not cause internal bleeding as aspirin does. This combination builds up the bodies. tolerance to pain.

PAIN RELIEF
Concentrated extract of White Willow Bark.

BODILY INFLUENCE; Analgesic, Anodyne, Anti-inflammatory.
SPECIFIC CONDITIONS: Pain, Headache, Muscle pain, Arthritis, Bursitis, Gout, Sore muscles.

White Willow bark is the original source of aspirin. Salicyclic acid was extracted out and made synthetically. Latest studies have shown that aspirin is so dangerous to consume that if it was a new product coming out of the market today, they would never allow it to be released. You can hemorrhage 1 to 2 tsp. Of blood by just taking one aspirin. Taken on a daily basis, you can cause a stomach ulcer, or causing the blood to become so thin you can become a bleeder. White Willow bark is safe to take even in a concentrated form.

PARASITES
Pumpkin seeds, Black Walnut, Cascara Sagrada, Violet leaves, Chamomile, Mullein, Marshmallow, Slippery Elm.

BODILY INFLUENCE: Laxative-mild, Parasiticide.
SPECIFIC CONDITIONS: Constipation, Parasites, Prostate problems, Toxic bowel, Worms/parasites-expels.

According to the Center for Disease Control in Atlanta, Georgia, one out of every 4 individuals in the U.S. has one or more parasitic involvement. They also have said that 55% of all operations would be unecessary, if the doctor surgeon would only understand parasitic involvement.

PARASITES
Elecampane bark, Spearmint, Turmeric root, Ginger root, Garlic bulb, Clove bud.

BODILY INFLUENCE: Expectorant, Parasiticide, Stimulant.
SPECIFIC CONDITIONS: Parasites, Respiratory problems.

Much research has gone on to find ingredients that could be taken into the human body that will destroy parasites, but not harm the human body. Elecampane tops the list.

PARASITES

Diatomaceous earth, Wormwood, Black Walnut.

BODILY INFLUENCE: Expectorant, Parasiticide.
SPECIFIC CONDITIONS: Parasites,

Diatomaceous earth has been used by gardeners, spraying it on plants to kill parasites while feeding them nutrients at the same time.

PETS, ANIMALS (SEE GLANDULAR BALANCER)

PMS

Chinese herbs: Dong Quai root, Peony root, Bupleurum root, Hoelen palnt, Atractylodes rhizome, Codonopsis root, Alisma bark, Licorice root, Magnolia root, Ginger root, Peppermint leaves, Moutan root, Gardenia fruit, Cyperus, Vitamins A, C, B-1, B-2, Niacinamide, Calcium, Iron, Vitamin D, E, B-6, Folic acid, Vitamin B-12, Iodine, Magnesium, Zinc, Copper, Biotin, Pantothenic acid, Manganese, Chromium, Selenium, Potassium, Choline, Inositol, Bioflavonoids.

BODILY INFLUENCE: Anti-spasmodic, Hormonal, Nutritive.
SPECIFIC CONDITONS: Female problems, Menstrual cramps, PMS.

PMS is no joke. It takes a woman you love the most and can turn her into Mildred McNasty once a month. She can,t even stand herself when her hormones are out of balance. This combination would be best taken 10 days before the period. A women,s monthy cycle is an important cleansing period. During this time, a women,s nutrition is more important than other times in the month. Many women take on stress and experience overwork during their period. Nutritionalists world-wide have always recommended supplemental care and nourishment before and during the menstrual cycle. The cummilative effects of stress and muscle fatigue can create serious female disorders.

PMS

Dong Quai, White Willow bark, Uva Ursi, Valerian, Juniper Berries, Licorice, Black Cohosh, Cramp Bark, Ginger.

SPECIFIC CONDITIONS: Cramps, Bloating, Weight gain,

Backaches, Irritability, Nervousness, Tension, Migraine eadaches, Hot flashes, Ovarian problems, Uterine discomfort, Premenstrual syndrome.

Another natural combination to make life worth living. (SEE PMS ABOVE)

POTASSIUM/HERBAL

Kelp, Dulse, Watercress, Wild Cabbage, Horseradish, Horsetail.

BODILY INFLUENCE: Diuretic, Nervine, Nutritive, Sedative.
SPECIFIC CONDITIONS: Electrolyte balance, Blood pressure-high, Cancer, Circulation to the brain, Cysts, Dry skin, Hardened tissues, Irregular heart beat, Liver-sluggish, Muscle tone-lack of, Nervousness, Paralysis, Reflexes-poor, Skin disorders, Sodium-excess of, Thirst-excessive.

The cells are generally made of potassium and the bloodstream is generally made up of sodim. This is your electrolyte balance. Without potassium, your muscles would fail. This formula has in each capsule 42 mg. of high assimilable potassium through the synergistic action of all the other minerals that are found in this combination.

POTASSIUM

Potassium gluconte, Kelp, Alfalfa, Parsley.

BODILY INFLUENCE: Diuretic, Nervine, Nutrient, Sedative.
SPECIFIC CONDITIONS: Electrolyte balance, Blood pressure-high, Cancer, Circulation to the brain, Cysts, Dry skin, Hardened tissues, Irrregular heartbeat, Liver sluggish, Muscle tone, Nervousness, Paralysis, Reflexes, Skin disorders, Sodium excess, Thirst excessive.

By combining herbs and vitamins together synergistically you raise the assimilation of these nutrients when they were taken singly before. People die from lack of potassium.

PRENATAL

Black Cohosh, Butcher's Broom, Squaw Vine, Red Raspberry, Dong Quai.

BODILY INFLUENCE: Hormonal-female, Oxytocic.

SPECIFIC CONDITIONS: Birthing pain, Childbirth-tonic prior to, Dysmenorrhea, Hot flashes, Pregnancy-last 5 weeks.

This combination is designed for women to use in the last five weeks of pregnancy. It is designed to strengthen the uterus and to help with the elasticity to the pelvic and vaginal area in preparation for delivery. Midwives recommend expectant mothers in the fourth to fifth week before delivery, 9 per day and in the last 3 weeks to 12 per day. This is in addition to the supplements they are already taking. Along with prenatal classes, exercise and good diet, most of these mothers brag about delivery being practically bloodless and painless.

PROSTATE
Pygeum, Saw Palmetto, Stinging Nettle, Gotu Kola, Zinc.

BODILY INFLUENCE: Adaptogen, Anti-inflammatory, Astringent, Hormonal-prostate.
SPECIFIC CONDITIONS: Impotency, Prostate problems, Inflammation-prostate.

Saw palmetto has been a long time favorite in Europe. Millions of dollars of combinations like this are being sold in Europe proving its worth.

PROSTATE
Saw Palmetto, Broccoli, Zinc, Beta Carotene.

BODILY INFLUENCE: Anti-inflammatory, Glandular, Hormonal-prostate.
SPECIFIC CONDITIONS: Prostate problems, Hormones, Kidney, Bladder, Impotency, Inflammation-prostate.

Cruciferous vegetables such as broccoli have been proven to prevent and reverse cancer. By combining together herbs and vitamins, you many times increase the absorption factor.
(SEE PROSTATE ABOVE)

PROSTATE/BLADDER
Black Cohosh, Licorice, Kelp, Gotu Kola, Capsicum, Golden Seal, Ginger, Dong Quai.

BODILY INFLUENCE: Diuretic, Hormonal-prostate.
SPECIFIC CONDITIONS: Acne-male hormones, Lumbago,

Prostate problems, Urinary problems, Kidney infection, Bladder, Liver, Spleen, Hormone regulator, Urinary tract.

Male prostate problems are prevalent today. Again, lack of nutrition is one of the major problems. Another is one caused by poor nutrition and poor diet and without enough bulk and roughage in the diet. Consequently, we have poor bowel elimination and we cause ballooning and pockets in the area of the colon related to the prostate. The bowels must be taken care of with prostate problems. This combination is designed to feed, cleanse and restore integrity.

PROSTATE/BLADDER

Capsicum, Siberian Ginseng, Golden Seal, Ginger, Parsley, Uva Ursi, Marshmallow.

BODILY INFLUENCE: Adaptogen, Antibiotic, Bitter, Diuretic, Hormonal.
SPECIFIC CONDITIONS: Edema, Impotency, Prostate problems, Urinary infections.

This combination originated from Dr. Christopher and has had years of proven use.
(SEE PROSTATE/BLADDER ABOVE)

PROSTATE/BLADDER

Golden Seal, Parsley, Marshmallow, Ginger, Capsicum, Queen of the Meadow, Juniper Berries, Uva Ursi, Pan Pien Lien.

BODILY INFLUENCE: Adaptogen, Antibiotic, Bitter, Hormonal.
SPECIFIC CONDITIONS: Prostate, Hormones, Prostste problems, Kidney, Urinary infections, Impotency, Edema.
(SEE PROSTATE/BLADDER ABOVE)

SINUSES

Burdock root, Chinese Ephedra herb, Goldenseal root, Capsicum fruit, Parsley herb, Horehound herb, Althea root, Yerba Santa herb.

BODILY INFLUENCE: Antihistamine, Decongestant.
SPECIFIC CONDITIONS: Allergies-antihistamine, Asthma, Coughs, Eyes-itching, Hayfever-antihistamine, Sinusitis, Sinus

congestion, Wheezing, Colds-natural antihistamine, Runny nose, Sinus infection.

This combination can also be used for allergies and hayfever problems as well as sinusitis. This original formula was designed by Dr. John Christopher. It has a long and proven track record.

SKELETAL/CONNECTIVE TISSUE

White Oak Bark, Comfrey root, Wormwood, Pan Pien Lien, Scullcap, Black Walnut, Queen of the meadow, Marshmallow, Mullein.

BODILY INFLUENCE: Astringent, Bitter, Expectorant, Mucilant, Muscle relaxant, Stimulant.
SPECIFIC CONDITIONS: Bruises, Sore joints, Wasting, Weak connective tissue(i.e., muscle, cartilage, tendons.), Ligaments, Lower back pain, Discs, Muscle disorders

This combination was originally designed by Dr. John Christopher to take care of degenerative and debilitating problems brought on by accidents or aging.

SKIN   (SEE HAIR)

SKIN

Herbal concentrate: (Floro root, Chinese asparagus, Sweet orange peel, Red dates, Licorice root, Ginger), Marine protein complex, Acerola, d. Salina, L. Acidophilis, Grape seed concentrate, Grape skin concentrate, Aloe concentrate, Dahlulin™.

BODILY INFLUENCE: Antioxidant, Nutritive, Tonic.
SPECIFIC CONDITIONS: Skin disorders, Nutrient-skin, Youthfullness, Anti-aging, Tightens and tones skin internally.

This combination enhances circulation and also nourishes the hair, skin and nails, promotes new tissue growth and helps to detoxify the body. You're only as young as your skin looks, is very true.

SLEEP AID
Valerian, Scullcap, Hops.

BODILY INFLUENCE: Analgesic, Anti-spasmodic, Hypotensive, Nervine, Sedative.

SPECIFIC CONDITIONS: Alcoholism, Anxiety, Blood pressure-high, Drug addiction, Headache, Hyperactivity, Insomnia, Menstrual disorders, Nervous disorders, Nocturnal emissions, Pain-acute, Smoking-calms nerves, Stress, Bell's Palsy, Sleeping aid, Muscle tension, Herbal tranquilizer, Promotes safe sleep.

This combination is to promote a safe sound sleep. It is not like sleeping pills that people become dependent on. It could be used on a daily basis for any type of nervous condition.

SLEEP AID
Valerian, Hops, Wood Betony, Scullcap, Black Cohosh, Mistletoe, Pan Pien Lien, Capsicum, Lady's Slipper.

BODILY INFLUENCE: Analgesic, Anti-spasmodic, Calmative, Hypotensive, Nervine, Sedative.

SPECIFIC CONDITIONS: Alcoholism, Anxiety, Blood pressure-high, Nervousness, Strengthens nerves, Insomnia, Drug addiction, Headaches, Hyperactivity, Bell's Palsy, Sleep aid, Herbal tranquilizer.
(SEE SLEEP AID ABOVE)

SLEEP AID
Scullcap extract, Hops ext., Chamomile ext., Valerian ext., Passion flower, Kava Kava, Catnip.

BODILY INFLUENCE: Analgesic, Anti-spasmodic, Calmative, Hypotensive, Nervine, Sedative.

SPECIFIC CONDITIONS: Insomnia, Alcoholism, Anxiety, Blood pressure-high, Nervousness, Strengthens nerves, Drug addiction, Headaches, Hyperactivity, Bell's Palsy, Sleep aid, Herbal tranquilizer
(SEE SLEEP AID ABOVE)

STRESS

Chamomile flowers, Passion flowers, Hops flowers, Fennel seeds, Marshmallow root, Feverfew herb, Suma root, Astragalus root, Siberian Ginseng root, Ginkgo leaves, Gotu Kola herb, Schizandra fruit, Choline bitartrate, PABA, Wheat germ, Bee Pollen, Valerian root, Scullcap herb, Inositol, Hops flowers, Citrus bioflavonoids, Vitamins C, B-1, B-2, B-6, B-12, Folic acid, Biotin, Niacinamide and Pantothenic acid, Hops concentrate, Hops herb.

This is a combination of herbs and vitamins put together to meet the everyday demands put on us by the stress of everyday living. These herbs and vitamins will provide the necessary nutrients to replace those that have been expended coping with stressful everyday conditions.

THYROID

Kelp, Irish Moss, Parsley, Hops, Capsicum.

BODILY INFLUENCE: Antibiotic, Hormonal, Nervine, Nutritive.
SPECIFIC CONDITIONS: Allergies, Cold limbs, Convalescence, Debility, Epilepsy, Fatigue-low thyroid, Glandular swelling, Goiter, Obesity-low thyroid,   Blood pressure-low, Frigidity, Hair loss, Hyperactivity, Incoherent speech, Hypoactivity, Emotional, Cries easily.

This combination was originally put together by Dr. Stan Malstrom. It has been improved two times. The last time was by Master Herbalist, Larry Annis. Larry's research found that this formula could be taken in smaller doses with greater effectiveness with the addition of Hops. This combination is designed to be used for both overactive and underactive thyroid.

THYROID

Norwegian Kelp, Irish Moss, Parsley, Capsicum.

BODILY INFLUENCE: Antibiotic, Hormonal, Nervine, Nutritive.
SPECIFIC CONDITIONS: Allergies, Convalescense, Debility, Epilepsy, Fatigue, Thyroid-low, Goiter, Obesity, Swollen glands, Cries easily, Frigidity, Depression, Schizophrenia.
(SEE THYROID ABOVE)

THYROID

Kelp, Irish Moss, Parsley, Hops, Capsicum, Zinc and Manganese chelated in the amino acids Glutamine, Proline and Histidine.

BODILY INFLUENCE: Antibiotic, Hormonal, Nervine, Nutritive.
SPECIFIC CONDITONS: Fatigue, Obesity, Skin-lack of tone, Thyroid-low, Schizophrenia, Hair loss, Allergies, Cold limbs, Convalescence, Debility, Epilepsy, Glandular swelling, Goiter, Blood pressure-low, Frigidity, Hyperactivity, Hypoactivity, Incoherent speech, Emotional, Cries easily,

Dr. Harvey Ashmead has been given credit for this formula because of his research in mixing vitamins with herbs. This raises the assimilation 4 to 5 times what they were before. This is a chelated formula.

THYROID

Irish Moss, Kelp, Black Walnut, Parsley, Watercress, Sarsaparilla.

BODILY INFLUENCE: Aperitive, Hormonal, Mucilant, Nutritive.
SPECIFIC CONDITIONS: Allergies, Convalescence, Debility, Epilepsy, Fatigue-low thyroid, Goiter, Obesity, Swollen glands, Thyroid-low, Depression, Frigidity, Cries easily, Schizophrenia. (SEE THYROID ABOVE)

ULCERS

Golden Seal, Capsicum, Myrrh gum.

BODILY INFLUENCE: Antibiotic, Hemostat, Stomachic, Vulnerary.
SPECIFIC CONDITIONS: Bleeding-internal, Boils, Canker sores, Colitis, Gastritis, Halitosis, Hiatal hernia, Ulcer-stomach, Ulcerations, Ulcers-duodenal, Ulcers, Pyorrhea, Mouth and gum sores, Ulcers in and on the body and anywhere throughout the alimentary tract, Cancer, Crohn's disease.

Dr. Stan Malstrom originally put this formula together. This combination also aids in the common problems of digestion and also has the ability to stop bleeding ulcers.

ULCERS

Slippery Elm, Marshmallow, Plantain, Chamomile, Rose Hips, Bugleweed.

BODILY INFLUENCE: Astringent, Mucilant, Soothing, Vulnerary.
SPECIFIC CONDITIONS: Ulcers, Ulcerations, Colitis, Crohn's disease, Abdomen-inflammation of, Ulcerations-duodenal, Hemorrhoids, Hiatal hernia, Irritable bowel syndrome, Intestines-inflammation of, Heartburn, Cancer, Pyorrhea.

This combination was designed by Master Herbalist, Jeanne Burgess. It is designed to increase digestion, stop irritation and heal inflammed tissues wherever it is found in the body. It has saved many an individual from having surgery.

VAGINA

Squaw Vine, Chickweed, Slippery Elm, Comfrey root, Golden Seal, Yellow Dock, Mullein, Marshmallow.

BODILY INFLUENCE: Antibiotic, Hormonal, Mucilant, Nutirtive.
SPECIFIC CONDITIONS: Toxemia, Cysts, Endometriosis, Dry tract, Polyps, Uterine tumors, Discharge problems, Leucorrhea.
It can be used for douches or with cocoa butter to make vaginal suppositories.

NOTE: Melt cocoa butter in double boiler, add herb powder to make a thick dough-like consistency, cool sufficiently for handling, roll small finger-sized cylinders (on wax paper), let harden and refrigerate, then coat with vegetable oil before inserting,

WEIGHT CONTROL

Chickweed, Cascara Sagrada, Licorice, Safflowers, Parthenium, Black Walnut, Gotu Kola, Hawthorn, Papaya, Fennel, Dandelion.

BODILY INFLUENCE: Alterative, Diuretic, Laxative-mild, Parasiticide, Breaks down fat.
SPECIFIC CONDTIONS: Appetite-excessive, Constipation-mild, Edema, Fatigue, Obesity, Toxemia, Worms/parasites-expels, Weight loss, Helps the body digest and cleanse, Provides energy.

This combination was designed by LaDean Griffin and

probably is one of the most popular combinations and well known in the herbal world. Many people have made copies of this combination that are successful also. Some people call this Skinny Formula. This combination seems to be formulated so well that it is possible that it would be good food even for a thin or under-weight person to take.

WEIGHT CONTROL
Chickweed, Licorice, Saffron, Gotu Kola, Norwegian Kelp, Black Walnut, Dandelion, Fennel, Hawthorn, Echinacea, Angustifolia root, Papaya.

BODILY INFLUENCE: Alterative, Diuretic, Laxative, Parasiticide, Breaks down fat.
SPECIFIC CONDITIONS: Assists in weight control, Curbs appetite, Increases metabolism, Stimulates the thyroid to aid in weight loss, Obesity, Energy, Worms, Parasites.
(SEE WEIGHT CONTROL ABOVE)

WEIGHT CONTROL
Vitamins B-6, Lecithin, Apple cider vinegar, choline, Inositol, Vitamin F, Kelp, Calcium, Magnesium, Juniper Berries, Uva Ursi.

BODILY INFLUENCE: Digestant, Diuretic, Galactogogue.
SPECIFIC CONDITIONS: Edema, Obesity, Cholesterol, Kidneys, Bladder, Thyroid, Fatigue.
It helps with water retention, helps to dissolve fat and aids in digestion.
(SEE WEIGHT CONTROL ABOVE)

WEIGHT CONTROL
Brindall Berries, Gymnema leaves, Marshmallow, Psyllium.

BODILY INFLUENCE: Appetite suppressant, Sugar blocker, Breaks down fat.
SPECIFIC CONDITIONS: Weight loss, Appetite control, Fat metabolism, Blood sugar problems, Sugar craving, Obesity.
Brindall Berries triggers fatty acid oxidation preventing excess carbohydrates into fat and is a appetite suppressant. Psyllium expands 10 to 13 times its normal size when exposed to liquids giving us a bulking and fibrous agent preventing hunger pains

also. The Gymnema in this product can block absorption of up to 50% of dietary sugar calories. It also blocks the taste of sugar. It makes sweet things not taste as sweet.

WEIGHT CONTROL

Senna, Buckthorn, Peppermint, Caa Inhem, Uva Ursi, Orange peel, Rose Hips, Althea, Honeysuckle, Chamomile.

BODILY INFLUENCE: Digestant, Diuretic, Laxative, Nutritive, Parasiticide, Relaxant, Stimulant, Stomachic.
SPECIFIC CONDITIONS: Appetite suppressant, Constipation, Edema, Fatigue, Obesity, Toxemia, Parasites, Worms.

This combination is a good tasting herbal tea. It is so formulated, it could be used during your entire lifetime to provide good nutrition and normalcy. Many individuals who are not overweight, take this because it makes them feel better. Many people overweight or not have constipation and parasite problems and this combination covers both of those. It definitely helps with water retention by supporting the urinary system. Many people experience an increase in energy. It was not designed for children or pregnant women.

It tastes good, prevents fat deposits on your hips and also in your arteries.

WEIGHT LOSS

Ma Huang(Chinese ephedra), Salix Alba (White Willow bark, Fucus Vesiculosus(Kelp).

BODILY INFLUENCE: Astringent, Expectorant, Hormonal.
SPECIFIC CONDITIONS: Weight loss, Obesity, Curb appetite, Fatigue, Provides energy, Thermogenesis.

This formula was designed to create a conditon called Thermogenesis. Thermo meaning 'heat,' and genesis, meaning 'life.' It is designed to raise body temperature and provide more energy. There have been studies to show that if you raised normal body temperature (98.6) by 1 degree and hold for one full year you will lose weight.

HERBAL COMBINATIONS - CANADA

ENERGY/IMMUNE REJUVENATOR
Siberian Ginseng, Korean Ginseng, White Willow, Echinacea Purpurea, herbs, spices, Psyllium Hulls, Doedorized Garlic.

BODILY INFLUENCE: Adaptogen, Analgesic, Anodyne, Antibiotic, Anti-inflammatory, Blood purifier, Laxative, Mucilant, Nutritive, Stimulant, Tonic, Vermifuge.
SPECIFIC CONDITIONS: Longevity, Energy, Endurance, Depression, Fatigue, Mental & Physical exhaustion, Blood pressure-lowers, Sexual potency, vitality, Shock-counteract, Heart weakness, Exhaustion, Pain, Nervous system disorders, Sore muscles, Infection fighter, Blood purifier, Constipation, Diverticulitis.
    This combination is a blend of natural herbs that promote good health. Their nutritional benefit is improved when used in conjunction with proper exercise.

THYROID
Norwegian Kelp, Irish Moss, Parsley, Capsicum.

BODILY INFLUENCE: Antibiotic, Hormonal, Nervine, Nutritive.
SPECIFIC CONDITIONS: Thyroid gland, Metabolism, Glandular health, Blood circulation, Cellular structure, Allergies, Convalescence, Debility, Epilepsy, Fatigue-low thyroid, Cold limbs, Goiter, Obesity, Swollen glands, Cries easily, Frigidity, Depression, Schizophrenia.
    This herbal combination was originally put together by Dr. Stan Malstrom. This combination is designed to be used for both the overactive and underactive thyroid.

WEIGHT LOSS
Oriana bark, Kola nut, Cinnamon, Licorice root, Mate, Capsicum, Kelp.

BODILY INFLUENCE: Digestant, Laxative, Stimulant.
SPECIFIC CONDITIONS: Weight loss, Obesity, Hormone balance, Fitness, Constipation, Fat Burner.

This herbal combination is designed to keep energy levels up to the maximum while they are on a dietary program. Calories become weight, Energy burns calories.

WEIGHT LOSS/LAXATIVE

Senna, Buckthorn bark, Peppermint Leaves, Caa Inhem, Uva Ursi, Chickweed, Orange peel, Rose Hips, Althea root, Honeysuckle, Chamomile.

BODILY INFLUENCE: Digestant, Diuretic, Laxative, Nutritive, Parasiticide, Relaxant, Stimulant, Stomachic.
SPECIFIC CONDITIONS: Body cleanser, Weight loss, Appetite suppressant, Fat burner, energy, Cellulite, Digestive aid, Constipation, Edema, Fatigue, Obesity, Toxemia, Worms.

This combination is a good tasting herbal tea. It is so formulated that it could be used during your entire lifetime to provide good nutrition and normalcy. Many individuals who are not overweight, take this because it makes them feel better. Many people overweight have constipation and parasite problems and this combination covers both of these. It definitely helps with water retention by supporting the urinary system. Many people experience an increase in energy. It was not designed for children or pregnant women. It tastes good, prevents fat deposits on your hips and also in arteries.

WEIGHT LOSS

Buckthorn bark, Peppermint leaves, Caa Inhem, Uva Ursi, Chickweed, Orange peel, Rose Hips, Althea root, Honeysuckle, Chamomile.

(SEE WEIGHT LOSS ABOVE)

HERBAL LIQUID EXTRACTS

CHLOROPHYLL

Alfalfa in an isotonic solution of pure water soluble Chlorophyll delicately flavored with mint oil.

BODILY INFLUENCE: Alterative, Blood Builder, Deodorant, Nutritive, Tonic.
SPECIFIC CONDITIONS: Anemia-blood builder, Blood purifier, Body odor, Deodorant-internal, Pregnancy-prevents toxemia, Crohn's disease, Laryngitis, Blood detoxifier, Leukemia, Breath freshener, Multiple Sclerosis, Energy, Foot odors, Lactation, Liver, Iron absorption-influences, Hemorrhaging-blood transfusions, Diabetes, Digestive disorders, Hemorrhoids.

Chlorophyll is a popular blood purifier because of its high content of vitamin K, which aids in coagulation of the blood. Chlorophyll carries carbon dioxide as food to the cells of the plant and carries oxygen from its cells as waste to be discharged from its system, while hemoglobin carries the oxygen as food to the cells of the animal and carbon dioxide from the cells as waste to be discharged from the system. Because one of the liver's main function is the detoxification of the blood, Chlorophyll may assist and support the functions required by the liver in this major job.

BLOOD CLEANSER/DETOXIFIER/CANCER

Red Clover blossoms, Sheep Sorrel, Prickly Ash bark, Sarsaparilla root, Buckthorn bark, Burdock, Licorice root, Peach bark, Barberry bark, Echinacea purpurea, Cascara Sagrada, Rosemary in a bas of distilled water and glycerin.

BODILY INFLUENCE: Alterative, Antibiotic-mild, Anti-inflammatory, Blood Purifier, Diuretic, Laxative, Stimulant, Tonic.
SPECIFIC CONDITIONS: Cancer, Liver problems, Tumors, Lupus, Psoriasis, Multiple Sclerosis, Acne, Skin diseases.

This liquid extract combination of herbs supplies nutritional elements necessary for the healthy function of the liver, blood and lymphatic system, cleansing them of accumulated body waste and acquired toxins, supporting the immune blood balancing system.

COLD REMEDY

Peppermint, Elderberry, Sweet Orange Peel, Juniper berry, Catnip, Marigold flower, Angelica root, White Pine bark, Burdock, Peach bark, Elecampane, Licorice root in a base of honey, glycerin and distilled water.

BODILY INFLUENCE: Anti-inflammatory, Aromatic, Bitter, Blood purifier, Digestive, Diuretic, Expectorant, Nervine, Stimulant.

SPECIFIC CONDITIONS: Colds, Mucus-dissolves, Sinuses-drains, Digestive problems, Flu, Sore throat.

This herbal extract is beneficial in relieving the uncomfortable symptoms associated with colds and flu. It can help cleanse the body by liquifying the mucus thus draining the sinuses. It is also useful for a sensitive stomach and digestive problems. If taken frequently when a cold first starts, it will help cleanse the system thus, shortening the duration of the cold "nipping it in the bud" or help eliminate it altogether.

COUGHS

Chickweed, Licorice root, Juniper berries, Marshmallow, Mullein, Horehound, Capsicum in a base of distilled water and glycerin.

BODILY INFLUENCE: Anti-bacterial, Antibiotic, Anti-spasmodic, Astringent, Bitter, Expectorant, Nervine, Mucilant, Stimulant.

SPECIFIC CONDITIONS: Coughs, Coughs-hacking, Hoarseness, Throat-tight and scratchy.

This extract is designed to soothe the irritated throat from the tickling and irritation experienced during the common cold. It helps loosen a tight, scratchy throat and clear out the accumulating mucus. It helps to alleviate hoarseness and that hacking cough.

FLU/EPIDEMICS

Garlic, Gravel root, Marshmallow, White Oak bark, Black Walnut hulls, Mullein, Uva Ursi in a base of apple cider vinegar, glycerine and honey.

BODILY INFLUENCE: antibiotic, Anti-fungal, Astringent, Demulcent, Diuretic, Immuno-stimulant, Mucilant, Nervine, Nutritive, Parasiticide.

SPECIFIC CONDITIONS: Flu epidemics, AIDS, Immune system-stimulates, Colds, Fevers, Plague, Digestion.

This combination was originally put together by Dr. Christopher. He said, that the way we are destroying the environment around us, that we are weakening our bodies' immune system. He went on to say that the plagues were going to revisit us and this formula was needed to take care of us then. There have been people that have used this formula for the flu, viruses and even for AIDS.

MUCUS/EXPECTORANT
Garlic, Mullein, Fennel in a base of distilled water, glycerin and apple cider vinegar.

BODILY INFLUENCE: Antibiotic, Anti-fungal, anti-inflammatory, anti-spasmodic, Aromtaic, Demulcent, Digestant, Diuretic, Expectorant, Mucilant.
SPECIFIC CONDITIONS: Asthma, Mucus-loosens, Bronchitis, Congestion, Emphysema, Pneumonia.

Expectorants are designed to loosed and expel mucus relieving congestion. This opens up the breathing passages allowing the body to heal itself. It helps speedy recovery from pneumonia, emphysema and bronchitis.

PARASITES
Black Walnut hulls, Sage, Fennel, Male Fern in a base of distilled water and glycerin.

BODILY INFLUENCE: Bitter, Cathartic, Laxative, Parasiticide.
SPECIFIC CONDITIONS: Parasites, Laxative, Thyroid, Constipation, Fungus, Impetigo, Ringworm, Herpes.

In one case I know of, where parasites had completely eaten up the lining of the intestinal tract, this was the only product that could be effective and not irritate the lining. Other parasitic combinations were tried and only succeeded in causing violent vomiting, but in this formula the glycerin was soothing. It literally saved her life.

SINGLE CHINESE HERBS

ASTRAGALUS (Astragalus membranaceus)
A.K.A.,: Huang chi, Bak kay.

BODY INFLUENCE: Energy tonic, Diuretic, acts to inhibit sweating.
PART USED: Root.

It is most known for its effective application where lung and spleen problems appear. Astragalus has been an effective part of treating digestion ailments, increasing appetite and is good for enhancing control of diarrhea. It strengthens energy and resistance to weakness, colds, flu and disease. Astragalus finds useful application to ease chemotherapy and radiation side effects and inhibits the spreading of tumors. (See Astragalus in the SINGLE HERBS Section)

ATRACTYLODES
(Atractylodes alba, A. macrocephalae)
A.K.A.,: Bai zhu, Bak sut.

BODILY INFLUENCE: Energy tonic, diuretic, carminative.
PARTS USED: Root.

Atractylodes is one of the major plants used to nourish and strengthen the spleen and stomach. It is useful in treating any condition where fluid retention is a problem.

BUPLEURUM (Bupleurum falcatum)
A.K.A.,: Chai hu; Chai wu.

BODILY INFLUENCE: Anti-pyretic, Diaphoretic, Carminative, Alterative.
PART USED: Root.

This plant is known for its treatment quality for the liver, gall bladder and menstrual problems. It is known to stabilize emotional problems due to female discomforts during and prior to menstruation.

CHRYSANTHEMUM (Chrysanthemum morifolium)
A.K.A.,: Ja hua, Gook fah.

BODILY EFFECTS: Anti-pyretic, Carminative, Anti-spasmodic, Alterative, Tonic.
PART USED: Flowers.

Chrysanthemum is useful in treating colds, flu, fevers, headaches and pneumonia. It also calms anger and irritability.

CITRUS (Citrus reticulata)
A.K.A.,: Chen pi, Chen pay.

BODILY INFLUENCE: Carminative, Stimulant, Expectorant, Anti-tussive, Anti-emetic, Tonic.
PARTS USED: Aged Dried Peel.

The peel of Citrus, especially the Tangerine moves stagnant energy in the abdomen and strengthens the digestive tract. It is useful for the lungs in that the inner part of the part creates mucus and the peel helps to eliminate it.

CODONOPIS (Codonopis pilosulae)
A.K.A.,: Dang shen, Dong sum.

BODILY INFLUENCE: Energy tonic, Demulcent, Expectorant.
PARTS USED: Root.

This plant is used at times to substitute the qualities expected in Ginseng. It increases vital energy and overall blood improvement. It is given to help any condition acknowledged as general weakness, tiredness, anemia and poor appetite.

CORNUS (Cornus officinalis)
A.K.A.,: Shan zhu yu, San yu yok.

BODILY INFLUENCE: Astringent, Tonic.
PARTS USED: Fruit.

Cornus berries are astringent and this is called its essence, for treatment of a weak body and excessive loss of fluids in the body. It is helpful for incontinence, excessive sweating, night sweats and benefits weak backs and knees.

CYPERUS (Cyperus spp.,)
A.K.A.,: Xiang fu, Heung fu.

BODILY INFLUENCE: Carminative, Antis-spasmodic, Emmenagogue.
PARTS USED: Root.

Cyperus is a specific when there is distension and pain in the abdomen and and chest and is helpful in conditions such as gas, bloating, menstruation problems and digestive problems.

DIOSCOREA (Discorea batata, D. japonica)
A.K.A.,: Shan yao, Wai san.

BODILY INFLUENCE: Energetic tonic, Nutritive, Demulcent.
PARTS USED: Root.

This rhizome is effective in rejuvenating, by strengthening the digestive tract. It will help build up conditional weakness in the lungs and kidneys, as well as helping tiredness, poor digestion and fatigue. This plant is better known as Chinese Wild Yam.

DONG QUAI (Angelica sinensis)
A.K.A.,: Dang gui, Dong kway.

BODILY INFLUENCE: Blood tonic, Emmenagogue, Sedative, Analgesic, Laxative.
PARTS USED: Root.

There is a long history of this herb's benefit to women. It is considered the female Ginseng, for treating many female disorders. It helps promote circulation, stimulating the uterus and stopping pain in that area. It is also helpful where there is anemia and is usually given to women, but men may also benefit from taking this herb when there are signs of anemia.

EPHEDRA (Ephedra spp.,)
A.K.A.,: Ma huang, Ma wong.

BODILY INFLUENCE: Diaphoretic, Stimulant, Diuretic, Expectorant, Astringent.
PART USED: Above-ground portion.

Chinese Ephedra is a strong stimulant with an action like adrenaline. It is useful for about every bronchial condition, including asthma, bronchitis, wheezing and where there is difficulty in breathing. It is helpful in relieving colds, flu and fever, by its ability to cause sweating.

FU LING (Poria cocos)
A.K.A.,: Fu ling, Fuk ling.

BODILY INFLUENCE: Diuretic, Sedative, Tonic.
PART USED: Whole fungus.

Fu ling is a treasured North American mushroom called Tuckahoe, but more commonly known as Indian bread. Its mildness makes it very useful, especially with children and the elderly. For difficult urination, it is one of the best diuretics. It helps to calm the mind, aid digestion and relieve anxiety.

GARDENIA (Gardenia jasminoides)
A.K.A.,: Zhi zi, San jee jee.

BODILY INFLUENCE: Alterative, Anti-pyretic, Hemostatic.
PART USED: Fruit.

Gardenia is known as the 'happiness herb.' It is beneficial for restlessness, irritability, anger, hypertension and such ailments. It can also be used externally in a poultice to treat inflammation. It is useful for fevers, urinary tract infections, jaundice and insomnia.

GINSENG (Panax ginseng)
A.K.A.,: Ren shen, Yun sum.

BODILY INFLUENCE: Energy tonic, Rejuvenative, Demulcent, Stimulant.
PART USED: Aged root.

Ginseng helps build vitality, strengthens the body when there is low energy, increases longevity, resistance to disease and promotes tissue growth.
Refer to the section on Single Herbs.

HONEYSUCKLE (Lonicera japonica)
A.K.A.,: Jin yin hua, Gum nan fah.

BODILY INFLUENCE: Alterative, Febrifuge, Anti-biotic, Diuretic, Refrigerant, Diaphoretic.
PART USED: Flowers.

Honeysuckle is effective as a poultice in the treatment of wounds or open cuts, where there is danger of infection. It is good for inflammations in areas such as the intestines, urinary tract and reproductive organs. It is helpful in the treatment of fevers due to infection, working effectively as a natural anti-biotic for staph and strep infections.

HO SHOU WU (Polygonum multiflorum)
A.K.A.,: He shou wu, Ho sao wu.

BODILY INFLUENCE: Blood tonic, Astringent
PART USED: Root.

This plant is said to have mysterious properties and is often called Fo Ti (margeting name) in America It has been known to reverse the conditions thought to be true from aging. It has restored hair color and even enabled teeth to grow in elderly people. It builds blood in everyone, is helpful for wrinkles, is known as a tonic for the liver, kidneys and blood and increases sperm count in men. Refer to Single Herbs

JUJUBE (Zizyphus sativa)
A.K.A.,: Da zao, Dai jo.

BODILY INFLUENCE: Energy tonic, Expectorant, Nutritive, Sedative
PART USED: Fruit.

This plant is noted for its delicious giant red fruit and is used to strengthen the digestive system in general. It is also effective in treating exhaustion and nerves resulting from exhaustion and calming the emotions.

LYCII (Lycium chinensis)
A.K.A.,: Gou qi zi, Gay jee.

BODILY INFLUENCE: Blood and Nutritive tonic, Hemostatic, Anti-pyretic.
PART USED: Fruit.

The berry of this plant strengthens the blood, especially when there is anemia. It is effective in treating a variety of problems associated with the eyes. The berries are high in the ingredient beta-carotene. It is also helpful for sore backs, knees and legs.

PEONY (Paeonia lactiflorae)
A.K.A.,: Bai shao, Bal chuk.

BODILY INFLUENCE: Blood and Nutritive tonic, Emmenagogue, Anti-spasmodic, Astringent.
PART USED: Root.

Historically, this is a blood toner and general overall cleanser. It may be used for many conditions due to toxins in the blood. In combination with other herbs, Peony is given to act as a relaxant, reducing tension. It can be effective as a calming agent as well.

PUERARIA (Pueraria lobata)
A.K.A.,: Ge gen, Gwat gun.

BODILY INFLUENCE: Diaphoretic, Anti-spasmodic, Digestant, Demulcent, Tonic.
PART USED: Root.

Pueraria is also known as Kuzu root and is a common ingredient found in macrobiotic dietary cooking. It has been used effectively in the treatment of colds, fever, headache, colitis and other ailments. It has been found to be an effective remedy for the treatment of diabetes and hypoglycemia. It neutralizes acidity in the body, so it is helpful in relieving aches and pains.

REHMANNIA (Scrophulariaceae glutinosa)
A.K.A.,: Sheng di hauang, Sang day/when raw.

BODILY INFLUENCE: Blood and Nutritive Tonic, Hemostatic, Demulcent, Laxative, Alterative.
PARTS USED: Root, raw or prepared.

When eaten raw, Rehmannia will extract heat from the body and the blood. It is most effective to treat a high fever, clear thirst, irritability, constipation and chronic throat pain. Cooked Rehmannia will strengthen the blood. It is helpful as a prescription for female ailments. It also strengthens the bones and tendons.

REISHI   (Ganderma lucidum)
A.K.A.,: Ling zhi.

BODILY INFLUENCE: Rejuvenative, Anti-bacterial, Anti-viral, Anti-tumor, Immune tonic.
PART USED: Whole Mushroom.

The Reishi Mushroom has long term use with the Chinese Herbalist. It has a wide range of applications to the human system, including allergies, rheumatism, insomnia, hepatitis, liver diseases and viruses. It has been known as a life elixir because it revitalizes the entire system and is reputed for its ability to restore life.

SCHIZANDRA (Schizandra sinensis)
A.K.A.,: Wu wei zi, Ng way jee.

BODILY INFLUENCE: Astringent, Tonic, Sedative
PART USED: Fruit.

As a tonic, Schizandra strengthens the tissue and works to retain body energy. It is known as a calmer and helpful in treating forgetfulness. It contains mild adaptogens, which regulate body functions and enable the ability to handle stress. It is helpful with coughing, lung weakness, asthma, night sweats and prolonged diarrhea.

TENCHI   (Panax pseudoginseng)
A.K.A.,: Tien qi, San qi, Som chuk.

BODILY INFLUENCE: Tonic, Hemostatic, Emmenagogue.
PART USED: Root.

Because of its Ginseng-like strengthening abilities, Tenchi is called pseudo Ginseng. Its primary purpose is to stop bleeding and hemorrhaging. It is helpful in reduction of swelling, wounds and cuts. It also dissolves blood clots relieves pain and quickly promotes the circulation of blood.

ZIZYPHUS   (Zizyphus spinosa)
A.K.A.,: Suan zao ren, Shune cho yun.

BODILY INFLUENCE: Nervine, Sedative, Tonic, Astringent.
PART USED: Seed.

Zizyphus seeds help calm the mental and emotional changes, can relieve stress due to insomnia, nervous exhaustion and anxiety. It is a moistening, nurturing and strengthening herb which helps when energy is low and the blood needs cleansing. It is safe for children and treatment of the elderly.

CHINESE HERBAL COMBINATIONS

"This system of medicine (Chinese Herbology) is based on the most solid foundation of any system of medicine in the world. It is wholly based on natural laws. Man cannot pollute it; man cannot change it; man cannot improve upon it. Although it may be new in the Western world, one has to recognize that one-quarter of the world's population has been treated by this system of medicine for over four-thousand years. If it was not valid, then it would have died thousands of years ago."

J.R. Worsley, "Talking about Acupuncture in New York." College of Traditional Acupuncture Element Nooks Ltd., Great Britain, 1982), P. 15.

The great wonder of the Chinese Herbalist, has for centuries, been the interplay in nature between man and herbs. Over four thousand years has been elapsing while they built their skills and traditions to collect and hoard a vast treasure of knowledge concerning herbs and their benefits to mankind.

This expertise of collecting, mixing and working with nature's plant and animal kingdom has educated them through deep experience into the inner secrets of the rhythmic balance of nature, its ebb and flow. They have observed the universe about them being built on the principal of two opposing forces that control the forces of nature: the Yin and the Yang. It is believed by the Chinese that through this balance between the Yin and the Yang hangs the health of mankind, physical, mental and spiritual.

As modern research science and medicine began to realize the existence and importance of the sympathetic and parasympathetic nervous system, it was obvious that the ancient Chinese traditions and views that "disease will be the end result" when the balance of nature is interfered with or distracted, is in fact, true. The ancient Chinese cultural view of balancing the inner and the outer energy (the Yin and the Yang) has been renewed in the Western mind, realizing that an out-of-balance sympathetic and parasympathetic nervous system can produce stress-related problems such as high blood pressure, heart trouble, stomach problems, ulcers, insomnia, oxygen debts, headaches, etc.

Here in the West, we have educated ourselves to believe we must attack nature's warning signs, the disease, and ignore the underlying cause. The Western mind refuses to accept the blame of his wrong course of action as being the true underlying cause of his discomfort. When the pain factor or change in body chemistry and function cease to bring his problems to his attention, he returns to his old habits and ignores the underlying cause of his dis-ease. We, the Western mind, therefore, seek relief from pain or ask that we be assured that "all is well." This untimely thought has become the unconscious death parade as many self-inflicted robots walk blindly through a life of slow deterioration and through our mob psychology of following the crowd in life's fashions, "quick foods" etc. we suffer, by our choice, the loss of health and well being as we continue to believe that everything was normal and all is just an aging process.

Why Chinese herbs? They are to bring harmony to the whole physical man and overcome in us, the slow and painful realization that, for eons of time, we were on a long, long journey of no return, only to awaken at that final moment of life with no recourse, surprised to find that the magic pill, the needle, that potion that was to bring us utopia and take away our pain or hide us there in front of the big wide screen dulling our senses to the end. There was no utopia, no beautiful ever after, we had heard the pied piper blowing his tempting flute and all we, like sheep, following until it was too late, the agony of everlasting misery with drug dependence and the premature end was upon us?

In the Chinese herbal health philosophy, we find that individuals are placed in a type category or constitution - wood, fire, metal, earth, water, heat, energy - these are basic, from there it is decided where to place them, either stressed-type or a weakened-type person. If one has this basic understanding, they can better choose the herbs or herbal combinations adaptable for their health, or as the Chinese Herbalist would say, best suited for body balancing.

The Chinese further work on the premise that all form of life are motivated by a vital life-force, an essential energy force called Chi. Chi also means "breath" and "air" and is similar to the Hindu concept of Prana. Chi is invisible, tasteless, odorless, and formless. Chi, in spite of this, fills the whole universe. Chi is transferable and transmutable: digestion extracts Chi from food and drink and transfers it to the physical being: breathing extracts Chi from air and transfers it to the lungs. When these two forms meet in the bloodstream, they transmute to form human-chi, which then circulates throughout the body as vital energy. It is the quality, quantity, and balance of your chi that determines your state of health and span of life. The Chinese consider that optimum health is a natural and harmonious balance among the vital energies within the human being, as well as between those of the human being and the external environment.

The Chinese teach that the Chi, through our eating, is extracted from the medicinal plant and goes directly from the plant energies to its bodily organ of affinity, for which they were prescribed. There they work to restore the diseased organ to its original tissue tone and natural functions, in the process redressing the attendant imbalances of vital energy.

Constitutional therapy is a useful approach to better health derived from the Chinese concept that one should base treatment on the nature of the person rather the nature of the diseases they suffer.

The Constitutional Type is a reflection of how a person goes through life.

CONSTITUTIONAL CHINESE THERAPY

The seven constitutional types relate as follows:
Water - Kidney/Bladder
Fire - Heart/Cardiovascular
Wood - Liver/Gall bladder
Heat/Dryness - Lymphatic/Fluids
Metal - Lungs/Respiratory
Earth - Stomach/Spleen
Energy/Immune system

The Thyroid type includes both the Water and Fire constitution.

The Adrenal type includes both the Wood and Heat/Dryness constitution.

The Pituitary type includes just the Metal constitution.

The Gonadal type includes both the Earth and the Energy constitution.

Chinese Herbology says that there is yet a stressed and a weakened type for each constitution. For each constitution (Wood, Fire, Metal, Earth, Water, Heat and Energy), there is a stressed and a weakened person.

Some people fall into one category or the other, and it is through observation of those individuals that we recognize the validity of the basic concept of Constitutional Typing. Most people show a tendency towards one of these behavioral types, even if they have some characteristics of each.

The Chinese observe similarities between these natural products of nature and qualities in human beings.

Chinese thinking tends to view the body as part of the whole. They seek to build and strengthen the body as a whole. As a result, they have developed herb combinations designed to strengthen or "tonify" various types of people.

The Chinese constitutional formulas are nutritional supplements designed to feed and support different types of people.

Hence, they might say that a person with fire-like behavior and fire-like health problem has an excess of the fire element. They don't intend this to mean that the person has too much fire. It is just a way of describing an observation. In Western terminology, it can be said that this person is hyper-active or Type A behavior.

TYPE A BEHAVIOR (Needs reducing formulas)

A person who is ambitious, driven, goal oriented, always busy, pushing against deadlines, worrying about satisfying both superiors and those working beneath, eating too fast, drinking too much, and sleeping too little.

TYPE B BEHAVIOR (Needs enhancing formulas)

A person who is relaxed, taking things as they come, leaving room for pleasure and leisure, allowing others to take on the burden of deadlines or of satisfying demands of impatient individuals, taking time with meals, and sleeping longer hours. This means layed back or underactive or hypoactive.

Constitution therapies are not drug therapies; they are a type of nutritional therapy used to balance the body.

LIVER

CHINESE NAME: TIAO HE
CHINESE TRANSLATION: WOOD REDUCING -
MEDIATE HARMONY
CONSTITUTIONAL TYPE: WOOD-STRESSED

TIAO HE (Wood stressed)
Bupleurum & Peony Twelve Combination:
    Bupleurum root, Zhishi fruit, Peony root, Scute root, Pinellia rhizome, Cinnamon twig, Dang Gui root, Fushen plant, Atractylodes rhizome, Panax Ginseng root, Ginger rhizome, Licorice root.

BODILY INFLUENCE: Anti-depressant, Carminative, Cholagogue, Diaphoretic, Hepatic, Laxative, Nervine.

SPECIFIC CONDITIONS: Allergies-food, Anemia, Anger-excessive, Backache, Depression, Diarrhea-support liver, Dysmenorrhea, Food poisoning, Gallstones, Gastric ulcer, Hangover, Hepatitis, Hypochondria, Hypoglycemia, Insomnia, Irritability, Liver problems-acute, Menstrual disorders, Migraine headache, Morning sickness, PMS, Skin condition-inflammation, Stress, Supports gall bladder, intestines and stomach.

    This is a liver herbal combination used to relieve acute nervous tension and depression and to encourage an overall sense of well being by nutritionally building health. It improves the general circulation, function of the gall bladder and liver function relieving liver congestion. Cold hands and feet, fatigue, tension in the chest and allergies are benefited the most in using this combination. As one author has said, " it has a calming effect on the spirit."

BLOOD PURIFIER

CHINESE NAME: BU XUE
CHINESE TRANSLATION: INCREASE WOOD-NOURISH THE BLOOD
CONSTITUTIONAL TYPE: WOOD-WEAKENED

BU XUE (Wood weakened)
Dang gui & Peony Eighteen Combination:
   Ganoderma plant, Dang Gui root, Peony root, Lycium fruit, Bupleurum root, Curcuma root, Cornus fruit, Salvia root, Ho Sho Wu root, Atractylodes rhizome, Ligustrum fruit, Alisma rhizome, Astragalus root, Ligusticum rhizome, Rehmannia root, Panax Ginseng root, Cyperus root.

BODILY INFLUENCE: Adaptogen, Alterative, Antispasmodic, Blood Purifier, Diuretic, Emmenagogue, Hepatic, Immuno-stimulant, Stimulant, Tonic-Liver.

SPECIFIC CONDITIONS: Alcoholism, Anemia-builds liver, Appetite-loss of, Blurred vision, Cirrhosis, Cramps, Deafness and loss of sight, Dizziness, Dysmenorrhea, Eyes-dry, Fatigue, Gall bladder-weakened, Hepatitis, Jaundice, Immune deficiency, Infertility, Leukemia, Liver problems-chronic, Menstrual disorders, Menstrual disorders-long cycle, Mood swings, Morning sickness, Nausea-chronic, Polyps, Postpartum depression.

   This is a liver herbal combination to relieve and strengthen a chronic weakened liver, providing nutrition to aid the circulatory system, exerting a soothing effect on the spirit and body, overcoming blood deficiencies and hormone imbalance associated with chronic liver dysfunction. This combination works to enhance immune response and to restore blood circulation when there is physical damage to organs induced by injury, chemicals or disease. It is an antioxidant, acts as a cell restorer, is calming, relieves muscle cramping, improves urine flow, increases menstrual flow and works to help one think clearly.

INFLAMMATION/FEVER

CHINESE NAME: QUING RE
CHINESE TRANSLATION: CLEAR THE HEAT
CONSTITUTIONAL TYPE: HEAT/DRYNESS-STRESSED

QING RE (Heat/Dryness stressed)
Forsythia & Schizonepta Eighteen Combination:
Vitex fruit, Licorice root, Carthamus flowers, Coptis rhizome, Lonicera flowers, Philodendron bark, Scute root, Siler root, Forsythia fruit, Bupleurum root, Platycodon root, Dang Gui root, Ligusticum rhizome, Arctium seed, Schizonepeta herb, Peony root, Chrysanthemum flowers, Gardenia fruit.

BODILY INFLUENCE: Alterative, Analgesic, Anti-inflammatory, Diuretic.
Laxative, Sedative.

SPECIFIC CONDITIONS: Anemia, Chipping nails, Colds-with fever/inflammation, Depression, Ear infections, Eyes-dry, Eyes-irritation of, Fever-with chills, Flu, Gallstones, Gum inflammation, Headache, Hemorrhoids, Hepatitis, Immune deficiency, Inflammation, Insomnia, Menopause, Mouth sores, Night sweats, Pain, PMS, Ribs, Shoulder and wrist pain, Skin eruptions, Sore throat, TMJ, Toxic blood.

This combinations aids in reducing fever, pain and helps alleviate inflammation. This is a blood purifier, a detoxifier and has a laxative effect, increases urine flow, is soothing to inflamed tissues and has an overall calming effect. It is said to have an antibiotic effect, speeds up fat metabolism, relieves headaches and aids vision.

HYPOGLYCEMIA/DIABETES

CHINESE NAME: BU YIN
CHINESE TRANSLATION: NOURISH THE YIN
CONSTITUTIONAL TYPE: HEAT/DRYNESS
WEAKENED

BU YIN (Heat/Dryness Weakened)
Rehmannia & Ophiopogon Sixteen Formula:
Dendrobium herb, Eucommia bark, Rehmannia root, Ophiopogon root, Trichosanthes root, Pueraria root, Anemarrhena rhizome, Achyranthes root, Hoelen plant, Asparagus root, Mouton root bark, Alisma rhizome, Philodendron bark, Cornus fruit, Licorice root, Schizandra fruit.

BODILY INFLUENCE: Antipyretic, Bulk laxative, Carminative, Demulcent, Diuretic, Expectorant, Stimulant, Tonic-General.

SPECIFIC CONDITIONS: Blurred vision, Constipation, Cough-dry, Diabetes-build pancreas, Dysuria, Fatigue-extreme, Fever, Heart problems, Hot and tingly hands, Hot hands and feet, Hot flashes, Hypertension, Hypoglycemia, Inflammation, Insomnia, Kidney problems, Memory problems, Menopause, Night sweats, Skin-burning, Skin-dry, Sore throat, Thirst, Tinnitus.

This is an herbal combination that seeks to normalize a great many problems associated with metabolic processes such as sugar metabolism and menopause. It tends to moisten the body to overcome excessive dryness of the throat, skin and bowels, normalizing hormone imbalances, aiding feverish feelings and relieving depression. It soothes inflamed tissues, increases blood circulation, stimulates adrenal activity, strengthens kidney function, increasing urine flow.

STRESS/NERVES

CHINESE NAME: AN SHEN
CHINESE TRANSLATION: FIRE QUENCHING -
PACIFY THE SPIRIT
CONSTITUTIONAL TYPE: FIRE-STRESSED

AN SHEN (Fire stressed)
Fushen & Dragon Bone Sixteen Combination:
Dragon bone, Oyster shell, Albizzia bark, Polygonum stem, Fushen plant, Polygala root, Acorus rhizome, Panax Ginseng root, Saussurea root, Zizyphus seed, Curcuma root, Haliotis shell, Coptis rhizome, Cinnamon bark, Licorice root, Ginger rhizome.

BODILY INFLUENCE: Antispasmodic, Carminative, Diuretic, Nervine, Relaxant, Sedative, Stomachic.

SPECIFIC CONDITIONS: Angina pain, Backache-low, Chest distress, Convulsions, Dizziness, Drug withdrawal-eases, Emotional problems, Excitability, Flushing, Fright-excessive, Headache, Heart palpitations, Hyperventilation, Incoherent speech, Indigestion, Insomnia, Irritability, Mental illness, Moles on the body, Neurosis, Nervous disorders, Paranoia, Restlessness, Stress.
This is an anti-stress, soothing combination with a natural occuring source of calcium and minerals. It has a calming, regulating effect on the muscles, circulatory system and nerves, mirroring anti-stress vitamin supplements and many Western nervine formulas. It relieves muscle spasms that are anxiety caused, being that it is a natural tranquilizer, it relaxes the internal system to overcome anxiety, fear and agitated energy.

HEART STIMULANT

CHINESE NAME: YANG XIN
CHINESE TRANSLATION: NOURISH THE FIRE-
NURTURE THE HEART
CONSTITUTIONAL TYPE: FIRE-WEAKENED

YANG XIN (Fire weakened)
Biota & Zizyphus Eighteen Formula:

Schizandra fruit, Dang Gui root, Cistanche herb, Biota seed, Succinum, Ophiopogon root, Cuscuta seed, Lycium fruit, Panax Ginseng root, Polygonum rhizome, Hoelen plant, Dioscorea root, Astragalus root, Lotus seed, Polygala root, Acorus rhizome, Zizphus seed, Rehmannia root.

BODILY INFLUENCE: Adaptogen, Anti-depressant, Cardiotonic, Carminative, Diuretic, Sedative.

SPECIFIC CONDITIONS: Anemia, Angina pains, Anxiety, Back pain, Confusion, Depression, Digestion, Digestion-weak, Emotional problems, Exhaustion-nervous, Heart palpitations, Heart-supports, Heart weakness, Impotency, Insomnia, Memory problems, Night sweats, Nervous disorders, Restlessness, Sex drive-lack of, Skin-dry, Urination-frequent.

This is an energizing, invigorating combination, increasing vitality and heat (possibly relating to hypothyroidism). It improves digestion thus increasing the nourishment available to the nervous and circulatory systems resulting in a sense of well-being. It is a nerve and heart tonic relieving depression allowing the body to respond faster to stress. It increases strength, overcomes chronic nervous disorders, increases oxygen utilization and improves confused thinking and mental frustration. It helps with insomnia, especially a condition of "waking up every hour or two."

ANTI-GAS/DIGESTIVE SYSTEM

CHINESE NAME: XIAO DAO
CHINESE TRANSLATION: DISPEL EARTH-CLEAR
THE CONGESTION
CONSTITUTIONAL TYPE: EARTH-STRESSED

XIAO DAO (Earth stressed)
Agastache & Shenqu Sixteen Combination:
Agastache herb, Magnolia bark, Shenqu tea, Crataegus fruit, Oryza seed, Hoelen plant, Panax Ginseng root, Pinellia rhizome, Saussurea root, Gastrodia rhizome, Citrus peel, Atractylodes rhizome, Cadamon fruit, Platycodon root, Ginger rhizome, Licorice root.

BODILY INFLUENCE: Anti-inflammatory, Carminative, Diuretic, Laxative, Stimulant, Stomachic.

SPECIFIC CONDITIONS: Abdominal bloating, Anxiety, Appetite-lack of, Bowel-sluggish, Circulation-poor, Cold limbs, Congestion-general, Diarrhea, Digestion-sluggish, Digestive aid, Difficulty in rising, Fatigue after eating, Food allergy, Foul belching, Gas-relieves, Gastroenteritis, Headaches, Indigestion, Intestinal pains, Morning sickness, Motion sickness, Nausea, Obesity, Stomachaches, Sweet cravings, Worry-excessive.

This combination is helpful in cases of acute indigestion and to loosen and disperse the mucus (or phlegm) and toxins from the digestive tract. The herbs in this combination help encourage the normal function of the circulatory, urinary and digestive systems. The herbs are mildly laxative thus, helping with elimination which helps with weight loss. It helps to relieve bloating, gas, nausea and relieves intestinal pains.

ULCERS/COLITIS

CHINESE NAME: WEN ZHONG
CHINESE TRANSLATION: ENHANCE EARTH
WARM THE CENTER
CONSTITUTIONAL TYPE: EARTH-WEAKENED

WEN ZHONG (Earth weakened)
Ginseng & Licorice Eighteen Formula:
Panax ginseng root, Astragalus root, Atractylodes rhizome, Hoelen plant, Dioscorea root, Lotus seed, Galanga rhizome, Pinellia rhizome, Chaenomeles fruit, Magnolia bark, Saussurea root, Dang Gui root, Citrus peel, Dolichos seed, Licorice root, Ginger rhizome, Zanthoxylum fruit, Cardamon fruit.

BODILY INFLUENCE: Adaptogen, Anti-inflammatory, Antiseptic, Carminative, Demulcent, Immuno-stimulant, Stimulant, Stomachic, Tonic-digestive.

SPECIFIC CONDITIONS: Abdomen-inflammation of, Aches, Anorexia, Appetite-poor, Arthritis, Assimilation of foods-improves, Chills, Circulation-poor, Cold limbs, Colitis, Cramps-stomach, Depression, Diarrhea, Digestion, Edema, Fatigue, Flu, Hemorrhoids, Hernias, Hiatal hernia, Hunger-unusual, Indigestion, Leg cramps, Menstrual cramps, Skin-dry, Skin-sallow, Ulcers, Uterus-prolapsed, Worry-excessive.

This is a combination for poor digestion, being an overall strengthening formulation that works as a nutritional support for the digestive and circulatory systems. It works as a general tonic whose function is to rejuvenate the body, enhance the production of digestive fluids and enzymes, helping to increase blood circulation and boost immune response. The herbs are antiseptic and work to reduce inflammation. This formulation stimulates digestion, is a blood builder and an infection fighter. It relieves inflammation and infection of the gastrointestinal tract, helps with poor muscle tone and cramping in the legs.

ALLERGY/LUNG

CHINESE NAME: XUAN FEI
CHINESE TRANSLATION: METAL REDUCING-
VENTILATE THE LUNGS
CONSTITUTIONAL TYPE: METAL-STRESSED

XUAN FEI (Metal stressed)
Pinellia & Citrus Sixteen Combination:
  Citrus peel, Pinellia rhizome, Ma Huang herb, Fritillaria
bulb, Bamboo sap, Bupleurum root, Hoelen plant,
Platycodon root, Xingren, Morus root bark, Magnolia bark,
Tussilago flowers, Ophiopogon root, Schizandra fruit,
Ginger rhizome, Licorice root.

BODILY INFLUENCE: Anti-depressant, Antihistamine,
Decongestant, Diaphoretic, Diuretic, Expectorant,
Stimulant, Stomachic.

SPECIFIC CONDITIONS: Asthma-acute attack,
Breathing-shallow, Bronchial congestion, Bronchitis, Colds,
Congestion-respiratory, Cough-chronic, Croup, Edema,
Emphysema, Grief-excessive, Headache, Indigestion, Lungs-
fluid in, Lungs-supports, Muscle tension, Sinus congestion,
Sore throat, Tuberculosis, Wheezing.
  This is a combnation for acute congestion of the
respiratory tract, known in Western herbology as an
expectorant combination used to treat bronchitis and the
respiratory system. The herbs work to increase blood
circulation and dilate the bronchioles. This combination
also induces sweating, increases the flow of lymphatic fluids
and decreases the thickness while increasing the production
of mucosal fluid. This formula's purposes are as a
decongestant for the lungs and sinuses, acting as a diuretic
and also helps to strengthen those experiencing over-
whelming grief.

LUNG HEALER

CHINESE NAME: FU LEI
CHINESE TRANSLATION: METAL SUPPORTING-
SUPPORT THE WEAK
CONSTITUTIONAL TYPE: METAL-WEAKENED

FU LEI (Metal weakened)
Anemarrhena & Astragalus Sixteen Formula:

Astragalus root, Aster root, Qinjiao root, Platycodon root, lycium bark, Ophiopogon root, Dang Gui root, Panax Ginseng root, Anemarrhena root, Bupleurum root, Blue Citrus peel, Schizandra fruit, Atratylodes rhizome, Citrus peel, Pinellia rhizome, Licorice root.

BODILY INFLUENCE: Anti-inflammatory, Antiseptic, Antispasmodic, Antitussive, Anti viral, Expectorant, Immuno-stimulant, Stimulant, Tonic-general.

SPECIFIC CONDITIONS: Asthma, Bronchial spasms, Bronchitis-chronic, Chest tightness, Cold limbs, Colds or Flu-frequent, Constipation, Cough-chronic, Debility, Dizziness, Edema, Emphysema, Fever, Muscle tone-lack of, Pain in limbs, Pneumonia, Prostate-swelling of, Respiratory infection-chronic, Strengthens the Thin and Weak, Sweating, Thirst, Urine-scant, Weakness-general, Weight gain, Wheezing.

This combination helps to nutritionally build and strengthen the respiratory and circulatory systems and enhances the immune system in cases of chronic lethargy. It is used for purposes of cleansing the lungs through blood-purifying and an immune-building properties. This combination is a tonic formula used to enhance the body's response to stress. The herbs work to stimulate blood circulation, relieve muscle spasms, soothe inflamed tissues and fight infections, especially chronic weaknesses of the respiratory system. It clears lungs and bronchials, relieves discomfort of emphysema, alleviates the tightness in the chest, improves appetite, normalizes blood sugar and helps relieve negativity.

KIDNEY/BLADDER/PROSTATE

CHINESE NAME: QU SHI
CHINESE TRANSLATION: ELIMINATE MOISTURE-
CLEAR THE DAMPNESS
CONSTITUTIONAL TYPE: WATER-STRESSED

QU SHI (Water stressed)
Alisma & Hoelen Sixteen Combination:
  Stephania root, Hoelen plant, Morus root bark, Chaenomeles fruit, Astragalus root, Atractylodes rhizome, Magnolia bark, Polyporus plant, Areca peel, Akebia stem, Cinnamon twig, Pinellia rhizome, Ginger rhizome, Citrus peel and Licorice root.

BODILY INFLUENCE: Analgesic, Anti-inflammatory, Antiseptic, Carminative, Diuretic, Stimulant, Stomachic.

SPECIFIC CONDITIONS: Apathy, Arthritis, Backache, Bloating-GI tract and limbs, Breast inflammation, Colitis, Diarrhea, Digestive problems, Dizziness, Edema, Fatigue, Hypertension, Indigestion, Joint pain, Kidney problems, Nephritis, Obesity, Pain in limbs, Prostate-infection of, Prostate-swelling of, Supports kidney and urinary tract, Urinary tract infection, Urination-burning, Urine-scanty.

  This is a combination that provides nutritional support for the urinary system. It is a diuretic formula for kidney problems and used to relieve water retention in the legs and lungs. The herbs work to increase the flow of urine, relieve pain and inflammation and fight urinary tract infections. The herbs also soothe and moisten inflamed tissues, increase blood flow and reduce lymphatic congestion. Being a diuretic, it relieves joints that ache, enhances urinary system function and helps reduce inflamation of the prostate.

KIDNEY/BONE

CHINESE NAME: JIAN GU
CHINESE TRANSLATION: STRENGTHEN WATER-
STRENGTHENS THE BONES
CONSTITUTIONAL TYPE: WATER-WEAKENED

JIAN GU (Water weakened)
Eucommia & Achyranthes Eighteen Formula:
   Eucommia bark, Cistanche herb, Rehmannia root,
Morinda root, Drynaria rhizome, Achranthes root, Hoelen
plant, Dipsacus root, Lycium, Dioscorea root, Ligustrum
fruit, Cornus fruit, Dang Gui root, Panax Ginseng root,
Astragalus root, Epimedium herb, Liquidamber fruit and
Atractylodes.

BODILY INFLUENCE: Adaptogen, Analgesic, Astringent,
Stimulant.

SPECIFIC CONDITIONS: Adrenal exhaustion, Anemia,
Arthritis, Asthma, Backache, Bladder infection, Bone
fractures, Bones-weak and brittle, Fatigue, Hair-graying of,
Impotency, Infertility, Insomnia, Kidney infection, Kidney-
chronic weakness, Legs-heavy, Memory-poor, Nocturnal
emissions, Osteoporosis, Paranoia, Sex drive-low, Spine
disorders, Tinnitus, Urination-frequent, Urine-incontinent,
Weak knees.
   This herb strengthens the lower body, improves calcium
assimilation, relieves adrenal exhaustion and makes life
more enjoyable. It is a kidney tonic formula, which also
helps low back pain, infection in the urinary tract, prostrate
problems and other problems related to chronic kidney
weakness. It is an invigorating herbal combination that
nutritionally enhances the body's response to all weakening
agents, including time. This combination encourages the
normal functioning of the circulatory system and because of
its tonic quality, enhances the body's response to stress and

aging. The combination works to strengthen and rejuvenate the structure of the body, particularly the bones, connective tissue and sexual organs. These herbs help increase blood circulation, reduce inflamed tissues in the urogenital system and increase calcium absorption.

ANTI-DEPRESSANT

CHINESE NAME: JIE YU
CHINESE TRANSLATION: REGULATE CHI - RELIEVE THE DEPRESSION
CONSTITUTIONAL TYPE: ENERGY-STRESSED

JIE YU (Energy stressed)
Bupleurum & Cyperus Eighteen Combination:
    Perilla leaves, Saussurea root, Gambir twig, Bamboo sap, Bupleurum root, pinellia rhizome, Aurantium peel, Zhishi fruit, Ophiopogon root, Cyperus rhizome, Platycodon root, Ligusticum rhizome, Dang Quai root, Panax Ginseng root, Hoelen plant, Coptis rhizome, Ginger rhizome, Licorice root.

BODILY INFLUENCE: Anti-depressant, Anti-inflammatory, Diuretic, Expectorant, Nervine, Polarity-corrects, Sedative, Stimulant.

SPECIFIC CONDITIONS: Abdominal bloating, Abdominal pain, Adrenal glands-supports, Anxiety, Asthma, Breast lumps, Cold hands and feet, Depression, Dizziness, Dysmenorrhea, Energy-normalizes, Fatigue-w/depression, Energy stressed, General congestion, Headache, Hiccoughs, Hypersensitivity, Inner tension, Insomnia and fears, Loose stool, Lung congestion, Menopause, Mental negativity, Morning sickness, Nervous, Neurosis, Phlegm-sinus and lung, PMS, Postpartum depression, Tinnitus.
    These herbs support the nervous, urinary, respiratory and female reproductive systems. This is a general purpose formula

for aiding the energy flow through the body with specific indications of head-related problems. It is for "failing" energy when the reserves of the body have those sinking feelings of gloom and depression, with loss of vitality, weak digestion, fatigue and congestion. It moves energy toward the head and from the internal organs outward. In this way, the body's spirits are raised, the organs are no longer sinking which results in the expelling of toxins and allows repressed emotions like anger and sadness to leave. It helps with sinus and lung conditions by dispeling phlegm.

IMMUNE BUILDER

CHINESE NAME: SHENG MAI
CHINESE TRANSLATION: GENERATE CHI GENERATE THE PULSE
CONSTITUTIONAL TYPE: ENERGY-WEAKENED

SHENG MAI (Energy weakened)
Astragalus & Ganoderma Eighteen Formula:
  Astragalus root, Panax Ginseng root, Dang Gui root, Rehmannia root, Epimedium leaf, Ganoderma plant, Cucommia bark, Lycium fruit, Peony root, Polygala root, Ligustrum fruit, Schizandra fruit, Atractylodes rhizome, Hoelen plant, Achyranthes root, Ophiopogon root, Citrus peel, Licorice root.

BODILY INFLUENCE: Adaptogen, Immune stimulant, Nervine, Polarity-corrects, Stimulant, Tonic-general.

SPECIFIC CONDITIONS: Aging, Anorexia, Backache, Baldness, Chills, Cold limbs, Colds-frequent, Depression, Emotional problems, Epstein-Barr virus, Exhaustion, Fatigue, Hemorrhoids, Immune deficiency, Impotency, Memory problems, Menstrual flow-scant, Muscles-weak, Palpitations, Polarities-corrects, Poor health-chronic, Pulse-increases, Recovery from trauma, Supports Immune system, Sweating-excessive, Weak legs, Weakness-general.

This combination is a general tonic formula that works to stimulate immune response by enhancing the body's response to stress, improving blood circulation and promoting healing of trauma and chronic degenerative conditions. This is another general purpose formula for building the Chi (energy) of the body, working like Spirulina or Bee Pollen to correct the polarity of the body's energy field. This combination is used for fatigue and a depleted immune system due to infections caused by drug and radiation therapies and viruses.

ANTI-VIRAL/VIRUSES

Dandelion root, Purslane herb, Indigo herb and root, Thlaspi herb, Bupleurum root, Scute root, Pinellia rhizome, Ginseng root, Cinnamon twig, Licorice root.

BODILY INFLUENCE: Anti-viral.

SPECIFIC CONDITIONS: AIDS, Candida albicans, Canker sores-internal, Cold sores-to prevent, Epstein-Barr virus, Fever blisters, Flu, Herpes Simplex, Kidneys, Liver, Mononucleosis, Shingles.

Scientific studies show these herbs to be valuable in strengthening the immune system to counteract the physical/emotional stress that pollution, fatigue and depleted diet put on the body. This combination is a virus-fighting immune system stimulant and may benefit those who have used a lot of antibiotics for chronic viral infections. This combination helps glandular inflammation and protects the liver.

ENERGY/VITALITY

Ma Huang herb concentrate, Dong Quai root, Ho Shou Wu root, Astragalus root and Siberian Ginseng root.

BODILY INFLUENCE: Antihistamine, Stimulant.

SPECIFIC CONDITIONS: Appetite suppressant, Depression and fatigue-outwits, Energy-gives super, Longevity, Memory-improves, No-doze effect, Stamina, Sugar cravings, Weight loss.
CAUTION: Do not use if you have high blood pressure.

In the Oriental system of health, "Chi" is the term for vitality. This is a combination of five herbs that, according to Chinese herbology, is designed to move trapped vitality out from the center of the body. In other words, it disperses "stuck" energy forces from the center of the body outward.

IMMUNE ENHANCER

Barley Grass juice powder, Wheat Grass juice powder, Asparagus powder, Astragalus root, Broccoli powder, Cabbage powder, Ganoderma herb, Parthenium root, Schizandra fruit, Siberian Ginseng root, Myrrh Gum, Pau D.Arco bark, Vitamin A, C E, Zinc, Selenium, Panax Ginseng, Dang Gui root, Rehmannia root, Epimedium leaf, Eucommia bark, lycium fruit, Peony root, Polygala root, Ligustrum fruit, Atractylodes rhizome, Hoelen plant, Achyranthes root, Ophiopogon root, Citrus peel, Licorice root, Dandelion root, Purslane herb, Indigo herb and root, Thlaspi herb, Bupleurum root, Scute root, Pinellia rhizome, Cinnamon twig.

BODILY INFLUENCE: Immuno-stimulant.

SPECIFIC CONDITIONS: Immune system weakness.

This combination of key immune system herbs contain vital antioxidants and equally vital anti-viral herbs for an optimum immune-boosting effect which enhances the body's response from stress due to a system weakened by free radicals.

PARASITE-CLEANSE

Caprylic acid, Black Walnut hulls, Red Raspberry leaves, Pau D'Arco bark, Pumpkin seeds, Cascara Sagrada bark, Violet leaves, Chamomile flowers, Mullein leaves, Marshmallow root, Slippery Elm bark, Elecampane root, Spearmint leaves, Turmeric root, Ginger root, Garlic bulb, Clove flowers.

BODILY INFLUENCE: Anti-parasitic.

SPECIFIC CONDITIONS: Parasites.

This is a special 10-day herbal food specialty dietary program to help the body rid itself of parasitic involvement. This combination of herbs is designed to help expel parasites from the body. This combination contains Caprylic acid which has been beneficial in destroying the Candida Albicans fungus. It is beneficial to first cleanse the bowel to remove old matter and then to use this program for three weeks with a 10 day wait between each sequence.

LIVER CLEANSE

Bupleurum root, Zhishi fruit, Peony root, Scute root, Pinellia rhizome, Cinnamon twig, Dang Gui root, Fushen plant, Atractylodes rhizome, Panax Ginseng root, Ginger rhizome, Licorice root, Gentian root, Irish Moss plant, Cascara Sagrada bark, Golden Seal root, Slippery Elm bark,

Fenugreek seeds, Safflowers flower, Myrrh Gum, Yellow Dock root, Parthenium root, Black Walnut hulls, Barberry bark, Dandelion root, Uva Ursi leaves, Chickweed herb, Catnip herb, Cyani flowers, Buckthorn bark, Capsicum fruit,Turkey Rhubarb root, Couch Grass herb, Red Clover tops, Psyllium, Burdock.

BODILY INFLUENCE: Laxative, Alterative, Anti-parasitic.

SPECIFIC CONDITIONS: Constipation, Sinus problems, congestion, parasites, headaches, liver problems.

This is a 10-day nutritional program to help the body achieve 'Tiao He' - balance and harmony. It's a combination of Chinese nutritional and Western herbal expertise. This is designed to support the cleansing mechanisms of the body by targeting the intestinal, digestive and circulatory systems. This is a good spring cleaning whole-body cleansing program designed to cleanse metabolic wastes and mucus by increasing bowel eliminations.

WEIGHT LOSS

Ma Huang herb concentrate, Dong Quai root, Ho Shou Wu root, Astragalus root, Siberian Ginseng root, White Willow bark, Valerian root, Lettuce leaves, Capsicum fruit, Irish Moss, kelp plant, Black Walnut hulls, Parsley herb, Water Cress, Sarsaparilla root, Iceland Moss, Chromium, Red Clover tops, Yarrow flowers, Horsetail herb, Brindall berries, Marshmallow root, Gymnema leaves, Psyllium hulls, Chickweed herb, Cascara Sagrada bark, Licorice root, Safflower flower, Parthenium root, Gotu Kola herb, Hawthorn berries, Papaya fruit, Fennel seeds, Dandelion root.

BODILY INFLUENCE: Stimulant.

SPECIFIC CONDITIONS: Weight control.

CAUTION: Do not use this product if you have high blood pressure, diabetes, or heart disease. May cause heart palpitations, dizziness, insomnia, acts like natural speed. Discontinue use if adverse symptoms occur.

Thermogenesis is a process for increasing the metabolic burning of fat. The body uses Thermogenesis with exercise and good eating habits to help keep a healthy weight level. The principle of losing weight is a very simple one: just use up more energy than you take in. If the rate at which the body uses energy can be increased, weight loss will come more readily. Thermogenesis is the process of raising body temperature to speed up the body's metabolism, which increases the burning of fat. There is a working formula for guidance so as to use this in a safe controlled manner. There is so much energy expended per degree of body temperature raised.

HERBS DURING PREGNANCY

Most herbs can be taken throughout pregnancy with no ill effects. Many herbs are helpful during pregnancy, especially just before childbirth. Helpful herbs would include those to alleviate nausea, morning sickness, pain, and the like.

We are providing a list of herbs that can be used safely during pregnancy.

Use these herbs in the gentlest way as hot relaxing teas, capsules or tinctures.

- **Bilberry:** will fortify vein and capillary support, aids in kidney function and is a mild diuretic for bloating.
- **Blue Cohosh:** stops and eliminates false labor pains; for final weeks of pregnancy, to ease and/or induce labor.
- **Burdock Root:** helps prevent water retention and jaundice in the baby.
- **Chamomile:** aids digestive and bowel problems and relaxes for good sleep.
- **Echinacea:** aids the immune system to help prevent colds, flu and infections.
- **Ginger Root:** excellent for morning sickness.
- **Lobelia:** helps to relax the mother during delivery and helps speed up the delivery of the placenta.
- **Nettles:** will guard against excessive bleeding as it has vitamin K in it; it will improve kidney function and help prevent hemorrhoids.
- **Peppermint:** after the first trimester, may be used to help digestion, soothe the stomach and overcome nausea. It is an over-all body strengthener and cleanser.
- **Red Raspberry:** it is an all-around excellent herb to use for pregnancy. It is a uterine tonic, anti-abortive, and helps prevent infection. Aids in preventing cramps and anemia. Prevents excessive bleeding during and after labor and will facilitate the birth process by stimulating contractions.
- **Wild Yam:** for pregnancy pain, nausea or cramping and will lessen miscarriage.
- **Yellow Dock:** aids in iron assimilation and will help to prevent infant jaundice.

Many herbalists strongly recommend that some herbs NOT be taken during pregnancy.

NOTE: The herbs listed below should not be taken except by the recommendation of your herbalist and then only in COMBINATIONS.

- **Black Cohosh**: use only the final weeks of pregnancy; will ease and /or induce labor.
- **False Unicorn**: use only the final weeks of pregnancy; will ease and/or induce labor.
- **Golden Seal**: large amounts can cause uterine contractions.
- **Pennyroyal**: this herb can cause abortion; may be used in final weeks.

NOTE: The following herbs are LAXATIVE in nature and should be used sparingly or in combinations.

Aloe Vera
Barberry
Buckthorn
Cascara Sagrada
Mandrake
Rhubarb
Senna

Strong laxatives should be used with discretion as it causes cramping and stomach griping.

CAUTION: The following herbs to avoid during pregnancy:

- **Angelica**: can cause uterine contractions.
- **Cinchona**: Cinchona and its alkaloids should be avoided in pregnancies because of their oxytocic effects.
- **Coffee**: avoid caffeine, as it irritates the uterus; excessive amounts in some sensitive individuals can cause premature birth or miscarriage.
- **Eucalyptus oil**: This oil should be avoided during pregnancy as it is difficult to eliminate through the kidneys.
- **Juniper**: a too strong vaso-dilating, diuretic effect.
- **Lovage**: causes uterine contractions.
- **Ma Huang (Ephedra)**: This herb should be avoided during pregnancy as it has too strong of an anti-histamine effect.
- **Male Fern**: too strong a vermifuge.
- **Mistletoe**: can cause uterine contractions.

- **Mugwort:** stimulates uterine contractions and can be toxic in large doses.
- **Pennyroyal:** can cause abortion.
- **Poke root:** This herb should be avoided during pregnancy as it is a powerful emetic.
- **Rue:** can cause abortion.
- **Shepherds Purse:** too astringent; may be used for after-birth bleeding.
- **Tansy:** can cause uterine contractions.
- **Wild Ginger:** an emmenagogue that causes uterine contractions.
- **Wormwood:** stimulates uterine contractions and can be toxic in large doses.
- **Yarrow:** a strong astringent and mild abortifacient.

HERBS FOR CHILDREN

Children can take herbs without adverse effects in most cases. Obviously, the dosages for medicinal herbs must be reduced since the child is smaller than an adult. A rule for determining dosage is to calculate the dosage according to the body weight of the child. Preschool children take approximately 1/4 an adult dosage. From age five through ten, 1/2 the adult dosage is sufficient. Early teens take 3/4's the adult dosage. When the growing child reaches adult size (sometime between the ages of 16 and 21), then full doses can be used.

Many herbalists urge that children take nutrient herbs throughout the growing years to help build strong bodies. These nutrient herbs can usually be taken in relatively large amounts with no ill effects whatsoever.

The recommended food herbs include:
Alfalfa, Barley, Rose Hips, Dandelion, Bee Pollen, Capsicum, Garlic, Horsetail, Kelp, Papaya, Red Raspberry, Slippery Elm, Spirulina, Thyme.

Scullcap, Gotu Kola, and Eyebright are also popular as diet supplements to aid learning and studying during school age years. Many herbalists recommend that children take a calcium rich herb combination for growing bodies and bones.

It is often difficult to give needed medicinal herbs to infants and small children because the children are unable to swallow the capsules. The herb powder is sometimes so bitter that it cannot be added to food and still be palatable. Some mothers have used bananas, applesauce, or peanut or almond butter to hide the bitter taste of the herbs. When the taste is so bitter that it cannot be hidden, the herb can be taken through enemas or as suppositories in the rectum.

Although some of the aromatic herbs are very delicious and many are high in nutritive value, the only herbs to be cautious about giving to children are the hormone herbs. Ginseng, Damiana and Black Cohosh should not be given to children before they reach puberty. Also, some of the strong laxative herbs and herb combinations should be used sparingly. Cascara Sagrada is one herb that can have strong laxative effects for children, but we need to emphasize that herbal laxatives are no more habit forming than eating a bowl full of prunes. In fact, the herbal laxative combinations are put together to help rebuild and restore the natural muscular action in the colon.

INFANT CARE

NOTE: For further information on infant care, see section on infant enemas.

Colds/Chest Congestion: There are liquid herbal combinations for coughs and colds that are very effective. Homeopathics are effective for both children and adults. For more information, refer to *The Vitamin and Health Encyclopedia*, by Dr. Jack Ritchason.

Room Deodorizer and Disinfectant: When using a humidifier or vaporizer, add 5 to 10 drops (Tea tree oil, Eucalyptus oil) to water. This will aid in congestion when used while the baby is sleeping and will help sterilize and kill germs that may exist in the bedroom.

Cradle Cap: Mix equal amounts of Tea Tree and olive oil, massaging it into the scalp, then washing it out with a natural, organic vegetable based soap.

Diaper rash: Tea Tree oil and Tei Fu oil are very strong volatile oils and should be diluted by 1/2 before being used on babies tender skin. Use such things as Vitamin A oil, vitamin E oil or olive oil. For infants in diapers, Aloe Vera gel is a good solution for skin care.

Always washing the baby in a natural, organic based vegetable soap can certainly take care of the majority of those problems. Washing the babies clothes and bedcoverings in natural and organic laundry compounds will help take care of more of the problems. Using harsh laundry detergents with chlorine bleaches in them can cause the skin irritations and cause lung irritations when the child is breathing the smell coming from them. If soaking diapers, add a natural disinfectant and soak the diapers overnight.

Diarrhea/Loose bowel: Red Raspberry tincture is very effective. Carob powder, bananas and even Slippery Elm can help with loose bowels.

Ear Infections: An antibiotic herbal tincture can be used. Garlic oil has been used when diluted in 1/2 with such oils as Vitamin E, A or olive oil. Tea Tree and Tei Fu oil also can be used when diluted as above. Put a small amount in ear and apply as needed.

Fever: An enema with warm water will generally break a fever immediately. SEE SECTION ON ENEMAS. A cooling bath in warm water making sure the baby does not get a chill, keeping the room warm and covering the baby immediately after bath also helps in bringing down a fever.

Gas/Flatulence/Indigestion: Using a tincture of Catnip and Fennel would be beneficial. Shake the bottle thoroughly before using.

Jaundice: If the mother is nursing, she can use herbal liver combinations which will generally clear this up quickly.

Mouth sores/Thrush: This is Candida Albicans in the mouth. This problem could have started at birth from a mother who had a yeast infection. It also could be caused by the child being given multiple doses of antibiotics. Homeopathic Candida drops are beneficial. Acidophilis should be used on a daily basis and L-Lysine should be added to the diet. Caprylic acid should be used also and for future infections of any kind, natural herbal antiobitics should be used. Vitamin A, C and zinc should be used also.

Nasal congestion: Apply Tea Tree oil under nasal passages. Keep away from the hands of the child so as not to get into the eyes. If it gets into the eyes, flush with clear water immediately.

Parasite/worms: Black Walnut extract. Garlic oil internally. In an enema, garlic oil can be a great addition.

Sore throat/Tonsils: Use liquid cold remedies, Chlorophyll and Rose hips. Massage or apply Tei Fu oil or lotion on the throat and cover, keeping warm.

Teething: A drop of Peppermint oil or Lobelia extract applied to the gums can be helpful. The most effective teething remedy we know of is Homeopathic Chamomile. Homeopathics have no toxic effect and can be used frequently. Applying ice temporarily can also help. This can be done by giving the child ice chips to suck on.

GLOSSARY TERMS

ABORTIFACIENT: a substance that induces abortion, premature expulsion of the fetus.

ABSCESS: a localized collection of pus and liquefied tissue in a cavity.

ABSORB: to take in as through pores; to neutralize an acid.

ACIDOPHILUS: lactobacillus acidophilus bacteria, also called "friendly colonic flora".

ADAPTOGEN: an agent that increases resistance to stress.

ADRENALINE: a hormone secreted by the adrenal glands that produces the "fight or flight" response. Also called epinephrine.

ADSORB: attachment of a substance to the surface of another material.

ALKALOID: highly active plant constituent contain nitrogen atoms.

ALTERATIVE: cleansing, stimulating efficient removal of waste products, chemistry.

AMENORRHEA: absence or suppression of menstruation.

AMINO ACIDS: a group of nitrogen-containing chemical compounds that form the basic structural units of proteins.

ANALGESIC: relieves pain.

ANAPHRODISIAC: subdues sexual desire.

ANDROGEN: hormones that stimulate male characteristics.

ANESTHETIC: deadens sensation and reduces pain.

ANODYNE: reduces pain.

ANTAGONIST: oppose action of other medicines.

ANTHELMINTIC: (See parasiticide)

ANTACID: an agent that neutralizes acidity, especially in the stomach and duodenum.

ANTI-BACTERIAL: destroys or stops the growth of bacterial infections.

ANTI-BILIOUS: reduces biliary or jaundice condition.

ANTIBIOTIC: destroys or inhibits the growth of micro-organisms.

ANTI-CATARRHAL: eliminates mucus conditions.

ANTI-DEPRESSANT: relieves symptoms of depression.

ANTIDOTE: a substance that neutralizes or counteracts the effects of a poison.

ANTI-EMETIC: lessons nausea and prevents or relieves vomiting.

ANTI-FUNGAL: destroying or preventing the growth of fungi.

ANTI-GALACTAGOGUE: prevents or decreases secretion of milk.

ANTI-HEMORRHAGIC: stops bleeding and hemorrhaging.

ANTI-HISTAMINE: neutralizes the effects of histamine in an allergic response.

ANTI-INFLAMMATORY: counteracting or diminishing inflammation or its effects.

ANTI-LITHIC: agent that prevents or relieves calculi (stones).

ANTI-MICROBIAL: destroys or prevents the growth of micro-organisms.

ANTI-NEOPLASTIC: preventing the development, growth or proliferation of malignant cells.

ANTI-OXIDANT: a agent that prevents free radical or oxidative damage to body tissue and cells.

ANTI-PERIODIC: preventing regular recurrences of a disease or symptoms, as in malaria.

ANTI-PHLOGISTIC: an agent reducing inflammation.

ANTI-PYRETIC: agent that reduces fever.

ANTI-RHEUMATIC: agent that prevents or relieves rheumatism.

ANTISCORBUTIC: preventing or relieving scurvy.

ANTISEPTIC: an agent that combats and neutralize pathogenic bacteria, and prevents infection.

ANTI-SPASMODIC: agent that prevents or relieves spasms.

ANTI-SYPHILITIC: agent that cures or relieves syphilis or venereal diseases.

ANTI-THROMBOTIC: prevents blood clots.

ANTI-SCORBUTIC: cures or prevents scurvy.

ANTI-TOXIC: neutralizes a poison from the system.

ANTI-TUSSIVE: inhibits the cough reflex helping to stop coughing.

ANTI-VIRAL: opposing the action of a virus.

APERIENT: mild laxative without purging.

APERITIVE: herbs that stimulate the appetite.

APHRODISIAC: an agent that stimulates sexual desire.

AROMATIC: agent that contains volatile, essential oils which aids digestion and relieves gas.

ASTRINGENT: an agent that has a constricting or binding effect, i.e. one that checks hemorrhages or secretions by coagulation of proteins on a soft surface.

ATHEROSCLEROSIS: a process in which fatty substances (cholesterol and triglycerides) are deposited in the walls of medium to large arteries, eventually leading to blockage of the artery.

ATONIC: without normal tension or tone.

AYURVEDIC: a traditional system of Indian medicine, which literally means "a science of life."

BACTERICIDE: destroys bacteria.

BILIRUBIN: the breakdown product of the hemoglobin molecule of red blood cells.

BITTER: stimulates secretions of digestive and encouraging appetite.

BLOOD CLEANSER: an agent that cleanses the blood.

BLOOD PURIFIER: an agent that cleanses the blood as well as enhancing the blood by increasing the nutrient value.

BROMELAIN: the protein-digesting enzyme found in pineapple.

CALMATIVE: gently calms nerves.

CANDIDA: yeastlike fungi.

CANDIDA ALBICANS: the fungus responsible for monilial infections, such as thrush, vaginitis and sometimes systemic infection.

CARDIAC: heart tonic or restorative.

CARMINATIVE: relieves intestinal gas pain and distension; promotes peristalsis.

CARBUNCLE: painful infection of the skin and subcutaneous tissues with production and discharge of pus and dead tissue, similar to a boil (faruncle) but more severe and with a multiple sinus formation; usually caused by *Staphylococcus aureus*.

CATAPLASM: another name for poultice.

CATARRH: inflammation of a mucous membrane, especially of the nose and throat, with a discharge.

CATHARTIC: a strong laxative which causes rapid evacuation.

CELL PROLIFERATOR: enhances the formation of new tissue to speed the healing process.

CHOLAGOGUE: stimulates bile flow from the gall bladder and bile ducts into the duodenum.

CHRONIC: designating a disease showing little change or of slow progression; opposite of acute.

CIMCIFUGA: means 'to drive away bugs, neutralizes rattlesnake bites, scorpion stings.'

COLIC: spasmodic pain effecting smooth muscle, such as the intestines, gall bladder, or urinary tract.

COLITIS: inflammation of the colon.

CONDIMENT: improves the flavor of food.

CONVALESCENCE: the period of recovery after the termination of a disease or an operation.

COUNTERIRRITANT: causing irritation in one part to relieve pain in another part.

CYST: an abnormal lump or swelling, filled with fluid or semi-solid cheesy material, in any body organ or tissue.

CYSTITIS: inflammation of the inner lining of the bladder. It is usually caused by a bacterial infection.

DEBILITY: weakness of tonicity in functions or organs of the body.

DEMENTIA: senility; loss of mental function.

DEMULCENT: softens and soothes damaged or inflamed surfaces, such as the gastric mucous membranes.

DEOBSTRUENT: removes body obstructions.

DEPURATIVE: cleans or purifies blood by promoting eliminative functions.

DERMATITIS: inflammation of the skin evidenced by itching, redness, and various skin lesion, sometimes due to allergy.

DETERGENT: cleansing to wounds, ulcers or skin itself.

DIAPHORETIC: causes perspiration and increases elimination through the skin.

DIGESTIVE: aids digestion, usually by providing enzymes from various sources.

DISCUTIENT: an agent that causes the dispersal of a tumor or any pathologic accumulation.

DISINFECTANT: destroys the cause of infection.

DIURETIC: increases the secretion and flow of urine.

DIVERTICULI: pathological sac-like out pouchings of the wall of the colon.

DOCTRINE OF SIGNATURES: theory that the appearance of a plant indicates its inherent properties.

DRASTIC: a very active cathartic which produces violent peristalsis.

DROPSY: generalized edema in cellular tissue or in a body cavity.

DYSMENORRHEA: painful or difficult menstruation.

DYSPEPSIA: imperfect or painful indigestion; not a disease in itself but symptomatic of other diseases or disorders.

DYSPNEA: sense of difficulty in breathing, often associated with lung or heart disease.

EDEMA: accumulation of fluid in tissues (swelling).

EMETIC: a substance that causes vomiting.

EMMENAGOGUE: a substance that facilitates and regularizes menstrual flow. (avoid in pregnancy).

EMOLLIENT: softens and soothes inflamed tissue; softens and protects the skin.

ENERVATE: to deprive of strength, vigor, etc.; to weaken physically and mentally.

ENTERITIS: inflammation of the small intestine.

EPSTEIN-BARR VIRUS: the virus that causes infectious mononucleosis and that is associated with Burkitt's lymphoma and nasopharyngeal cancer.

ESTROGEN: hormone that exert female characteristics.

EXPECTORANT: encourages the loosening and removal of phlegm from the respratory tract.

FARUNCLE: another name of r a boil that involves a hair folicle.

FEBRIFUGE: (see anti-pyretic)

FISTULA: an abnormal passage between two internal organs, or from an organ to the surface of the body.

GALACTOGOGUE: agent that promotes the flow of milk.

GASTRITIS: inflammation of the stomach and intestinal tract.

GIARDIA: a genus of flagellate protozoa some of which are parasitic in the intestinal tract of man and domestic animal; transmitted by ingestion of cysts in fecally contaminated water and food; interfere with the absorption of fats; boiling water inactivates them.

GINGIVITIS: inflammation of the gums.

GLAUCOMA: a condition in which the pressure of the fluid in the eye is so high that it causes damage.

HEMATURIA: blood in the urine.

HEMOLYTIC: a substance which destroys red blood cells.

HEMORRHOIDS: distended veins in the lining of the anus.

HEMOSTATIC: herbs that stop bleeding.

HEPATIC: herbs that support and stimulate the liver, gall bladder and spleen, and increase the flow if bile.

HIATAL, HIATUS, HERNIA: displacement of the upper part of the stomach into the thorax through the esophageal hiatus of the diaphragm.

HOMEOSTASIS: equilibrium of internal environment.

HYDRAGOGUE: promotes watery evacuation of the bowels.

HYPERGLYCEMIA: an abnormal concentration of sugar in the blood.

HYPERTENSIVE: used to increase blood pressure.

HYPOTENSIVE: used to reduce blood pressure.

IATROGENIC: literally, "physician induced." This terms can be applied to any medical condition, disease, or other adverse occurrence that results from medical treatment.

IMMUNO-STIMULANT: enhances and increases the body's immune (defense) mechanism.

INCONTINENCE: the inability to control urination or defecation.

INDOLENT: sluggish; causing little or no pain.

INTERFERON: a potent immune-enhancing substance that is produced by the body's cells to fight off viral infection and cancer.

IRRITANT: induces a local inflammation.

JAUNDICE: a condition caused by elevation of bilirubin in the body and characterized by a yellowing of the skin.

LAXATIVE: a substance that stimulates bowel movements.

LETHARGY: a feeling of tiredness, drowsiness, or lack of energy.

LITHOTRIPTIC: an agent that dissolves urinary calculi (stones).

LYMPH: fluid contained in lymphatic vessels, which flows through the lymphatic system to be returned to the blood.

MALABSORPTION: impaired absorption of nutrients most often a result of diarrhea.

MENORRHAGIA: excessive loss of blood during menstrual periods.

METABOLISM: a collective term for all of the chemical processes that take place in the body.

MONTMORILLONITE: lake clays used in nutrition as a source of trace minerals.

MUCILAGE, MUCILANT: complex sugar molecules that are soft and slippery and protect mucous membranes and inflamed tissues.

MUCUS: the slick, slimy fluid secreted by the mucous membranes. Mucus acts as a lubricant and mechanical protector of the mucous membranes.

MYELIN SHEATH: a white fatty substance that surrounds nerve cells to aid in nerve impulse transmission.

NARCOTIC: causes stupor and numbness.

NAUSEANT: produces vomiting.

NEPHRITIS: inflammation of the kidney; the glomeruli, tubules and interstitial tissue may be affected.

NERVINE: strengthens functional activity of nervous system; may be stimulants or sedative.

NEURALGIA: pain along a nerve.

NUTRITIVE: pertaining to the process of assimilating food; having the property of nourishing.

OXYTOCIC: agent that stimulates contractions accelerating childbirth.

PARASITICIDE: an agent that kills parasites and worms.

PARKINSON'S DISEASE: a chronic nervous disease. A slowly progressive, degenerating nervous system disease characterized by restin tremor, pill rolling of the fingers, a masklike facial expression, shuffling gait, and muscle rigidity and weakness.

PARTURIENT: stimulates uterine contraction which induce and assist labor.

PECTORAL: healing to problems in the bronchio-pulmonary area.

PERISTALSIS: the alternate contraction and relaxation of the walls of a tubular structure by means of which its contents are moved onward, characteristic of the intestinal tract, ureter, etc.; a milking action.

PHLEGM: thick mucus especially from the respiratory tract.

PRECURSOR: starts a chain reaction which accelerates growth.

PROPHYLACTIC: any agent or regimen that contributes to the prevention of infection and disease.

PROSTAGLANDIN: hormone-like substance that has a wide range of functions including acting as chemical messenger and causing uterine contractions.

PUNGENT: penetrating or sharp to the taste.

PURGATIVE: causes watery evacuation of intestinal contents.

PUTREFACTION: decomposition of organic matter, especially proteins, by the action of bacteria, resulting in the formation of foul-smelling compounds.

RUBEFACIENT: stimulates blood flow to the skin, causing local reddening.

REFRIGERANT: agent that produces coolness or reduces fever.

RELAXANT: relaxes nerves and muscles; relieves tension.

RESOLVENT: that which reduces inflammation or swelling.

RESTORATIVE: an agent that is effective in the regaining of health and strength; restores normal physiological activity.

SAPONINS: active plant constituents, producing a lather in water.

SCROFULA: tuberculosis inflammation of lymph nodes of the neck in children.

SEDATIVE: quieting, an agent that exerts a soothing or tranquilizing effect; sedatives may be general, local, nervous or vascular.

SIALAGOGUE: an agent that stimulates the secretion of saliva.

SOPORIFIC: inducing sleep.

STIMULANT: increases internal heat, dispels internal chill and strengthens metabolism and circulation.

STOMACHIC: strengthens stomach function.

STYPTIC: contracting a blood vessel; stopping a hemorrhage by astringent action.

SUDORFIC: causing perspiration; see Diaphoretic.

SYNERGISTIC: the simultaneous action of two or more substances whose combined effect is greater than the sum of each working alone.

SYSTEMIC: relating to or affecting the entire body.

TAENIFUGE: agent that expels tapeworms.

TANNIN: active plant constituents that combined with proteins; stringent.

TAPEWORM: any of several ribbonlike worms that infest the intestines of invertebrates, including man.

TONIC: restoring, nourishing and supporting for the entire body; a substance that exerts a gentle strengthening effect on the body.

TOXIN: a poisonous substance of animal or plant origin.

UREMIA: toxic condition associated the renal insufficiency produced by the retention in the blood of nitrogenous substances normally excreted by the kidney.

VASOCONSTRICTOR: an agent that narrows blood-vessel openings, restricting the flow of blood through them.

VASODILATOR: causes relaxation of blood vessels.

VERMIFUGE: expels or repels intestinal worms.

VULNERARY: assists in healing of wounds by protecting against infection and stimulating cell growth.

BIBLIOGRAPHY

Abehsera, Michel, *The Healing Clay*. Carol Publishing Group, Secaucus, NJ, 1990, 124 pgs.

Aikman, Lonnelle, *Nature's Healing Arts: From Folk Medicine to Modern Drugs*. National Geographic Society, 1977, 200 pgs.

Austin, Phyllis, Thrash, Agatha M., M.D., and Thrash, Calvin L. Jr., M.D., *Natural Remedies: A Manual*. Yucci Pines Institute, Seale, Al, 1983, 282 pgs.

Balch, James F. , M.D., and Balch, Phyllis A., C.N.C., *Prescription for Nutritional Healing*. Avery Publishing Group Inc., Garden City Park, NY, 1990, 368 pgs.

Balch, Phyllis A., C.N.C., and Balch, James F., M.D., *Prescription for Cooking and Dietary Wellness*. P.A.B. Publishing, Inc., Greenfield, Indiana, 1987, 317 pgs.

Blake, Steve N.D.Sc, *Globalherb*. Computer Software, Compress IBM PC, Felson, CA, 1993.

Bridge, Ivy, *Ivy's Bridge to Better Health*. Ivy Herbs & Health Foods, Tustin, CA, 1991, 94 pgs.

Buchman, Diane Dincin, *Herbal Medicine*. Wings Books, Avenel, NJ, 1979, 310 pgs.

Budwig, Johanna Dr., *Flax Oil as a True Aid Against Arthritis, Heart Infarction, Cancer and Other Diseases*. Apple Publishing Co., Vancouver, British Columbia, Canada, 1992, 59 pgs.

Bullock, Shelia, *Historical Uses Series, Health Food Handbook*. Shelia Bullock, Naturally Yours, Dallas, TX, 1992, 29 pgs.

Bullock, Shelia, Historical Uses Series, *Herbs Nutrition for Plants, Pets and People*. Naturally Yours, Dallas, TX, 31 pgs.

Canning, Peggy M.A., *Exotic Supplements*. Margaret H. Canning, Vista, CA, 43 pgs.

Castleman, Michael, *The Healing Herbs*. Rodale Press, Emmaus, Penn., 1991, 436 pgs.

Chai, Mary Ann P. *Herb Walk Medicinal Guide*. The Gluten Co., Provo, UT, 1978.

Christopher, John R. M.D., Dr. Christopher's Three Day Cleansing Program. *Mucusless Diet and Herbal Combinations*. Christopher Publications, Springville, UT, 1969, 28 pgs.

Christopher, John R. M.D., *School of Natural Healing*. Christopher Publications, Springville, UT, 1976, 651 pgs.

Coon, Nelson, *Using Plants for Healing*. Rodale Press, Emmaus, PA, 1978.

Culpepper, Nicholas, *Complete Herbal*. Bloomsbury Books, London, England, 1992, 349 pgs.

Farwell, Edith Foster, *A Book of Herbs*. The White Pine Press, Piermont, NY, 1979.

Gerson, Scott MD., *The Ancient Indian Healing Art*. Element Books Limited, Rockport, MA, 1993, 115 pgs.

Goulart, Frances Sheridan, *The Grey Gourmet*. Thornwood Books, 1980.

Griffin, La Dean, *Is Any Sick Among You?*. Bi-World Publishers, Provo, UT, 1974, 228 pgs.

Griffin, La Dean, *Herbs to the Rescue*. Bi-World Publishers, Provo, UT, 1978, 35 pgs.

Heinerman, John, *The Science of Herbal Medicine*. Bi-World Publishers, Orem, UT, 1979, 318 pgs.

Hobbs, Christopher, *Echinacea: The Immune Herb*. Botanica Press, Capitola, CA, 1990, 40 pgs.

Hobbs, Christopher, *Foundations of Health: The Liver & Digestive Herbal*. Botanica Press, Capitola, CA, 1992, 322 pgs.

Hobbs, Christopher, *Ginko: Elixir of Youth*. Botanica Press, Capitola, CA, 1991, 80 pgs.

Hobbs, Christopher, *Usnea: The Herbal Antibiotic and other Medicinal Lichens*. Botanica Press, Capitola, CA, 1986, 20 pgs.

Hoffman, David, *The New Holistic Herbal*. Element Books Limited, Inc., Rockport, MA, 1991, 284 pgs.

Holmstead, Bruce and Lorena, *Herb Librarian*. Computer Software, Compress IBM PC., Holmstead Partners, 1993.

Hutchens, Alma R., *A Handbook of Native American Herbs*. Shambhala Publications, Inc., Boston, Mass., 1992, 256 pgs.

Hutchens, Alma R., *Indian Herbalogy of North America*. Shambhala Publications Inc., Boston, Mass., 1973, 382 pgs.

Hylton, William H., ed., *The Rodale Herb Book*. Rodale Press. Emmaus, PA., 1975.

Jensen, Bernard, D.C., Ph.D., *Garlic Healing Powers*. Bernard Jensen, Publisher, Escondido, CA, 1992, 87 pgs.

Jensen, Bernard, D.C., Ph.D., *Herbs: Wonder Healers*. Bernard Jensen, Publisher, Escondido, CA, 1992, 120 pgs.

Jensen, Bernard, D.C., Ph.D., *Herbal Handbook*. Bernard Jensen Enterprises, Escondido, CA, 1988, 55 pgs.

Johnston, Ingeborg M., C.N., and Johnston, James, Ph.D., *Flaxseed (Linseed) Oil and the Power of Omega-3*. Keats Publishing, Inc., New Canaan, CO, 1990, 32 pgs.

Keith, Velma J., and Gordon, Monteen, *The How To Herb Book*. Mayfield Publishing, Pleasant Grove, UT, 1984, 256 pgs.

Kloss, Jethro, *Back to Eden*. Lifeline Books, Santa Barbara, CA, 1975.

Krochmal, Arnold and Connie, *A Guide to the Medicinal Plants of the United States*. Quandrangle Books, NY. 1973.

Krochmal, Connie, *A Guide to Natural Cosmetics*. Thornwood Books, Springville, UT, 225 pgs.

Kuts-Cheraux, A.W., B.S., M.D., N.D., *Naturea Medicina and Naturopathic Dispensatory*. Antioch Press, Yellow Springs, Ohio, 1953, 430 pgs.

Lad, Vasant Dr., *The Science of Self Healing*. Lotus Press, Santa Fe, NM, 1984, 175 pgs.

Ley, Beth M., *Natural Healing Handbook*. Christopher Lawrence Communications, Lee Fargo, North Dakota, 1990, 320 pgs.

Ley, Beth M., *Castor Oil: It's Healing Properties*. B. L. Publications, 1989, 31 pgs.

Lucas, Richard M., *Herbal Health Secrets*. Parker Publishing, West Nyack, NY, 1983, 226 pgs.

Lucus, Richard M., *Miracle Medicine Herbs*. Parker Publishing Co., West Nyack, NY, 1991, 203 pgs.

Lust, John, *The Herb Book*. Bantum Books, New York, NY, 1991, 659 pgs.

Malstrom, Dr. Stan, *Herbal Remedies 2-Revised*. Bi-World Publishers, Orem UT, 1975, 40 pgs.

Miesse, Frank Ph.D., *Chinese Herbs Made Easy*. Woodland Hills Health Books, Provo, UT, 20 pgs.

Millet, Edward Milo, *Herbal Aid: Herbs for Building Health and Vitality, Vol. I, II, III*. Thornwood Books, Springville, UT, 1980

Mills, Simon Y. M.A., *The Dictionary of Modern Herbalism*. Healing Arts Press, Rochester, Vermont, 1988, 222 pgs.

Mindell, Earl, R.Ph.D., Ph.D., *Earl Mindell's Herb Bible*. Simon & Schuster, New York, 1992, 300 pgs.

Moulton, LeArta, *Herb Walk*. The Gluten Co., Provo, UT 1979.

Mowery, Daniel B., Ph.D., *Milk Thistle*. American Institute of Health and Nutrition, 1991, 18 pgs.

Mowrey, Daniel B., Ph.D., *New Hope for Liver Health*. American Institute of Health and Nutrition, 1991, 24 pgs.

Mowrey, Daniel B., Ph.D., *Next Generation Herbal Medicine*. Cormorant Books, Lehi, UT, 1988, 157 pgs.

Mowrey, Daniel B. Ph.D., *Proven Herbal Blends*. Keats Publishing, Inc., New Canaan, Conn, 1986, 46 pgs.

Mowrey, Daniel B., Ph.D., *The Scientific Validation of Herbal Medicine*. Cormorant Books, 1986, 316 pgs.

Murray, Michael T. Murray, N.D., *The Healing Power of Herbs*. Prima Publishing, Rocklin, CA, 1992, 246 pgs.

Nature's Guide To Healthy Plants and Natural Formulas. Woodland Books, Provo, UT, 1994, 41 pgs.

Nebelkopf, Ethan, *The New Herbalism: A Self-Help Guide.* Bi-World Publishers, Orem, UT, 1979, 35 pgs.

Nickell, J.M., *Botanical Ready Reference.* Enos Publishing Co., Banning, CA, 1976, 275 pgs.

O'Brien, James Edmond, *Nature's Healing Herbs.* Globe Communications Corp., Boca Raton, FL., 1994, 66 pgs.

Ody, Penelope, *The Complete Medicinal Herbal.* Dorling Kindersley, Inc., New York, NY, 1993, 192 pgs.

Olsen, Cynthia B., *Austrailian Tea Tree Oil First Tea Tree Oil First Aid Handbook .* Kali Press, Fountain Hills, AZ, 1991, 31 pgs.

Passwater, Richard PH.D., *Evening Primrose Oil.* Keats Publishing Inc., New Canaan, Conn., 1981, 30 pgs.

Passwater, Richard PH.D., *The New Superantioxidant Plus.* Keats Publishing, New Canaan, Conn., 1992, 46 pgs.

Pedersen, Mark, *Nutritional Herbology.* Pedersen Publishing, Bountiful, UT, 1987, 377 pgs.

Pedersen, Mark, *Nutritional Herbology. Volume II.* Pedersen Publishing, Bountiful, UT, 1989, 125 pgs.

Pitkanen, A.L., *Tropical Fruits.* Renan Prevost, Publisher, Lemon Grove, CA, 1967, 232 pgs.

Reader's Digest, *Magic and Medicine of Plants.* The Reader's Digest Association, Pleasantville, N.Y., 1986, 464 pgs.

Rector-Page, Linda G., N.D.,Ph.D, *Healthy Healing: An Alternative Healing Printing Reference.* Griffin Printing, 1985, 373 pgs.

Rector-Page, Linda, N.D., Ph.D., *How To Be Your Own Herbal Pharmacist.* Linda Rector-Page, Publisher, 1991, 204 pgs.

Reed, Daniel P., *Chinese Herbal Medicine.* Shambhala, Boston, Mass., 1993, 174 pgs.

Rodale's, *Illustrated Encyclopedia of Herbs.* Rodale Press, Emmaus, Penn., 1987, 545 pgs.

Rose, Jeanne, *Herbs & Things.* Workman Publishing Co., New York, NY, 1972, 323 pgs.

Royal, Penny C., *Herbally Yours. Bi-World Publishers Inc.,* Provo, UT, 128 pgs.

Santillo, Humbart B.S., M.D., *Natural Healing With Herbs.* Hohm Press, Prescott, AZ, 1984, 375 pgs.

Schechter, Steven R. N.D., *Fighting Radiation & Chemical Pollutants.* Vitality Ink, Encinitas, CA, 1988, 294 pgs.

Scheer, James F., *Royal Jelly Health and Life Enhancer Better Nutrition.* 1993, 38 pgs.

Shaffer, Willa, *Wild Yam Birth Control Without Fear*. Woodland
Health Books, Provo, UT, 1986, 8 pgs.

Talbert, Lee Ph.D., and Pauly, Michelle M., Bilberry. *American
Institute of Health and Nutrition*, 1991, 13 pgs.

Tenney, Deanne, *Natural Health Guide*. Woodland Health Books,
Provo, UT, 1992, 98 pgs.

Tenney, Deanne, *Nature's Guide To Healthy Plants and Natural
Formulas in Canada. 3rd Edition*, Woodland Health Books,
Provo, UT, 1994, 18 pgs.

Tenney, Louise, M.H., *Nutritional Guide With Food Combining*.
Woodland Health Books, Provo, UT, 1991, 237 pgs.

Tenney, Louise, *Today's Herbal Health, 3rd Edition*. Woodland
Books, Provo, UT, 1992, 377 pgs.

Thrash, Agatha, M.D. & Thrash,Calvin, M.D., *Charcoal*. New
Lifestyle Books, 1988, 108 pgs.

Tierra, Leslie L. AC., *The Herbs of Life*. The Crossing Press,
Freedom, CA, 1992, 250 pgs.

Tierra, Michael C.A.,N.D., *Planetary Herbology*. Lotus Press, Twin
Lakes, WI., 485 pgs.

Tierra, Michael C.A., N.D., *The Way of Herbs*. Pocket Books,
New York, NY, 1980, 378 pgs.

Towler, Solala, *The Way of Chinese Medicine (A Patient's Guide)*.
Quan Yin Enterprises, Inc., Portland, OR, 1990, 17 pgs.

Vogel, Dr. A., *The Swiss Nature Doctor's Secrets of Therapeutic
Medicine*. Keats Publishing, Inc., New Canaan,Conn.,
1990, 24 pgs.

Wagner, Eugene S. Ph.D., and Hunt, Gerald L., *Ginkgo Biloba*.
American Institute of Health and Nutrition, 1992, 20
pgs.

Wallach, J.D., DVM, N.D., and Ma Lan, M.D., M.S., *Lets Play
Doctor*. Wholistic Publications, Rosarito Beach, Baja,
CA, Mexico, 1989, 203 pgs.

Weiss, Jennifer and Burnett, Vena, *Colon Cleansing: The Best Kept
Secret*. Jennifer Weiss and Vena Burnett, Auburn, CA,
1989, 117 pgs.

Willard, Terry Ph.D., *Reishi Mushroom*. Sylvan Press, Issaquah,
WA, 1990, 167 pgs.

Willard, Terry Ph.D., *The Wild Rose Scientific Herbal*. Wild Rose
College of Natural Healing Ltd., Calgary, Alberta,
Canada, 1991, 416 pgs.

Willard, Terry Ph.D., *Textbook of Modern Herbology. Revised
Edition*, C.W. Progressive Publishing Group Inc., Calgary,
Alberta, Canada, 389 pgs.

Wood, Linden, "NBS-AV," *Nature's Field*, July/August 1994, Provo, UT, Page 9.

Wood, Matthew, *Seven Herb Plants As Teachers*. North Atlantic Books, Berkeley, California, 1986, 124 pgs.

Yeung, Him-Che, O.M.D., Ph.D., *Handbook of Chinese Herbs and Formulas Vol 1*. Him-Che Yeung, Los Angeles, CA, 1983, 710 pgs.

Yeung, Him-Che O.M.D.,PhD., *Handbook of Chinese Herbs and Formulas Vol II*. Him-Che Yeung, Los Angeles, CA 1983, 399 pgs.

Yoder, Jonas, *Herbs Natural Alternatives*. A Handbook of Food and Herb Supplements. 15 pgs.

INDEX

combination for, 269

Aspirin, 26, 97, 250

Asthma, 6, 8, 11, 12, 18, 20, 21, 24, 29, 30, 34, 38, 46, 53, 56, 61, 63, 64, 66, 67, 70, 73, 78, 80, 81, 84, 86, 88, 94, 99, 100, 102, 104, 109, 111, 119, 120, 125, 129, 133, 135, 136, 137, 139, 140, 143, 145, 148, 151, 155, 156, 158, 164, 167, 168, 182, 186, 214, 215, 217, 218, 222, 230, 231, 238, 239, 240, 246, 247, 249, 255, 262, 339, 343; herb combination for, 269

Astragalus, 14, 335

Atherosclerosis, 92, 104, 114

Athlete's foot, 8, 30, 43, 62, 89, 94, 194, 230, 233

Atractylodes, 335

Backaches, 11, 13, 46, 55, 61, 62, 67, 123, 124, 150, 180, 184, 192, 235

Bad breath, 5, 6, 12, 16, 62, 84, 86, 149, 150, 155, 164, 200, 201, 218

Barberry, 15, 370

Barley, 17

Basil, 19

Bayberry, 19

Bedsores, 8, 156, 254

Bedwetting, 27, 37, 52, 66, 84, 118, 122, 123, 128, 143, 145, 148, 159, 164, 180, 209, 219, 234, 235

Bee pollen, 21

Bee's Royal Jelly, 23

Bell's Palsy, 6, 122, 133

Berberine, 15

Beta carotene, 5, 224

Bilberry, 24, 369

Biousness, 218

Bioflavonoid, 25

Birch, 25, 26

Birth control, 31, 32, 248, 249

Birth Defects; prevention, 131

Bistort, 26

Bites, 43, 84, 137, 199, 207; poisonous, 29, 77

Black walnut, 30

Black birch, 25

Black Cohosh, 2, 28, 33, 370

Blackberry, 27

Bladder, problems, 4, 6, 16, 19, 26, 34, 36, 37, 51, 53, 64, 66, 70, 73, 74, 109, 120, 122, 128, 133, 145, 159, 164, 170, 179, 194, 199, 214, 222, 226, 234, 237, 238, 241; infection, 14, 33, 41, 66, 77, 109, 111, 124, 129, 180, 192, 207, 223, 235, 244; stones, 25, 107, 123, 124, 192; herb combination for, 303, 304, 360; urinary, 31

Bleeding, 4, 8, 20, 26, 27, 38, 39, 43, 46, 56, 64, 67, 75, 102, 104, 128, 145, 149, 151, 158, 174, 180, 219, 226, 243, 244, 251, 344; internal 109, 122, 209

Blessed Thistle, 31, 69

Blisters, 72, 73, 110, 11

Bloating, 337

Blood builder, 13, 20, 21, 77, 164, 225

Blood circulation, 25, 29, 32, 62, 75, 78, 97, 99, 110

Blood cleanser, 8, 16, 26, 29, 33, 41, 43, 46, 55, 64, 73, 77, 82, 95, 135, 148, 164, 170, 184, 194, 209, 211, 225, 260, 331

Blood clots, 6, 42, 94, 105, 114, 117, 151, 152, 203

Blood disorders, 53, 77, 102, 128, 160, 207

Blood poisoning, 41, 55, 56, 77, 86, 95, 137, 145, 148, 180, 216, 218

Blood pressure, 6, 11, 13, 14, 15, 16, 18, 21, 23, 29, 33, 37, 46, 49, 51, 60, 62, 66, 73, 75, 90, 95, 103, 104, 106, 110, 116, 117, 124, 125, 147, 148, 153, 158, 164, 166, 174, 201, 215, 217, 218, 219, 225, 237, 246, 248; herb combination for, 270, 271

Blood purifier, 6, 16, 18, 22, 26, 32, 36, 40, 41, 43, 52, 55 - 58, 66, 68, 73, 74, 76, 77, 78, 95, 96, 158 - 160, 163, 167, 168, 180, 185, 186, 194, 199, 209, 210, 211, 212, 228, 241, 249; herb combination for, 271, 272, 273, 351

Blood sugar, 85, 101, 116, 155, 163, 228, 249

Blue vervain, 33

Blood vessels, 123

Blue Cohosh, 32, 369